Emergency and Critical Care of Small Animals

Editor

ELISA M. MAZZAFERRO

VETERINARY CLINICS OF NORTH AMERICA: SMALL ANIMAL PRACTICE

www.vetsmall.theclinics.com

November 2020 • Volume 50 • Number 6

ELSEVIER

1600 John F. Kennedy Boulevard ● Suite 1800 ● Philadelphia, Pennsylvania, 19103-2899
http://www.vetsmall.theclinics.com

VETERINARY CLINICS OF NORTH AMERICA: SMALL ANIMAL PRACTICE Volume 50, Number 6
November 2020 ISSN 0195-5616, ISBN-13: 978-0-323-73362-5

Editor: Stacy Eastman
Developmental Editor: Nicole Congleton

Veterinary Clinics of North America: Small Animal Practice (ISSN 0195-5616) is published bimonthly by Elsevier Inc., 360
Park Avenue South, New York, NY 10010-1710. Months of issue are January, March, May, July, September, and
November. Business and Editorial Offices: 1600 John F. Kennedy Blvd., Ste. 1800, Philadelphia, PA 19103-2899.
Customer Service Office: 3251 Riverport Lane, Maryland Heights, MO 63043. Periodicals postage paid at New York,
NY and additional mailing offices. Subscription prices are $348.00 per year (domestic individuals), $705.00 per year
(domestic institutions), $100.00 per year (domestic students/residents), $451.00 per year (Canadian individuals),
$876.00 per year (Canadian institutions), $488.00 per year (international individuals), $876.00 per year (international
institutions), $100.00 per year (Canadian students/residents), and $220.00 per year (international students/residents).
To receive student/resident rate, orders must be accompanied by name of affiliated institution, date of term, and the *sig-
nature* of program/residency coordinator on institution letterhead. Orders will be billed at individual rate until proof of status
is received. Foreign air speed delivery is included in all *Clinics* subscription prices. All prices are subject to change without
notice. **POSTMASTER:** Send address changes to *Veterinary Clinics of North America: Small Animal Practice*, Elsevier
Health Sciences Division, Subscription Customer Service, 3251 Riverport Lane, Maryland Heights, MO 63043. Customer
Service (orders, claims, online, change of address): Elsevier Periodicals Customer Service, Elsevier Health Sciences Di-
vision Subscription **Customer Service 3251 Riverport Lane Maryland Heights, MO 63043. Tel: 1-800-654-2452
(U.S. and Canada); 314-447-8871 (outside U.S. and Canada). Fax: 314-447-8029. E-mail: journalscustomerser-
vice-usa@elsevier.com (for print support); journalsonlinesupport-usa@elsevier.com (for online support).**
Reprints. For copies of 100 or more of articles in this publication, please contact the Commercial Reprints Department,
Elsevier Inc., 360 Park Avenue South, New York, NY 10010-1710. Tel.: 212-633-3874; Fax: 212-633-3820; E-mail:
reprints@elsevier.com.

Veterinary Clinics of North America: Small Animal Practice is also published in Japanese by Inter Zoo Publishing
Co., Ltd., Aoyama Crystal-Bldg 5F, 3-5-12 Kitaaoyama, Minato-ku, Tokyo 107-0061, Japan.

Veterinary Clinics of North America: Small Animal Practice is covered in *Current Contents/Agriculture, Biology and Environmental Sciences, Science Citation Index, ASCA, MEDLINE/PubMed (Index Medicus), Excerpta Medica, and BIOSIS.*

Contributors

EDITOR

ELISA M. MAZZAFERRO, MS, DVM, PhD
Diplomate, American College of Veterinary Emergency and Critical Care; Staff Criticalist, Cornell University Veterinary Specialists, Stamford, Connecticut, USA; Adjunct Associate Clinical Professor, Emergency and Critical Care, Cornell University Hospital for Animals, Ithaca, New York, USA

AUTHORS

ANUSHA BALAKRISHNAN, BVSc
Diplomate, American College of Veterinary Emergency and Critical Care; Cornell University Veterinary Specialists, Stamford, Connecticut, USA

HEIDI L. BARNES HELLER, DVM
Diplomate, American College of Veterinary Internal Medicine (Neurology); Owner, Barnes Veterinary Specialty Services, LLC

MANUEL BOLLER, Dr med vet, MTR
Diplomate, American College of Veterinary Emergency and Critical Care; Senior Lecturer, Emergency and Critical Care, Melbourne Veterinary School, The University of Melbourne, Melbourne, Victoria, Australia

ANDREW G. BURTON, BVSc
Diplomate, American College of Veterinary Pathologists, Clinical Pathologist, IDEXX Laboratories, Inc., North Grafton, Massachusetts, USA

CHRISTOPHER G. BYERS, DVM, CVJ
Diplomate, American College of Veterinary Emergency and Critical Care; Diplomate, American College of Veterinary Internal Medicine (Small Animal Internal Medicine); Omaha, Nebraska, USA

DANIEL L. CHAN, DVM
Diplomate, American College of Veterinary Emergency and Critical Care; Diplomate, European College of Emergency and Critical Care; Diplomate, American College of Veterinary Nutrition; Professor, Department of Clinical Science and Services, The Royal Veterinary College, University of London, North Mymms, Hertfordshire, United Kingdom

ARMELLE M. DE LAFORCADE, DVM
Diplomate, American College of Veterinary Emergency and Critical Care; Tufts University, Cummings School of Veterinary Medicine, North Grafton, Massachusetts, USA

THOMAS EDWARDS, DVM, MS, LTC, VC
Diplomate, American College of Veterinary Emergency and Critical Care; Chief, Research Support Division, U.S. Army Institute of Surgical Research, JBSA Fort Sam Houston, San Antonio, Texas, USA

DANIEL J. FLETCHER, PhD, DVM
Diplomate, American College of Veterinary Emergency and Critical Care; Associate Professor of Emergency and Critical Care, Department of Clinical Sciences, Cornell University College of Veterinary Medicine, Ithaca, New York, USA

J.D. FOSTER, VMD
Diplomate, American College of Veterinary Internal Medicine (Small Animal Internal Medicine); Nephrology/Urology, Internal Medicine, Friendship Hospital for Animals, Washington, DC, USA

ROBERT GOGGS, BVSc, PhD, MRCVS
Diplomate, American College of Veterinary Emergency and Critical Care; Diplomate, European College of Veterinary Emergency and Critical Care; Assistant Professor, Emergency and Critical Care, Department of Clinical Sciences, Cornell University College of Veterinary Medicine, Ithaca, New York, USA

ANTHONY L. GONZALEZ, DVM
Diplomate, American College of Veterinary Emergency and Critical Care; Staff Criticalist, Cornell University Veterinary Specialists, Stamford, Connecticut, USA; Adjunct Assistant Clinical Professor, Emergency and Critical Care, Cornell University College of Veterinary Medicine, Ithaca, New York, USA

KARL E. JANDREY, DVM, MAS
Diplomate, American College of Veterinary Emergency and Critical Care; Professor, Clinical Small Animal Emergency and Critical Care, Department of Surgical and Radiological Sciences, School of Veterinary Medicine, University of California, Davis, Davis, California, USA

KENDON W. KUO, DVM, MS
Diplomate, American College of Veterinary Emergency and Critical Care; Assistant Clinical Professor, Emergency and Critical Care, Department of Clinical Sciences, College of Veterinary Medicine, Auburn University, Auburn, Alabama, USA

GREGORY R. LISCIANDRO, DVM
Diplomate, American Board of Veterinary Practitioners; Diplomate, American College of Veterinary Emergency and Critical Care; President, International Veterinary Point-of-Care Ultrasound Society, Co-owner, Emergency and Critical Care, Hill Country Veterinary Specialists, CEO, FASTVet.com, Spicewood, Texas, USA

ELISA M. MAZZAFERRO, MS, DVM, PhD
Diplomate, American College of Veterinary Emergency and Critical Care; Staff Criticalist, Cornell University Veterinary Specialists, Stamford, Connecticut, USA; Adjunct Associate Clinical Professor, Emergency and Critical Care, Cornell University Hospital for Animals, Ithaca, New York, USA

MAUREEN McMICHAEL, DVM, MEd
Diplomate, American College of Veterinary Emergency and Critical Care; Professor, Emergency and Critical Care, Department of Clinical Sciences, College of Veterinary Medicine, Auburn University, Auburn, Alabama, USA

ALEXANDRA PFAFF, MedVet
Diplomate, American College of Veterinary Emergency and Critical Care; Tufts University, Cummings School of Veterinary Medicine, North Grafton, Massachusetts, USA

JENNIFER PRITTIE, DVM
Diplomate, American College of Veterinary Emergency and Critical Care; Diplomate, American College of Veterinary Internal Medicine (Small Animal Internal Medicine); The Animal Medical Center, New York, New York, USA

MARC R. RAFFE, DVM, MS
Diplomate, American College of Veterinary Anesthesia and Analgesia; Diplomate, American College of Veterinary Emergency and Critical Care; Director, VACCA LLC

ELIZABETH A. ROZANSKI, DVM
Diplomate, American College of Veterinary Internal Medicine; Diplomate, American College of Veterinary Emergency and Critical Care; Tufts University, Cummings School of Veterinary Medicine, North Grafton, Massachusetts, USA

NICOLE SPURLOCK, DVM
Diplomate, American College of Veterinary Emergency and Critical Care; Animal Specialty Emergency Center, Los Angeles, California, USA

CARISSA W. TONG, BVM&S, MRCVS
Resident, Emergency and Critical Care, Cornell University Veterinary Specialists, Stamford, Connecticut, USA

RACHEL MATUSOW WYNNE, DVM, MS
Diplomate, American College of Veterinary Ophthalmologists; Staff Ophthalmologist, Cornell University Veterinary Specialists, Stamford, Connecticut, USA; Adjunct Assistant Clinical Professor of Ophthalmology, Cornell University College of Veterinary Medicine, Ithaca, New York, USA

Contents

the respiratory system and the clinical recognition, stabilization, and initial diagnostic planning for small animal patients that present for respiratory emergencies.

Small animal ocular emergencies vary from relatively benign to potentially vision or life threatening, with significant overlap in clinical signs. Careful ophthalmic examination in dim light conditions with a bright light source and competent patient head restraint are crucial to properly diagnosing ocular disease. Adjunctive ophthalmic diagnostic testing should be performed to rule out corneal ulceration, glaucoma, and dry eye before empiric topical antibiotic or steroid medications are prescribed. Most emergency cases present because of ocular redness, cloudiness, discomfort, apparent bulging, or vision loss; categorizing differential diagnoses on this basis can be helpful to the emergency clinician.

Hospitalized companion animals have increased susceptibility for hospital-acquired/nosocomial infections. Veterinarians have a responsibility to ensure adequate infection control, biosecurity, and biosafety within veterinary hospitals. Through elimination of pathogens and substitution of hazards, as well as implementation of engineering and administrative controls and the use of personal protective equipment, veterinary teams can dramatically reduce unintentional disease transmission.

Albumin is among the most important proteins and plays a significant role in maintenance of colloid osmotic pressure, wound healing, decreasing oxidative damage, carrying drugs and endogenous substances, and coagulation. Hypoalbuminemia is common in acute and chronic illnesses. Replenishment of albumin can be in the form of fresh frozen, frozen or cryopoor plasma, or in the form of human or canine albumin concentrates. Infusion of human albumin concentrate to healthy and critically ill dogs can induce acute and delayed hypersensitivity reactions. Death has been reported. Therefore, allogenic transfusion in the form of plasma products or canine albumin concentrate is recommended.

Canine parvoviral enteritis is one of the most common causes of morbidity and mortality in dogs worldwide. Tests can detect viral antigen in feces, and characteristic decreases in total leukocyte, neutrophil, and lymphocyte counts can increase the index of suspicion in affected cases and can be used to prognosticate morbidity and mortality. The standard of care for infected animals includes IV crystalloid and sometimes colloid fluids, antiemetics, broad-spectrum antibiotics, and early enteral nutrition. Vaccination induces protective immunity in most dogs. Vaccination, along with limiting exposure in young puppies, is the most effective means of preventing parvoviral enteritis in dogs.

Immune-mediated hemolytic anemia is a common hematologic disorder in dogs. Disease management involves immunosuppression using glucocorticoids, potentially in combination with other medications such as azathioprine, cyclosporine, or mycophenolate mofetil. Therapeutic drug monitoring may enhance the utility and maximize the safety of cyclosporine and mycophenolate mofetil. The disease is proinflammatory and prothrombotic. Antithrombotic drug administration is therefore essential, and anticoagulant therapy should be initiated at the time of diagnosis. Additional therapies include red blood cell transfusion to support blood oxygen content. Future therapies may include therapeutic plasma exchange, anti-CD20 monoclonal antibodies, and complement inhibitors.

Hypercoagulable tendencies may develop in critically ill dogs and to a less known extent, cats. Although the use of antithrombotics is well-established in critically ill people, the indications and approach are far less well-known in dogs and cats. The goal of this article was to review the relevant CURATIVE guidelines, as well as other sources, and to provide recommendations for critically ill patients with directions for future investigation.

Therapy with human intravenous immunoglobulin (hIVIG) as an immunomodulator in veterinary patients results in effective but transient immunosuppression, and may be viable as part of a multidrug strategy against immune-mediated thrombocytopenia and autoimmune cutaneous disease. Efficacy of hIVIG against other veterinary autoimmune diseases is questionable. Veterinary patients tolerate hIVIG therapy well, with few infusion reactions documented. Veterinary clinical trials of hIVIG are limited, and more work is needed to determine the true efficacy and risk of hIVIG administration in companion animals.

Traumatic injuries in small animals are a common cause for presentation to emergency departments. Severe traumatic injury results in a multitude of systemic responses, which can exacerbate initial tissue damage. Trauma resuscitation should focus on the global goals of controlling hemorrhage, improving tissue hypoperfusion, and minimizing ongoing inflammation and morbidity through the concept of "damage-control resuscitation." This approach focuses on the balanced use of blood products, hemorrhage control, and minimizing aggressive crystalloid use. Although these tenets may not be directly applicable to every veterinary patient with trauma, they provide guidance when managing the most severely injured subpopulation of these patients.

Viscoelastic testing, such as thromboelastography or thromboelastometry, is performed on whole-blood samples, which include both soluble plasma factors as well as blood cells and platelets bearing tissue factor and phospholipid. This methodology allows identification of fibrinolysis and can provide analysis of platelet function. Viscoelastic testing has become increasingly accessible and popular in emergency and critical care settings in recent years and can provide important information for the diagnosis and management of patients with hemostatic disorders. This article discusses the principles and interpretation of viscoelastic testing, application to small animal emergency and critical care medicine, and potential advantages and disadvantages.

Over the past couple of decades, a component of veterinary critical care was simply to ensure that nutritional support formed some part of the treatment plan. Great emphasis was made on early placement of feeding tubes in critically ill veterinary patients to facilitate enteral feeding. Progress has been made on techniques for nutritional provision, establishing feasibility of nutritional interventions in various patient populations and establishing that nutritional support does have an important role in veterinary critical care. Some refinement of appropriate caloric targets in critically ill animals has decreased complications relating to overfeeding, but further work is required to establish optimal feeding regimes.

Seizures are common in veterinary patients and control is critical to the overall patient health. The benzodiazepine class of drugs (diazepam, midazolam, and lorazepam) often are the drug class of choice; however, levetiracetam and propofol also have been gaining favor as anticonvulsant drugs for acute seizure management. After cessation of seizures, practitioners then can discuss long-term seizure control on a case-by-case basis with clients.

The practice of creating and maintaining general anesthesia using intravenous anesthetic drugs is defined as total intravenous anesthesia. Total intravenous anesthesia produces general anesthesia by selective drug properties that fulfill the 3 elements of anesthesia. Total intravenous anesthesia has potential application in veterinary emergency and critical care medicine. This article reviews the theory and application of total intravenous anesthesia and identifies possible application in emergency and critical care medicine.

Cageside Ultrasonography in the Emergency Room and Intensive Care Unit

Gregory R. Lisciandro

Global Focused Assessment with Sonography for Trauma (FAST) and point-of-care ultrasonography carry the potential to screen for and monitor conditions rather than traditional means without ultrasonography. Advantages include being point of care, cageside, low impact, rapid, safe, and radiation sparing, and requiring no shaving and/or minimal patient restraint. Moreover, information is real time for free fluid and soft tissue abnormalities of the abdomen, heart, and lung, which are missed or only suspected by physical examination, basic blood and urine testing, and radiography. A standardized approach with recording of patient data is integral to a successful Global FAST program.

VETERINARY CLINICS OF NORTH AMERICA: SMALL ANIMAL PRACTICE

SERIES OF RELATED INTEREST

Veterinary Clinics of North America: Exotic Animal Practice
https://www.vetexotic.theclinics.com/

THE CLINICS ARE NOW AVAILABLE ONLINE!
Access your subscription at:
www.theclinics.com

Preface

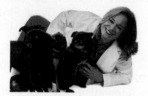

Elisa M. Mazzaferro, MS, DVM, PhD
Editor

Emergency and critical care has been my passion for more than 2 decades. The fast pace and quick thinking involved in a dynamic rapidly changing patient and hospital environment are exciting but can pose some challenges for the small animal practitioner. With that in mind, we must familiarize ourselves with the improvements in technology, science, and medicine in order to raise our standard of care and hopefully improve patient outcomes.

For this issue of *Veterinary Clinics of North America: Small Animal Practice*, I have invited content experts to discuss the latest information on a variety of older and some newer topics related to emergency and critical care. This issue reviews and discusses updates on canine parvoviral enteritis, ophthalmologic emergencies, therapies for immune-mediated hemolytic anemia, transfusion medicine, nutritional support of the critical patient, resuscitative strategies in trauma, and review of respiratory emergencies. Newer concepts and therapies, such as implementation of biosecurity in a veterinary practice, albumin therapy in the critically ill patient, use of antithrombotic agents, viscoelastic monitoring, extracorporeal therapies for toxin and other illnesses, cage-side ultrasound, and total intravenous anesthesia, are also discussed in detail. Finally, if all else fails, the latest update on evidence-based strategies for cardiopulmonary resuscitation is discussed.

A number of colleagues from Cornell University Veterinary Specialists, Cornell University Hospital for Animals in Ithaca, and the American Colleges of Veterinary Emergency and Critical Care and Internal Medicine have dedicated valuable time and efforts so that we can continue to grow as an emergency and critical care profession. I thank you. I hope the information provided here will allow us to save lives, one patient at a time.

Vet Clin Small Anim 50 (2020) xiii–xiv
https://doi.org/10.1016/j.cvsm.2020.08.002
0195-5616/20/© 2020 Published by Elsevier Inc.

vetsmall.theclinics.com

Sincerely,

Elisa M. Mazzaferro, MS, DVM, PhD
Cornell University Veterinary Specialists
880 Canal Street
Stamford, CT 06902, USA

E-mail address:
emazzaferro@cuvs.org

Update on Cardiopulmonary Resuscitation in Small Animals

Manuel Boller, Dr med vet, MTR[a],*, Daniel J. Fletcher, PhD, DVM[b]

KEYWORDS

- Cardiopulmonary resuscitation • Cardiopulmonary arrest • Basic life support
- Advanced life support • Postcardiac arrest care • Dog • Cat

KEY POINTS

- For dogs and cats that experience cardiopulmonary arrest (CPA), survival is best in patients with perianesthetic CPA and other acute, reversible causes, but poor in all other animals; cardiopulmonary resuscitation (CPR) is the only treatment for CPA.
- To reduce death because of in-hospital CPA in dogs and cats, a comprehensive strategy is necessary that includes preventive and preparedness measures, basic life support, advanced life support, and postcardiac arrest critical care.
- Optimal implementation of each of these elements is required to improve overall survival from CPA.
- The Reassessment Campaign on Veterinary Resuscitation initiative completed an exhaustive literature review and generated a set of evidence-based, consensus CPR guidelines.

INTRODUCTION

Cardiopulmonary arrest (CPA) is the acute cessation of ventilation and systemic perfusion, which leads to discontinuation of tissue oxygen delivery and death if not quickly reversed. Common causes in small animals include anesthetic overdose, trauma, asphyxiation, and exacerbation of severe critical illnesses, such as sepsis. Despite reported resuscitation rates (ie, return of spontaneous circulation, ROSC) suggesting that the heart can be restarted in approximately 40% to 50% of dogs and cats treated with cardiopulmonary resuscitation (CPR), only a small percentage of all affected animals survive to hospital discharge.[1–5] That percentage varies from 0% to 19% among studies, with most survivors occurring among dogs and cats that experience CPA during anesthesia. In fact, a recent study found a 15-fold increase in the odds for survival

[a] Melbourne Veterinary School, The University of Melbourne, Melbourne, Victoria, Australia; [b] Department of Clinical Sciences, Cornell University College of Veterinary Medicine, DCS Box 31, Ithaca, NY 14853, USA
* Corresponding author. Melbourne Veterinary School, Faculty of Veterinary and Agricultural Sciences, The University of Melbourne, 250 Princes Highway, Werribee, Victoria 3030, Australia.
E-mail address: manuel.boller@unimelb.edu.au

Vet Clin Small Anim 50 (2020) 1183–1202
https://doi.org/10.1016/j.cvsm.2020.06.010
0195-5616/20/© 2020 Elsevier Inc. All rights reserved.

to discharge in small animals with CPA during anesthesia when compared with other causes of CPA.[5]

A broad strategy is necessary to minimize mortality owing to CPA, and several opportunities exist to optimize outcomes.[6] Recognition of animals at imminent risk and the quick implementation of preventative interventions can reduce the number of animals experiencing CPA. Should CPA occur, then preparedness of the resuscitation team is required for an early and effective response. High-quality basic (BLS) and advanced life support (ALS) serve to limit organ injury and to increase the likelihood of ROSC. Finally, provision of individualized post-cardiac arrest (PCA) care is the indispensable final step. To optimize patient survival, knowledge gained from medical science on how to best perform the above steps needs to be integrated in educationally efficient strategies and then implemented well in clinical practice.[7] Nearly 10 years ago, the Reassessment Campaign on Veterinary Resuscitation (RECOVER) conducted a systematic review of literature on the following topics and generated evidence- and consensus-based clinical guidelines to provide a clear basis for training and practice of CPR[8,9]: Preparedness and prevention,[10] BLS,[11] ALS,[12] monitoring,[13] and PCA care.[14] This article presents key aspects of these guidelines and provides updates based on emerging medical science.

PREVENTION, PREPAREDNESS, AND EARLY RECOGNITION

In dogs and cats, CPA occurs predominantly as a consequence of progressive systemic illness or trauma while hospitalized, or in relation to events (eg, anesthesia) within the hospital. This environmental context permits fast recognition of patients at risk of CPA and quick, efficient intervention to prevent CPA. Anticipating scenarios that could lead to a CPA allows formulation of a monitoring plan, leading to early recognition of CPA in at-risk patients. Evidence from human hospitals suggests that such an approach increases the likelihood of early recognition of a patient's worsening condition before an actual deterioration or CPA occurs and decreases the incidence of in-hospital CPA.[15]

Minimizing the time interval between occurrence of CPA and initiation of CPR is important. Hence, veterinary practices must be well equipped for early recognition of and quick response to CPA (**Box 1**).

Proficiency in CPR skills and knowledge can best be achieved via didactic training (eg, lectures or online courses), hands-on practice, and opportunities to debrief on simulated and real CPR scenarios.[10,16] Refresher training should occur at least once every 6 months.[17,18] Staff should be familiarized with the resuscitation environment, which includes a crash cart and clearly visible cognitive aids. The crash cart should contain all necessary drugs and equipment and should be routinely audited to ensure availability of all required materials.[19] Cognitive aids, such as a CPR algorithm and a dosing chart, may help in conducting tasks according to guidelines.[20] Debriefing sessions held immediately after each CPR event allow critical reflection on team performance, improve future resuscitation efforts, and may serve as refresher training.[21,22]

Prompt recognition of CPA is the precondition for early initiation of CPR. In all acutely unresponsive patients, CPA should be rapidly ruled out. In nonanesthetized patients, CPA is recognized simply by the presence of unconsciousness and lack of breathing. To rule out CPA, a brief, focused physical examination of 10 to 15 seconds' duration, including evaluation of airway, breathing, and circulation (ABC), has been advocated in any unresponsive patient. However, because of frequent false positives associated with pulse palpation, the circulation assessment is not recommended in

---

Box 1
Preparedness and prevention key recommendations

CPR training
  Both didactic and hands-on training are essential
  Refresher training should be done at least every 6 months

Crash cart
  Available in central location
  Regularly stocked and audited

Cognitive aids
  CPR algorithm, drug, and dosing charts
  Personnel should be trained in their use

Diagnosis of CPA
  Standardized ABC assessment in any acutely presenting or decompensating patient
  ABC assessment should take no longer than 15 seconds
  CPA: Unconscious, apneic patient
  If there is any doubt whether the patient is in CPA, CPR should be started without delay

---

the current guidelines. In anesthetized patients, unconsciousness and apnea are not reliable indicators of CPA, and changes of end-tidal CO_2 ($ETCO_2$), electrocardiogram (ECG), and direct arterial blood pressure may, in combination, form the basis for quick recognition of CPA.[23] If any doubt of the presence of CPA persists, CPR should be started immediately rather than allowing further delays to pursue additional assessments. This recommendation is based on evidence that even short delays in initiating CPR may reduce the likelihood of successful resuscitation, whereas the risks of performing CPR on a patient not in CPA are small.[24]

BASIC LIFE SUPPORT

Once CPA is recognized, the first action to be taken is to call for help and to initiate BLS measures as quickly as possible. Well-performed BLS is of utmost importance because it is the CPR measure most relevant for blood flow generation (**Box 2**). BLS starts with immediate initiation of external chest compressions followed by ventilation.

Chest Compressions

During untreated CPA, blood flow ceases, leading to exhaustion of cellular energy stores, compromise of organ function, ischemic organ injury with time, and reperfusion injury upon reinstitution of tissue blood flow after ROSC. Thus, early effective reinstitution of tissue blood flow through high-quality chest compressions is of fundamental importance. However, experimental studies in dogs and swine suggest that even well-executed closed-chest CPR may only lead to a cardiac output of 25% to 40% of normal.[25–27] Poor-quality chest compressions will likely produce much lower cardiac output.

Although understudied in dogs and cats, experimental data and anatomic considerations suggest that chest compressions are best administered with the dog or cat in either left or right lateral recumbency, with a compression depth of one-third to one-half the laterolateral width of the chest and at a compression rate of 100 to 120 per minute with 50% of the cycle devoted to compression (see **Box 2**).[25,28] Visual or acoustic prompts, such as a flashing light, a metronome, or a song at the correct tempo (eg, the Bee Gees' "Stayin' Alive"), improve adherence to correct compression

---

Box 2
Basic life support key recommendations

Chest compression technique
  Most patients in lateral recumbency
  Rate of 100 to 120 compressions per minute regardless of species or size
  Compress one-third to one-half the width of the chest
  Allow full recoil of the chest between compressions
  Minimize interruptions and delays in starting compressions
  Rotate compressor after every 2-minute cycle of CPR

Chest compression posture
  Lock elbows and interlock hands
  Stack hands to form 1 focal compression point
  Shoulders directly above hands
  Bend at waist and use core muscles
  Avoid leaning

Chest compression point
  Medium and large round-chested dogs: over widest portion of the chest
  Keel-chested dogs: directly over the heart
  Small dogs and cats: directly over the heart, consider 1-handed technique
  Flat-chested dogs (eg, bulldogs): dorsal recumbency, hands on sternum

Ventilation
  Intubated patient (preferred technique)
    Ten breaths per minute simultaneously with compressions
    One-second inspiratory time
    Approximately 10 mL/kg tidal volume
  Mouth to snout
    Close patient's mouth tightly
    Make seal over both nares with mouth
    Deliver 2 quick breaths with 1-second inspiratory time
    30:2 technique: 30 chest compressions, 2 quick breaths, immediately resume compressions

---

rates.[29,30] Leaning on the chest between compressions must be avoided to permit full elastic recoil of the chest. Disallowing full reexpansion of the thorax between compressions increases intrathoracic pressure, compromises venous return to the chest and heart, and in turn reduces cerebral and myocardial blood flow.[31,32] Chest compressions should be administered without interruption in cycles of 2 minutes because pauses were shown to be associated with worsened outcome.[33,34] Interruptions in compressions should be avoided and be of minimal duration, because it takes a significant time (ie, 60 seconds) of continuous chest compressions to build up maximum coronary perfusion pressure.[35] Coronary perfusion pressure in turn is a critical determinant of myocardial blood flow, and a value of at least 20 mm Hg is generally required to achieve ROSC.[36] To minimize pauses, establishment of vascular access and endotracheal intubation should be conducted during ongoing chest compressions, if feasible. Moreover, ECG analysis or pulse palpation should occur in a scheduled 3- to 5-second pause at the end of each 2-minute cycle of CPR. After that pause, a different team member should take over chest compressions to avoid rescuer fatigue and the associated effects on chest compression depth, rate, and leaning.

Blood flow during CPR is generated in a fundamentally different way compared with spontaneous circulation. Two distinct models, the thoracic and the cardiac pump theories, have been postulated to describe how chest compressions may lead to systemic blood flow.[37] The cardiac pump theory suggests that the cardiac ventricles are diminished in their volume through direct compression, leading to a pressure increase in the ventricles, the opening of the pulmonic and aortic valves, and provision of blood flow to the lungs and the tissues driven by the resulting pressure gradients. In contrast to the selective ventricular pressure increase occurring with the cardiac pump, the thoracic pump theory proposes that external chest compressions increase the pressure in all intrathoracic structures, which leads to a marked pressure increase in the low-compliance arterial system, whereas such a pressure increase is diminished in the high-compliance venous compartment of the circulation. The resulting arteriovenous pressure gradient drives tissue perfusion. In either model, the negative intrathoracic pressure from passive recoil of the chest during the decompression phase increases venous return of blood from extrathoracic to intrathoracic vessels. In accordance with these concepts, the recommended compression point on the thorax varies with the animal's size and chest conformation (see **Box 2**).

In medium- to large-breed, round-chested dogs, such as Labradors or Rottweilers, it is likely the thoracic theory predominates. It is therefore recommended to locate the chest compression point at the widest point on the lateral thoracic wall to maximize peak intrathoracic pressure (**Fig. 1**A). Conversely, in keel-chested dogs, such as sighthounds, a compression point located directly over the heart is preferable, because the cardiac pump mechanism likely predominates (**Fig. 1**B). In those dogs in which the chest is wider than tall (eg, English bulldogs, French bulldogs, basset hounds), hand position over the midsternum with the animal in dorsal recumbency should be considered

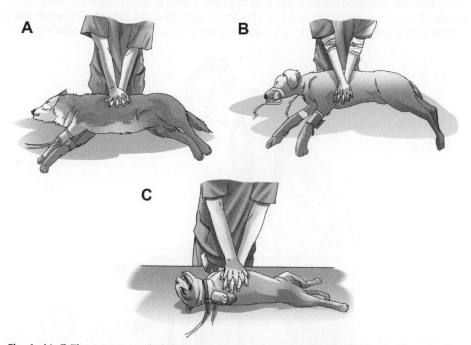

Fig. 1. (*A-C*) The recommended chest compression point varies with the chest conformation of the animal in medium- to large-breed dogs: (*A*) compress over the widest point of the chest in round-chested dogs (eg, Labrador retriever); (*B*) compress over the heart in keel-chested dogs (eg, greyhound); (*C*) compress over the midsternum with the animal in dorsal recumbency in flat-chested dogs (eg, English bulldog). (*From* Fletcher, DJ, Boller, M. Cardiopulmonary Resuscitation in the Emergency Room. In: Drobatz KJ, Hopper K, Rozanski E, Silverstein DC, eds. Textbook of Small Animal Emergency Medicine. Hoboken, NJ: John Wiley and Sons, Inc.; 2019:965-973; with permission.)

(**Fig. 1**C). Because considerable compression force is required for larger dogs, rescuer posture is important to maintain sufficient compression depth and rate. Compressors should position their hands on top of one another such that a focal compression point results, with their shoulders vertically above this compression point, and their elbows locked (**Fig. 2**). With this posture, the core muscles will generate the compression force, which will extend endurance compared with using triceps muscles alone. If the patient is on a table, a foot stool may be required to allow for optimal posture.

In most cats and small dogs, the cardiac pump theory may apply with the preferred chest compression point located directly over the heart. The same 2-handed technique as described for large dogs can be used. Alternatively, a single-handed technique can be used, whereby the compressing hand reaches around the sternum to compress the cardiac ventricles between the palm or thumb and opposing fingers (**Fig. 3**).

Ventilation

Although BLS is started with compressions first, ventilation should commence as soon as possible. If an endotracheal tube (ETT), a laryngoscope, and at least 2 rescuers are available, the animal should be intubated. To avoid interruption in chest compressions, intubation should occur in lateral recumbency during ongoing chest compressions. Inflation of the ETT cuff is essential to allow for effective alveolar ventilation during chest compressions. Securing the ETT with a tie to prevent accidental extubation during CPR is mandatory. Once intubated, animals should be ventilated at a rate of 10 breaths per minute with a short inspiratory time of approximately 1 second. A normal tidal volume

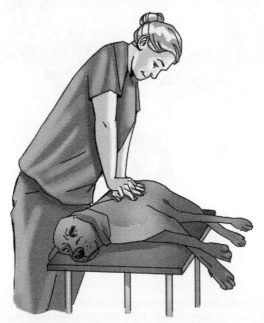

Fig. 2. Recommended rescuer posture for chest compressions in medium- to large-breed dogs: shoulders are positioned vertically above hands, the elbows locked, and the compression force is generated by bending at the waist and engaging the core muscles. (*From* Fletcher, DJ, Boller, M. Cardiopulmonary Resuscitation in the Emergency Room. In: Drobatz KJ, Hopper K, Rozanski E, Silverstein DC, eds. Textbook of Small Animal Emergency Medicine. Hoboken, NJ: John Wiley and Sons, Inc.; 2019:965-973; with permission.)

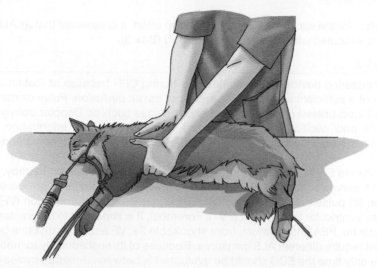

Fig. 3. Single-handed chest compressions using the cardiac pump approach in cats and small dogs. The stronger hand reaches around the sternum and compresses the heart between thumb/palm and the opposing fingers. The other hand stabilizes the position of the animal. (*From* Fletcher, DJ, Boller, M. Cardiopulmonary Resuscitation in the Emergency Room. In: Drobatz KJ, Hopper K, Rozanski E, Silverstein DC, eds. Textbook of Small Animal Emergency Medicine. Hoboken, NJ: John Wiley and Sons, Inc.; 2019:965-973; with permission.)

(eg, 10 mL/kg) should be targeted. Care should be taken not to hyperventilate the patient, because low arterial CO_2 tension leads to cerebral vasoconstriction, decreasing oxygen delivery to the brain, and because extensive positive pressure ventilation will compromise myocardial and cerebral blood flow and is harmful.[38]

If an ETT and laryngoscope are not readily available, intubation cannot be performed, or only a single rescuer is present, mouth-to-snout ventilation will provide adequate oxygenation and CO_2 removal. The recommended technique for mouth-to-snout ventilation in a dog or cat includes the closure of the animal's mouth with 1 hand, the extension of the neck so that it aligns with the back, the formation of a seal over the patient's nares with the rescuers mouth, and expiration into the animal's nares to inflate its chest. The breath should be continued until a normal chest excursion has occurred. An inspiratory time of approximately 1 second should be targeted. As an alternative, a tight-fitting face mask connected to a self-inflating resuscitation bag (eg, Ambu bag) can be used to deliver breaths in the nonintubated animal.

In either case, mouth-to-snout or bag-mask ventilation cannot be delivered while chest compressions are ongoing. Therefore, it is recommended that 30 chest compressions (at a rate of 100–120 compressions per minute) are administered alternating with 2 breaths. These sequences of compressions and breaths at a ratio of 30:2 should be continued for 2 minutes, followed by a short evaluation of the animal for signs of effective circulation, before resuming another 2-minute cycle of 30:2 CPR. Typically, 4 to 5 rounds of 30:2 CPR can be executed in a 2-minute cycle. Because the mouth-to-snout or bag-mask technique requires pauses in chest compressions, it should only be used when endotracheal intubation is not feasible.

ADVANCED LIFE SUPPORT

While BLS is ongoing, the resuscitation team should initiate ALS, which includes monitoring, drug treatment, and electrical defibrillation. Given the importance of high-quality BLS for the success of the resuscitation effort, it is essential that all ALS measures are executed without compromising BLS (**Box 3**).

Monitoring

Many monitoring devices are of limited use during CPR because of motion artifact, the lack of a sufficient arterial pulse, and poor tissue perfusion. Pulse oximetry and indirect blood pressure measurement with devices such as Doppler sphygmomanometers and oscillometric monitors do not provide valid information unless ROSC is restored. However, the use of ECG and capnography is recommended during CPR.

An accurate ECG rhythm diagnosis guides drug and defibrillation therapy. During CPR, this serves to identify which of the following arrest rhythms are present: (1) asystole, (2) pulseless electrical activity (PEA), (3) ventricular fibrillation (VF), or (4) pulseless ventricular tachycardia (PVT). Foremost, it is important to differentiate nonshockable (ie, PEA and asystole) from shockable (ie, VF and PVT) rhythms because these will require different ALS measures. Because of its susceptibility to motion artifact, the only time the ECG should be evaluated is between 2-minute cycles of CPR

Box 3
Advanced life support key recommendations

Monitoring
  Electrocardiogram
    Apply as soon as possible during CPR
    Determine rhythm diagnosis during intercycle pauses in compressions
  End-tidal carbon dioxide
    Target minimum of 15 mm Hg as an indicator of chest compression efficacy
    Sudden, marked increase indicates possible ROSC

Drug treatment
  Vasopressors (eg, epinephrine, vasopressin)
    Indicated for asystole, PEA, or refractory VF
    Divert blood from the periphery to core organs
    Repeat every other cycle of CPR (every 4 minutes)
    Use high-dose epinephrine only for prolonged CPR
  Vagolytics (eg, atropine)
    Indicated for asystole or PEA, especially if owing to high vagal tone
    Decrease parasympathetic tone
    One dose only
  Reversal agents (eg, naloxone, flumazenil, atipamezole)
    Administer in any patient treated with reversible drugs before CPA
  Intravenous fluids
    Use cautiously in euvolemic patients
    Administer in patients with known or suspected hypovolemia
  Corticosteroids
    Not recommended for routine use during CPR or after ROSC
    Consider low-dose hydrocortisone in patients after ROSC with refractory hypotension

Defibrillation
  Electrical defibrillation
    Treatment of choice for all patients with VF
    Continue chest compressions while charging
    Administer ONE shock
    Immediately resume chest compressions for 2 minutes after defibrillation
  Precordial thump
    Deliver a strong blow using the heel of the hand directly over the heart
    Minimal efficacy: use only if electrical defibrillation is not available

during a 3- to 5-second pause in chest compressions for rhythm check and patient evaluation. The resuscitation team leader should clearly announce the rhythm diagnosis to the group and invite other members to express differing opinion to minimize the risk of an inaccurate diagnosis. However, chest compressions should be resumed immediately and if any uncertainty regarding rhythm diagnosis persists, the respective discussion can be held during ongoing BLS in the subsequent 2-minute cycle of CPR.

$ETCO_2$ can be determined noninvasively and continuously during CPR and is generally feasible to use but requires endotracheal intubation. The presence of measurable $ETCO_2$ is indicative of correct ETT tube placement, but a consistently low value should be followed by visual verification of correct intubation.[39] Because $ETCO_2$ is correlated with cardiac output and alveolar ventilation, it can serve to estimate the adequacy of blood flow generated during CPR as long as ventilation is kept constant. A very low $ETCO_2$ value during CPR (eg, <10–15 mm Hg) was found to be associated with a reduced likelihood of ROSC.[3] A low $ETCO_2$ value requires action to be taken to improve the quality of chest compression or to investigate into and remove some other cause for low efficacy of CPR, such as hemorrhage or pneumothorax.[1,30] Because cardiac output substantially increases upon ROSC, a rapid increase in $ETCO_2$ can be observed; therefore, capnography is a suitable tool for early recognition of ROSC.[40]

Drug Treatment

During CPR, drugs are preferably administered by the intravenous (IV) or intraosseous (IO) route. Thus, establishing vascular access by peripheral or central venous or IO cannulation is required.[41] Depending on the arrest rhythm and the duration of CPA, administration of vasopressors, parasympatholytics, and anti-arrhythmics should be considered. In addition, a beneficial role for reversal agents (eg, naloxone, flumazenil, atipamezole), resuscitative IV fluids, and alkalinizing drugs (eg, sodium bicarbonate) may be present. **Table 1** lists common drugs and doses used during CPR.

Vasopressors are recommended to increase peripheral vascular resistance, thereby increasing central arterial pressure and thus coronary and cerebral perfusion pressures.[42] The catecholamine epinephrine causes peripheral vasoconstriction via stimulation of α_1 receptors, but also acts on β_1 and, to a lesser extent, on β_2 receptors. The α_1 effects have been shown to be the most beneficial during CPR.[43,44] Initially, low doses (ie, 0.01 mg/kg IV/IO every other cycle of CPR) are recommended because studies have shown that lower doses are associated with a higher survival to discharge in people, although more recent studies are more ambiguous regarding the optimal dosing.[45,46] After prolonged CPR, a higher dose (ie, 0.1 mg/kg IV/IO every other cycle of CPR) may be considered. Where no IV or IO access can be established, epinephrine may also be administered via the ETT (ie, 0.02 mg/kg low dose; 0.2 mg/kg high dose) by feeding a long catheter through the ETT and diluting the epinephrine 1:1 with isotonic saline or sterile water.[47]

Vasopressin is a peptide hormone that exerts its vasoconstrictive effects via activation of peripheral V1 receptors. It may be used interchangeably or in combination with epinephrine during CPR at a dose of 0.8 U/kg IV/IO every other cycle of CPR, but overall clinical evidence suggests that it will not purport survival benefit compared with epinephrine.[48,49] However, theoretic benefits of vasopressin over epinephrine include its efficacy in acidemic environments in which α_1 receptor responsiveness is diminished, and its lack of β_1 adrenoceptor stimulation, which increases myocardial oxygen consumption during arrest.[50]

The use of the anticholinergic atropine in CPR has been studied extensively.[51–53] The benefit of atropine administration in animals with nonshockable rhythms has

Table 1
Cardiopulmonary resuscitation drugs and doses

	Drug	Common Concentration	Dose/Route	Comments
Arrest	Epinephrine (low dose)	1 mg/mL (1:1000)	0.01 mg/kg IV/IO	Every other BLS cycle for asystole/PEA
			0.02–0.1 mg/kg IT	Increase dose 2–10× and dilute for IT administration
	Epinephrine (high dose)	1 mg/mL (1:1000)	0.1 mg/kg IV/IO/IT	Consider for prolonged (>10 min) CPR
	Vasopressin	20 U/mL	0.8 U/kg IV/IO	Every other BLS cycle
			1.2 U/kg IT	Increase dose for IT use
	Atropine	0.54 mg/mL	0.04 mg/kg IV/IO	Single dose
			0.15–0.2 mg/kg IT	Recommended for bradycardic arrests/known or suspected high vagal tone
				Increase dose for IT use
	Bicarbonate	1 mEq/mL	1 mEq/kg IV/IO	For prolonged CPR/PCA phase when pH <7.0
				Do not use if hypoventilating
Antiarrhythmic	Amiodarone	50 mg/mL	5 mg/kg IV/IO	For refractory VF/PVT
				Associated with anaphylaxis in dogs
	Lidocaine	20 mg/mL	2 mg/kg slow IV/IO push (1–2 min)	For refractory VF/PVT *only* if amiodarone is not available
Reversal agents	Naloxone	0.4 mg/mL	0.04 mg/kg IV/IO	To reverse opioids
	Flumazenil	0.1 mg/mL	0.01 mg/kg IV/IO	To reverse benzodiazepines
	Atipamezole	5 mg/mL	0.1 mg/kg IV/IO	To reverse α_2 agonists
Defibrillation (may increase dose once by 50%–100% for refractory VF/PVT)	Monophasic external		4–6 J/kg	Use copious amounts of electrode gel for external defibrillation
	Monophasic internal		0.5–1 J/kg	
	Biphasic external		2–4 J/kg	
	Biphasic internal		0.2–0.4 J/kg	

Abbreviation: CPR, cardiopulmonary resuscitation; IO, intraosseus; IT, intratracheal; IV, intravenous; PEA, pulseless electrical activity; PVT, pulseless ventricular tachycardia; VF, ventricular fibrillation.

been inconsistent, but there was no harm identified at a dose of 0.04 mg/kg. Atropine administration at that dose can therefore be considered. It is furthermore reasonable to administer atropine to all dogs and cats where asystole or PEA is thought to be associated with increased vagal tone. Atropine may also be administered via ETT (0.15–0.2 mg/kg).[54] Pharmacokinetic data suggest that a single dose of atropine is adequate.[54]

The most effective treatment of VF/PVT is electrical defibrillation, as discussed in detail later. However, dogs and cats with shockable rhythms refractory to defibrillation (ie, VF or PVT persist despite 5 or more defibrillation attempts) may benefit from amiodarone administration (2.5–5 mg/kg IV/IO).[55] Because the carrier (ie, polysorbate 80) used in some formulations of amiodarone may cause anaphylactic reactions and hypotension in dogs, animals should be closely monitored for signs of allergic reactions once ROSC is achieved.[56] If these signs occur, administration of diphenhydramine (2 mg/kg intramuscularly) and/or anti-inflammatory corticosteroids (eg, 0.1 mg/kg dexamethasone sodium phosphate IV) is warranted. Aqueous solutions of amiodarone do not appear to cause these reactions. Where amiodarone is unavailable, lidocaine (2 mg/kg slow IV/IO push) can be considered in dogs or cats with refractory VF. Although lidocaine has been shown to increase the defibrillation threshold in dogs in 1 study, benefit was evident in other studies, and in humans, the overall evidence suggests equivalence to amiodarone.[57–59]

In dogs and cats in which reversible anesthetic/analgesic drugs were recently administered, administration of the respective antagonists may be considered. Naloxone (0.04 mg/kg IV/IO) can be used to reverse opioids; flumazenil (0.01 mg/kg IV/IO) can be used for benzodiazepines, and atipamezole (0.1 mg/kg IV/IO) or yohimbine (0.1 mg/kg IV/IO) can be used for α_2 agonists such as medetomidine.

Resuscitative fluid therapy during CPR should be limited to those patients that are thought to be hypovolemic. CPA alone is not an indication for volume expansion therapy, and such an intervention may be harmful.[60–62] Because IV-administered fluid loading preferentially increases right atrial pressure, coronary and cerebral perfusion pressures and the respective tissue blood flow decrease.[61] In the presence of hypovolemia, however, intraarrest IV resuscitative fluid therapy will aid restoration of adequate circulating volume and increase the efficacy of chest compressions to improve tissue perfusion.

One veterinary prospective observational study showed an association between intraarrest administration of corticosteroids and an increased rate of ROSC in dogs and cats.[3] However, type and dose of steroids administered varied among animals, and the observational study design was unsuitable to demonstrate a cause-and-effect relationship. Two randomized controlled trials in humans with in-hospital cardiac arrest demonstrated improved ROSC, survival to discharge, and neurologically intact survival after the combined administration of vasopressin, epinephrine, and steroids (ie, methylprednisolone) when compared with epinephrine alone.[63,64] How this corresponds to benefit in dogs and cats, however, remains open. It is recognized, that even a single administration of high-dose corticosteroids can cause gastrointestinal bleeding in dogs, among other known side effects.[65,66] Because the documented risks of high-dose steroids outweigh their potential benefit, the routine use of steroids is not recommended in CPA patients.

Sodium bicarbonate (1 mEq/kg, once, diluted IV) administration may be considered with prolonged CPR (>10–15 minutes) whereby severe metabolic acidosis (eg, lactate) predictably leads to profound acidemia.[67] Inhibition of normal enzymatic and metabolic activity leading to reduced cardiac contractility and severe vasodilation can be the consequence.[55] As the metabolic acidosis may rapidly diminish upon ROSC, alkalinizing therapy should be reserved for patients with prolonged CPA or with documented severe acidemia (ie, pH <7.0) of metabolic origin.

Electrical Defibrillation

Electrical defibrillation is by far the most effective method to convert a shockable arrest rhythm to a perfusing rhythm. In adults, early electrical defibrillation in patients with VF as the primary arrest rhythm is associated with an increase in ROSC rates and survival to discharge.[68]

Defibrillators are described as monophasic if the current travels in 1 direction from 1 panel to the other, or biphasic if the current travels back and forth from 1 paddle to the other. The use of biphasic defibrillators is recommended because of their higher efficacy in terminating VF and their requirement for a lower current (and hence less myocardial injury). An initial dose of 4 to 6 J/kg should be used for external defibrillation with monophasic devices, whereas biphasic defibrillation should start at 2 to 4 J/kg. A subsequent shock can be delivered at an increased dose (ie, 50% higher), but subsequent doses should not be further increased.

It is important to minimize pauses during the defibrillation process. As soon as the VF/PVT is identified, chest compressions should resume until the defibrillator is charged. After shock administration, chest compressions should be resumed immediately for a full 2-minute cycle of CPR. The ECG is then assessed for the continued presence of a shockable rhythm requiring additional defibrillation.[69]

POST-CARDIAC ARREST CARE

In people with in-hospital cardiac arrest, two-thirds of those successfully resuscitated (ie, achieved ROSC) do not survive to hospital discharge but die during the postresuscitation phase.[70] Likewise, in 1 veterinary study, only 21% of dogs and cats that achieved any ROSC and 34% of those with ROSC of more than 20 minutes survived to hospital discharge.[5] Consequently, the PCA period offers an opportunity to save a significant number of lives (**Box 4**).

Rearrest early after ROSC is common, with 1 study reporting a median interval from ROSC to rearrest of 15 minutes.[3] The first goal of PCA care is therefore to support circulation and perfusion of vital organs (eg, brain and heart) and to assure normoxemia, thereby mitigating injury to these tissues and preventing rearrest. This initial support may include resuscitative fluid therapy, vasopressor infusions (eg, epinephrine), and continued ventilation and oxygen supplementation. With ROSC, the usual monitoring modalities (eg, pulse oximetry, Doppler sphygmomanometry) can be used to assess the cardiopulmonary function of the animal and guide treatment. An effort should be undertaken to identify and rapidly reverse clinically significant changes in electrolytes, glucose, acid-base status, hematocrit, oxygenation, and ventilation.

In general, patient outcome is influenced by comorbidities and events that led to CPA, the ischemic injury sustained during CPA, and the consequences of reperfusion. The clinical presentation of PCA is characterized by anoxic brain injury, postischemic myocardial dysfunction, the systemic response to ischemia and reperfusion, and persistent precipitating pathologic condition (eg, underlying disease processes).[71] Because these factors all vary between patients, the clinical picture in the PCA phase is highly variable, and a one-size-fits-all approach cannot be recommended. Rather, treatment should be titrated to critical care principles under consideration of the following specific PCA care elements.

Box 4
Postcardiac arrest care key recommendations

Respiratory optimization
  Ventilation
    Maintain normal $Paco_2$ (eg, 30–40 mm Hg)
    Mechanical ventilation required for persistent hypoventilation
  Oxygenation
    Titrate oxygen supplementation to maintain normoxemia (eg, Pao_2 80–100 mm Hg, SpO_2 94%–98%)
    Mechanical ventilation required for persistent hypoxemia nonresponsive to oxygen therapy

Hemodynamic optimization
  Target normotension or mild hypertension (mean arterial pressure 80–120 mm Hg, systolic arterial pressure 100–200 mm Hg)
  Treat hypovolemia with IV fluids
  Treat vasodilation with vasopressors
  Treat poor cardiac contractility with positive inotropes

Neuroprotective therapy
  Targeted temperature management (33°C–36°C) for 24 hours if comatose
  Slow rewarming (0.25°C–0.5°C per hour)
  Prevent hyperthermia/fever
  Treat seizures aggressively
  Mannitol (eg, 0.5 g–2 g/kg slow IV over 15–20 minutes) or 7% hypertonic saline (2–4 mL/kg IV over 15–20 minutes) for signs of increased intracranial pressure

---

Hemodynamic instability commonly occurs after ROSC. A strategy to achieve early hemodynamic optimization, similar to algorithms described for sepsis and septic shock, can be used in hemodynamically unstable small animals after CPA.[72,73] Resuscitation endpoints include a central venous oxygen saturation of at least 70% and normalization of lactate levels. Central venous pressure monitoring can be useful to limit the risk of pulmonary edema exacerbated by possible PCA left ventricular dysfunction and increased vascular permeability. Because autoregulation of cerebral blood flow can be impaired in the PCA phase, cerebral blood flow may depend more directly on cerebral perfusion pressure. Therefore, a higher mean arterial blood pressure goal than in septic patients should be targeted (eg, ≥80 mm Hg).[74]

Neuroprotective measures are of particular relevance to PCA patients, given the uniform exposure to cerebral hypoxia.[75] The maintenance of a core temperature below normal (ie, hypothermia) after ROSC improves neurologic outcome after CPA in humans and other species, including dogs and cats.[76–80] In humans, targeted temperature management with a core temperature goal of 33°C to 36°C (91.4°F–96.8°F) for at least 24 hours in patients that do not regain consciousness shortly after ROSC is recommended.[81] The current RECOVER guidelines suggest a temperature target of 32°C to 34°C (89.6°F–93.2°F) for 24 to 48 hours, but this may be revised to a more liberal temperature range in the new guidelines.[9] Although therapeutic hypothermia may not easily be administered in veterinary patients outside of critical care, individual reports demonstrate feasibility of the treatment in clinical practice.[82] In any case, post-ROSC dogs and cats are commonly hypothermic, and all that may be needed is not to actively rewarm these animals. In fact, current experimental evidence indicates that rapid active rewarming and hyperthermia after brain anoxia are harmful.[83,84] Aggressive, active rewarming should therefore be strictly avoided whether the patient is comatose or not, and passive rewarming should not surpass 1.0°C (1.8°F) per hour. Instead, a slower rewarming rate of 0.25°C to 0.5°C (0.45°F–0.9°F) per hour should be targeted. Seizures may occur in the PCA period and should be treated with diazepam (0.5 mg/kg IV/IO) and/or phenobarbital (4 mg/kg IV). Cerebral edema can occur early in the PCA period because of the lack of energy to power the Na/K-ATPase and accumulations of intracellular sodium, and because of loss of integrity of the blood-brain barrier.[85] Therefore, in patients that are persistently comatose and/or apneic after achieving ROSC, mannitol (0.5 g/kg IV) or 7% hypertonic saline (2–4 mL/kg IV) over 15 to 20 minutes is recommended.

Respiratory optimization is a third area of specific consideration for PCA care. To assure normal arterial oxygen tension (eg, Pao_2 80–100 mm Hg) and CO_2 (eg, $Paco_2$ 30–40 mm Hg), and to prevent respiratory arrest in the comatose PCA patient, positive pressure ventilation should be continued immediately after cardiac arrest and until stable spontaneous ventilation is achieved. Ventilation should be monitored using $ETCO_2$ or arterial blood gas analysis. Hyperoxia early during the reperfusion process should be avoided to reduce free radical production and subsequent exacerbation of neuronal injury.[86,87] Because hypoxemia is likewise harmful, it is reasonable to titrate supplemental oxygen to maintain normoxemia, such as an SpO_2 level of 94% to 96%.

Comorbidities are the most common reason for death in people after in-hospital cardiac arrest, followed by PCA neurologic injury and shock, and a similar relationship may be present in dogs and cats.[88] Accordingly, critical care management of the patient's precipitating disease process and concomitant organ dysfunctions (eg, ileus, acute kidney injury) is important but can be challenging. For that reason, referral to a specialty care facility with 24-hour critical care capability is reasonable for systemically ill PCA patients.

PROGNOSIS

Survival to hospital discharge in dogs and cats with CPA is an uncommon event, unless the CPA occurs under anesthesia. More recently reported survival to discharge rates of small animals undergoing CPR in academic veterinary hospitals ranges from 6% to 7% (dogs) and 7% to 19% (cats).[3,5] The inciting cause of cardiac arrest may be one of the most important prognostic factors. Among 15 dogs and 3 cats that survived to hospital discharge, only 3 animals had significant comorbidities.[89] Dogs and cats that experience CPA while in the care of the anesthesia service were 14.8 times as likely to survive to hospital discharge than those animals that were not.[5] Thus, prolonged CPR efforts (eg, >10–20 minutes) in the perianesthetic population are most rewarding.

Prognostication in animals that have achieved ROSC is understudied in the veterinary literature.[5] Such studies are complicated by the low percentage of survivors and the fact that most initially successfully resuscitated animals are euthanized (ie, 70% in 1 study)[5] for a variety of reasons, including economic considerations. In contrast, the post-ROSC criteria for withdrawal of life support because of a futile neurologic outcome have been extensively studied in people. Current recommendations (American Heart Association 2015) encourage a multimodal approach of neurologic prognostication using several criteria in conjunction and prescribe guidelines regarding timing.[81] A prognostication algorithm has been devised by the European Resuscitation Council.[90,91] According to this algorithm, the earliest time point for conclusive assessment is 72 hours after ROSC, whereby continued unconsciousness (ie, absence of pain response) in combination with bilaterally absent pupillary light response indicates an extremely poor neurologic prognosis. Other diagnostic modalities, such as electrophysiological measurements (ie, electroencephalogram, somatosensory evoked potentials), imaging (ie, MRI, computed tomography), and circulating biomarkers, can also be used after 72 hours or more. Taken together, neurologic prognostication during the first 1 to 3 days is not considered sufficiently accurate to predict a futile functional outcome in people. Although no data are available for dogs and cats, it is likely that adult animals with CPA-related anoxic brain injury recover along a similar timeline as humans do. It seems reasonable to think that euthanasia purely for the reason of a futile neurologic outcome in dogs and cats that remain unconscious during the first hours after ROSC is contrary to best evidence and may lead to a self-fulfilling prophecy. If comorbidities and pet owner wishes permit, it may be reasonable to allow animals a significant amount of time for neurologic recovery.

SUMMARY

CPA is associated with a high mortality, and CPR is the only treatment. To reduce the incidence of unexpected death owing to CPA, a cohesive strategy is necessary that includes well-implemented preventive and preparedness measures, BLS, and ALS, and PCA critical care titrated to the patient's needs.

DISCLOSURE

The authors have nothing to disclose.

REFERENCES

1. Kass PH, Haskins SC. Survival following cardiopulmonary resuscitation in dogs and cats. J Vet Emerg Crit Care 1992;2(2):57–65.
2. Wingfield WE, Van Pelt DR. Respiratory and cardiopulmonary arrest in dogs and cats: 265 cases (1986-1991). J Am Vet Med Assoc 1992;200(12):993–1996.
3. Hofmeister EH, Brainard BM, Egger CM, et al. Prognostic indicators for dogs and cats with cardiopulmonary arrest treated by cardiopulmonary cerebral resuscitation at a university teaching hospital. J Am Vet Med Assoc 2009;235(1):50–7.
4. McIntyre RL, Hopper K, Epstein SE. Assessment of cardiopulmonary resuscitation in 121 dogs and 30 cats at a university teaching hospital (2009-2012). J Vet Emerg Crit Care 2014;24(6):693–704.
5. Hoehne SN, Epstein SE, Hopper K. Prospective evaluation of cardiopulmonary resuscitation performed in dogs and cats according to the RECOVER guidelines. Part 1: prognostic factors according to Utstein-style reporting. Front Vet Sci 2019; 6:384.
6. Boller M, Boller EM, Oodegard S, et al. Small animal cardiopulmonary resuscitation requires a continuum of care: proposal for a chain of survival for veterinary patients. J Am Vet Med Assoc 2012;240(5):540–54.
7. Søreide E, Morrison L, Hillman K, et al. The formula for survival in resuscitation. Resuscitation 2013;84(11):1487–93.
8. Boller M, Fletcher DJ. RECOVER evidence and knowledge gap analysis on veterinary CPR. Part 1: evidence analysis and consensus process: collaborative path toward small animal CPR guidelines. J Vet Emerg Crit Care 2012; 22(Suppl 1):S4–12.
9. Fletcher DJ, Boller M, Brainard BM, et al. RECOVER evidence and knowledge gap analysis on veterinary CPR. Part 7: clinical guidelines. J Vet Emerg Crit Care 2012;22(Suppl 1):S102–31.
10. McMichael M, Herring J, Fletcher DJ, et al. RECOVER evidence and knowledge gap analysis on veterinary CPR. Part 2: preparedness and prevention. J Vet Emerg Crit Care 2012;22(Suppl 1):S13–25.

11. Hopper K, Epstein SE, Fletcher DJ, et al. RECOVER evidence and knowledge gap analysis on veterinary CPR. Part 3: basic life support. J Vet Emerg Crit Care 2012;22(Suppl 1):S26–43.

12. Rozanski EA, Rush JE, Buckley GJ, et al. RECOVER evidence and knowledge gap analysis on veterinary CPR. Part 4: advanced life support. J Vet Emerg Crit Care 2012;22(Suppl 1):S44–64.

13. Brainard BM, Boller M, Fletcher DJ, et al. RECOVER evidence and knowledge gap analysis on veterinary CPR. Part 5: monitoring. J Vet Emerg Crit Care (San Antonio) 2012;22(Suppl 1):S65–84.

14. Smarick SD, Haskins SC, Boller M, et al. RECOVER evidence and knowledge gap analysis on veterinary CPR. Part 6: post-cardiac arrest care. J Vet Emerg Crit Care 2012;22(Suppl 1):S85–101.

15. Smith GB. In-hospital cardiac arrest: is it time for an in-hospital 'chain of prevention'? Resuscitation 2010;81(9):1209–11.

16. Bhanji F, Finn JC, Lockey A, et al. Part 8: education, implementation, and teams: 2015 international consensus on cardiopulmonary resuscitation and emergency cardiovascular care science with treatment recommendations. Circulation 2015; 132(16 Suppl 1):S242–68.

17. Isbye DL, Meyhoff CS, Lippert FK, et al. Skill retention in adults and in children 3 months after basic life support training using a simple personal resuscitation manikin. Resuscitation 2007;74(2):296–302.

18. Mpotos N, Lemoyne S, Wyler B, et al. Training to deeper compression depth reduces shallow compressions after six months in a manikin model. Resuscitation 2011;82(10):1323–7.

19. Dyson E, Smith GB. Common faults in resuscitation equipment - guidelines for checking equipment and drugs used in adult cardiopulmonary resuscitation. Resuscitation 2002;55(2):137–49.

20. Hall C, Robertson D, Rolfe M, et al. Do cognitive aids reduce error rates in resuscitation team performance? Trial of emergency medicine protocols in simulation training (TEMPIST) in Australia. Hum Resour Health 2020;18(1):1.

21. Edelson DP, Litzinger B, Arora V, et al. Improving in-hospital cardiac arrest process and outcomes with performance debriefing. Arch Intern Med 2008; 168(10):1063–9.

22. Dine CJ, Gersh RE, Leary M, et al. Improving cardiopulmonary resuscitation quality and resuscitation training by combining audiovisual feedback and debriefing. Crit Care Med 2008;36(10):2817–22.

23. Moitra VK, Einav S, Thies KC, et al. Cardiac arrest in the operating room: resuscitation and management for the anesthesiologist Part 1. Anesth Analg 2018; 127(3):e49–50.

24. Bircher NG, Chan PS, Xu Y. Delays in cardiopulmonary resuscitation, defibrillation, and epinephrine administration all decrease survival in in-hospital cardiac arrest. Anesthesiology 2019;130(3):414–22.

25. Maier GW, Newton JR Jr, Wolfe JA, et al. The influence of manual chest compression rate on hemodynamic support during cardiac arrest: high-impulse cardiopulmonary resuscitation. Circulation 1986;74(6 Pt 2):IV51–9.

26. Weil MH, Bisera J, Trevino RP, et al. Cardiac output and end-tidal carbon dioxide. Crit Care Med 1985;13(11):907–9.

27. Voorhees WD, Babbs CF, Tacker WA Jr. Regional blood flow during cardiopulmonary resuscitation in dogs. Crit Care Med 1980;8(3):134–6.

28. Wolfe JA, Maier GW, Newton JR Jr, et al. Physiologic determinants of coronary blood flow during external cardiac massage. J Thorac Cardiovasc Surg 1988; 95(3):523–32.

29. Yeung J, Meeks R, Edelson D, et al. The use of CPR feedback/prompt devices during training and CPR performance: a systematic review. Resuscitation 2009; 80(7):743–51.

30. Kneba EJ, Humm KR. The use of mental metronomes during simulated cardiopulmonary resuscitation training. J Vet Emerg Crit Care 2020;30(1):92–6.

31. Yannopoulos D, McKnite S, Aufderheide TP, et al. Effects of incomplete chest wall decompression during cardiopulmonary resuscitation on coronary and cerebral perfusion pressures in a porcine model of cardiac arrest. Resuscitation 2005; 64(3):363–72.

32. Zuercher M, Hilwig RW, Ranger-Moore J, et al. Leaning during chest compressions impairs cardiac output and left ventricular myocardial blood flow in piglet cardiac arrest. Crit Care Med 2010;38(4):1141–6.

33. Edelson DP, Abella BS, Kramer-Johansen J, et al. Effects of compression depth and pre-shock pauses predict defibrillation failure during cardiac arrest. Resuscitation 2006;71(2):137–45.

34. Gundersen K, Kvaloy JT, Kramer-Johansen J, et al. Development of the probability of return of spontaneous circulation in intervals without chest compressions during out-of-hospital cardiac arrest: an observational study. BMC Med 2009;7:6.

35. Kern KB, Hilwig RW, Berg RA, et al. Importance of continuous chest compressions during cardiopulmonary resuscitation: improved outcome during a simulated single lay-rescuer scenario. Circulation 2002;105(5):645–9.

36. Kern KB. Coronary perfusion pressure during cardiopulmonary resuscitation. Best Pract Res Clin Anaesthesiol 2000;14(3):591–609.

37. Cipani S, Bartolozzi C, Ballo P, et al. Blood flow maintenance by cardiac massage during cardiopulmonary resuscitation: classical theories, newer hypotheses, and clinical utility of mechanical devices. J Intensive Care Soc 2019;20(1):2–10.

38. Aufderheide TP, Lurie KG. Death by hyperventilation: a common and life-threatening problem during cardiopulmonary resuscitation. Crit Care Med 2004;32(9 Suppl):S345–51.

39. Li J. Capnography alone is imperfect for endotracheal tube placement confirmation during emergency intubation. J Emerg Med 2001;20(3):223–9.

40. Sandroni C, De Santis P, D'Arrigo S. Capnography during cardiac arrest. Resuscitation 2018;132:73–7.

41. Beal MW, Hughes D. Vascular access: theory and techniques in the small animal emergency patient. Clin Tech Small Anim Pract 2000;15(2):101–9.

42. Michael JR, Guerci AD, Koehler RC, et al. Mechanisms by which epinephrine augments cerebral and myocardial perfusion during cardiopulmonary resuscitation in dogs. Circulation 1984;69(4):822–35.

43. Holmes HR, Babbs CF, Voorhees WD, et al. Influence of adrenergic drugs upon vital organ perfusion during CPR. Crit Care Med 1980;8(3):137–40.

44. Otto CW, Yakaitis RW, Redding JS, et al. Comparison of dopamine, dobutamine, and epinephrine in CPR. Crit Care Med 1981;9(9):640–3.

45. Vandycke C, Martens P. High dose versus standard dose epinephrine in cardiac arrest—a meta-analysis. Resuscitation 2000;45(3):161–6.

46. Vargas M, Buonanno P, Iacovazzo C, et al. Epinephrine for out of hospital cardiac arrest: a systematic review and meta-analysis of randomized controlled trials. Resuscitation 2019;145:151–7.

47. Pavlovic A, Popovic N, Bumbasirevic V, et al. Endotracheal administration of adrenaline in cardiopulmonary resuscitation of anaesthetized dogs. Acta Vet (Beogr) 2006;56(1):63–79.

48. Finn J, Jacobs I, Williams TA, et al. Adrenaline and vasopressin for cardiac arrest. Cochrane Database Syst Rev 2019;(1):CD003179.

49. Buckley GJ, Rozanski EA, Rush JE. Randomized, blinded comparison of epinephrine and vasopressin for treatment of naturally occurring cardiopulmonary arrest in dogs. J Vet Intern Med 2011;25(6):1334–40.

50. Lindner KH, Prengel AW, Pfenninger EG, et al. Vasopressin improves vital organ blood flow during closed-chest cardiopulmonary resuscitation in pigs. Circulation 1995;91(1):215–21.

51. DeBehnke DJ, Swart GL, Spreng D, et al. Standard and higher doses of atropine in a canine model of pulseless electrical activity. Acad Emerg Med 1995;2(12):1034–41.

52. Blecic S, Chaskis C, Vincent JL. Atropine administration in experimental electromechanical dissociation. Am J Emerg Med 1992;10(6):515–8.

53. Coon GA, Clinton JE, Ruiz E. Use of atropine for brady-asystolic prehospital cardiac arrest. Ann Emerg Med 1981;10(9):462–7.

54. Paret G, Mazkereth R, Sella R, et al. Atropine pharmacokinetics and pharmacodynamics following endotracheal versus endobronchial administration in dogs. Resuscitation 1999;41(1):57–62.

55. Jamme M, Ben Hadj Salem O, Guillemet L, et al. Severe metabolic acidosis after out-of-hospital cardiac arrest: risk factors and association with outcome. Ann Intensive Care 2018;8(1):62.

56. Cober RE, Schober KE, Hildebrandt N, et al. Adverse effects of intravenous amiodarone in 5 dogs. J Vet Intern Med 2009;23(3):657–61.

57. Sanfilippo F, Corredor C, Santonocito C, et al. Amiodarone or lidocaine for cardiac arrest: a systematic review and meta-analysis. Resuscitation 2016;107:31–7.

58. Dorian P, Cass D, Schwartz B, et al. Amiodarone as compared with lidocaine for shock-resistant ventricular fibrillation. N Engl J Med 2002;346(12):884–90.

59. Dorian P, Fain ES, Davy JM, et al. Lidocaine causes a reversible, concentration-dependent increase in defibrillation energy requirements. J Am Coll Cardiol 1986;8(2):327–32.

60. Fischer M, Hossmann KA. Volume expansion during cardiopulmonary resuscitation reduces cerebral no-reflow. Resuscitation 1996;32(3):227–40.

61. Voorhees WD 3rd, Ralston SH, Kougias C, et al. Fluid loading with whole blood or Ringer's lactate solution during CPR in dogs. Resuscitation 1987;15(2):113–23.

62. Gentile NT, Martin GB, Appleton TJ, et al. Effects of arterial and venous volume infusion on coronary perfusion pressures during canine CPR. Resuscitation 1991;22(1):55–63.

63. Mentzelopoulos SD, Malachias S, Chamos C, et al. Vasopressin, steroids, and epinephrine and neurologically favorable survival after in-hospital cardiac arrest: a randomized clinical trial. JAMA 2013;310(3):270–9.

64. Mentzelopoulos SD, Zakynthinos SG, Tzoufi M, et al. Vasopressin, epinephrine, and corticosteroids for in-hospital cardiac arrest. Arch Intern Med 2009;169(1):15–24.

65. Levine JM, Levine GJ, Boozer L, et al. Adverse effects and outcome associated with dexamethasone administration in dogs with acute thoracolumbar intervertebral disk herniation: 161 cases (2000-2006). J Am Vet Med Assoc 2008;232(3):411–7.

66. Rohrer CR, Hill RC, Fischer A, et al. Gastric hemorrhage in dogs given high doses of methylprednisolone sodium succinate. Am J Vet Res 1999;60(8):977–81.

67. Hopper K, Borchers A, Epstein SE. Acid base, electrolyte, glucose, and lactate values during cardiopulmonary resuscitation in dogs and cats. J Vet Emerg Crit Care 2014;24(2):208–14.

68. Chan PS, Krumholz HM, Nichol G, et al. Delayed time to defibrillation after in-hospital cardiac arrest. N Engl J Med 2008;358(1):9–17.

69. Callaway CW, Soar J, Aibiki M, et al. Part 4: advanced life support: 2015 International Consensus on Cardiopulmonary Resuscitation and Emergency Cardiovascular Care Science with treatment recommendations. Circulation 2015;132(16 Suppl 1):S84–145.

70. Peberdy MA, Kaye W, Ornato JP, et al. Cardiopulmonary resuscitation of adults in the hospital: a report of 14720 cardiac arrests from the National Registry of Cardiopulmonary Resuscitation. Resuscitation 2003;58(3):297–308.

71. Neumar RW, Nolan JP, Adrie C, et al. Post-cardiac arrest syndrome: epidemiology, pathophysiology, treatment, and prognostication. Circulation 2008; 118(23):2452–83.

72. Rivers E, Nguyen B, Havstad S, et al. Early goal-directed therapy in the treatment of severe sepsis and septic shock. N Engl J Med 2001;345(19):1368–77.

73. Gaieski DF, Band RA, Abella BS, et al. Early goal-directed hemodynamic optimization combined with therapeutic hypothermia in comatose survivors of out-of-hospital cardiac arrest. Resuscitation 2009;80(4):418–24.

74. Sundgreen C, Larsen FS, Herzog TM, et al. Autoregulation of cerebral blood flow in patients resuscitated from cardiac arrest. Stroke 2001;32(1):128–32.

75. Sekhon MS, Ainslie PN, Griesdale DE. Clinical pathophysiology of hypoxic ischemic brain injury after cardiac arrest: a "two-hit" model. Crit Care 2017; 21(1):90.

76. Busto R, Dietrich WD, Globus MY, et al. Small differences in intraischemic brain temperature critically determine the extent of ischemic neuronal injury. J Cereb Blood Flow Metab 1987;7(6):729–38.

77. Hossmann KA. Resuscitation potentials after prolonged global cerebral ischemia in cats. Crit Care Med 1988;16(10):964–71.

78. Kuboyama K, Safar P, Radovsky A, et al. Delay in cooling negates the beneficial effect of mild resuscitative cerebral hypothermia after cardiac arrest in dogs: a prospective, randomized study. Crit Care Med 1993;21(9):1348–58.

79. Leonov Y, Sterz F, Safar P, et al. Hypertension with hemodilution prevents multifocal cerebral hypoperfusion after cardiac arrest in dogs. Stroke 1992;23(1): 45–53.

80. Brodeur A, Wright A, Cortes Y. Hypothermia and targeted temperature management in cats and dogs. J Vet Emerg Crit Care 2017;27(2):151–63.

81. Callaway CW, Donnino MW, Fink EL, et al. Part 8: post-cardiac arrest care: 2015 American Heart Association guidelines update for cardiopulmonary resuscitation and emergency cardiovascular care. Circulation 2015;132(18 Suppl 2):S465–82.

82. Hayes GM. Severe seizures associated with traumatic brain injury managed by controlled hypothermia, pharmacologic coma, and mechanical ventilation in a dog. J Vet Emerg Crit Care 2009;19(6):629–34.

83. Hickey RW, Kochanek PM, Ferimer H, et al. Induced hyperthermia exacerbates neurologic neuronal histologic damage after asphyxial cardiac arrest in rats. Crit Care Med 2003;31(2):531–5.

84. Baena RC, Busto R, Dietrich WD, et al. Hyperthermia delayed by 24 hours aggravates neuronal damage in rat hippocampus following global ischemia. Neurology 1997;48(3):768–73.

85. Hayman EG, Patel AP, Kimberly WT, et al. Cerebral edema after cardiopulmonary resuscitation: a therapeutic target following cardiac arrest? Neurocrit Care 2018; 28(3):276–87.

86. Neumar RW. Optimal oxygenation during and after cardiopulmonary resuscitation. Curr Opin Crit Care 2011;17(3):236–40.

87. Roberts BW, Kilgannon JH, Hunter BR, et al. Association between early hyperoxia exposure after resuscitation from cardiac arrest and neurological disability. Circulation 2018;137(20):2114–24.

88. Witten L, Gardner R, Holmberg MJ, et al. Reasons for death in patients successfully resuscitated from out-of-hospital and in-hospital cardiac arrest. Resuscitation 2019;136:93–9.

89. Waldrop JE, Rozanski EA, Swanke ED, et al. Causes of cardiopulmonary arrest, resuscitation management, and functional outcome in dogs and cats surviving cardiopulmonary arrest. J Vet Emerg Crit Care 2004;14(1):22–9.

90. Sandroni C, Cariou A, Cavallaro F, et al. Prognostication in comatose survivors of cardiac arrest: an advisory statement from the European resuscitation council and the European society of intensive care medicine. Resuscitation 2014; 85(12):1779–89.

91. Cronberg T. Assessing brain injury after cardiac arrest, towards a quantitative approach. Curr Opin Crit Care 2019;25(3):211–7.

Small Animal Transfusion Medicine

Kendon W. Kuo, DVM, MS, Maureen McMichael, DVM, MEd*

KEYWORDS

- Transfusion • Red blood cells • Plasma • Platelets • Albumin • Hemolysis

KEY POINTS

- Transfusion medicine may be lifesaving.
- Pretransfusion compatibility testing may reduce the risk of transfusion reactions.
- Component therapy allows more efficient use of blood.
- Transfusion reactions range from mild to life threatening. Febrile nonhemolytic transfusion reactions are common but usually self-limiting.

INTRODUCTION

Transfusion medicine has progressed significantly since the first successful blood transfusion in 1665 between 2 dogs by Dr Richard Lower.[1] This article reviews the screening and selection of donors, ideal collection and storage, product selection, administration, and patient monitoring.

BLOOD DONORS

In our community blood bank, dogs are 1 to 8 years of age, greater than 23 kg, and provide 450 mL per donation. Cats are 1 to 10 years of age, greater than 4 kg, and provide 40 mL per donation. A detailed history is essential to assess donor health status and infectious disease risk. Animals who have received previous blood transfusions are unsuitable for donation. In 2015, The American College of Veterinary Internal Medicine (ACVIM) updated its consensus statement on canine and feline donor screening for blood-borne pathogens.[2]

BLOOD TYPES

Variations in inherited and acquired erythrocyte antigens may lead to blood incompatibility. As technologies improve, more erythrocyte antigens will continue to be discovered. Erythrocyte antigens are expressed on endothelial and epithelial cells, neurons,

Emergency and Critical Care, Department of Clinical Sciences, College of Veterinary Medicine, Auburn University, 1220 Wire Road, Auburn, AL 36849-5540, USA
* Corresponding author.
E-mail address: mam0280@auburn.edu

Vet Clin Small Anim 50 (2020) 1203–1214
https://doi.org/10.1016/j.cvsm.2020.07.001
0195-5616/20/© 2020 Elsevier Inc. All rights reserved.

and platelets, making the antigenicity of incompatible transfusions a systemic concern.[3] An in-depth review of erythrocyte antigens and antibodies provides excellent information on the topic.[4]

In dogs, the most recognized antigens are organized into the dog erythrocyte antigen (DEA) system. DEA 1 is the most important blood type clinically because it elicits a strong alloantibody response after sensitization and ~50% are DEA 1+. Without a previous transfusion, dogs are thought to have no clinically significant alloantibodies. In 2007, the *Dal* antigen was discovered after accidental sensitization of a *Dal*− Dalmatian given *Dal*+ blood.[5] In addition to Dalmatians, a high percentage of Doberman pinschers and shih tzus are *Dal*− and may be at risk of an acute, hemolytic transfusion reaction after sensitization with *Dal*+ blood. Most purebreds are *Dal*+, such as greyhounds, golden retrievers, Labrador retrievers, and German shepherd dogs. In 2017, *Kai 1* and *Kai 2* blood groups were discovered. The clinical importance of these alloantibodies needs to be determined. At present, a so-called universal donor in dogs is negative for DEA 1, DEA 3, DEA 5, and DEA 7, and positive for DEA 4. In humans, the concept of transfusing from a universal donor has never been shown to be superior and new research suggests that blood type matching may be more advantageous clinically than the use of universal donors.[6]

In cats, the major blood types are A, B, and rarely AB. Unlike dogs, cats produce clinically significant naturally occurring alloantibodies. Type A cats have lower titers of anti-B alloantibodies, but type B cats have high titers of anti-A alloantibodies, which can lead to severe acute hemolytic reactions, including death. Type AB cats do not produce either alloantibody. Another erythrocyte antigen, *MiK*, has been identified.[7] Although most cats are *MiK*+, *MiK*− cats may have naturally occurring alloantibodies, which can lead to hemolytic transfusion reactions. At present, there is no in-house typing system for *MiK* and no universal donor in cats.

LEUKOREDUCTION

Leukocytes in stored blood are associated with inflammation, ischemia-reperfusion injury, and transmission of infectious disease. Leukoreduction (LR) involves the removal of leukocytes from donated blood. Filtration at the time of collection (prestorage) is preferred because it removes leukocytes before they undergo apoptosis or necrosis, and before they can release breakdown products and inflammatory compounds such as histamine, plasminogen activator inhibitor-1, and myeloperoxidase.[8] Other benefits of prestorage LR include improved erythrocyte survival and reduced posttransfusion immunosuppression.[9]

LR products are becoming more available in veterinary medicine. In healthy dogs, LR eliminated the inflammatory response posttransfusion of autologous packed red blood cells (pRBCs).[10] There were lower concentrations of hemolysis, inflammatory cytokines, microparticles, and prothrombotic phospholipids along with higher 2,3-diphosphoglyceric acid (2,3-DPG) concentrations in LR pRBCs compared with non-LR pRBCs.[11–14] However, a study in healthy dogs showed an inflammatory response following transfusion of autologous 28-day-old pRBCs that was not attenuated by LR.[15] In a storage and simulated transfusion study, LR did not reduce phosphatidylserine expression, a recognized storage lesion.[16] In critically ill dogs, LR did not significantly reduce most markers of inflammation after transfusion of pRBCs stored for less than or equal to 12 days.[17] In 766 dogs, LR pRBCs had fewer acute transfusion reactions compared with non-LR pRBCs, but the difference was not statistically significant.[18] LR increases the cost of blood products by approximately $30 per unit and may increase processing time if blood is cooled before filtering.[19] For dogs, approximately 60 mL of blood is lost during filtration. For cats, an in-line neonatal filter is used and results in a loss of 8 mL.[20]

STORAGE

The storage of blood products increases availability, but detrimental changes termed storage lesion may occur. In veterinary medicine, older pRBCs had higher levels of some cytokines, free hemoglobin, prothrombotic phospholipid concentrations, and proinflammatory microparticles.[12,14,21,22] In a canine model of *Staphylococcus aureus*–induced septic pneumonia, dogs underwent massive exchange transfusion (80 mL/kg total) with either 7-day-old or 42-day-old stored pRBCs and fresh frozen plasma (FFP). Mortality in the older blood group was 100% compared with 33% in the fresh group. The older blood group also had increased in vivo hemolysis, cell-free hemoglobin levels, pulmonary hypertension, tissue damage, and gas exchange abnormalities.[23] However, in a retrospective study of 3095 dogs, duration of pRBC storage was not associated with survival in the population but did have a negative association in dogs with immune-mediated hemolytic anemia (hemolysis).[24] A retrospective study in 210 dogs found product age was not associated with survival but did increase the risk of transfusion-related hemolysis.[25] A study comparing LR pRBCs and non-LR pRBCs found that product age was associated with the risk of transfusion reaction but did not affect mortality.[18] In human medicine, several large trials failed to find a detrimental effect from the transfusion of older pRBCs.[26] The findings must be interpreted cautiously because the trials did not address whether transfusion of the oldest blood (35–42 days of storage) is safe. Finding the optimal balance between minimizing waste and storage time will likely vary between individual hospitals. A veterinary study reported that minimizing storage time of pRBCs was associated with greater wastage compared with the traditional first-in-first-out model, and therefore, increased hospital costs.[27]

BLOOD PRODUCTS

Component therapy conserves resources by allowing longer storage and more efficient usage. The use of multiple components (eg, pRBCs, FFP, platelets) adds significantly to dilution, hypothermia, acidosis, and anticoagulant effects compared with use of fresh whole blood. In contrast, by tailoring transfusion to specific needs, targeted transfusion of only the essential components may reduce the risk of transfusion-related adverse effects. The commonly available products, dosing, and further details are summarized in **Table 1**.

RED BLOOD CELLS

Whole blood or pRBCs are indicated for anemia. The optimal transfusion trigger is unknown but is likely multifactorial. Considerations include historical findings (eg, rate of anemia development, duration of anemia), clinical status (eg, mentation, capillary refill time, mucous membranes, pulse rate and quality, temperature), and biochemical variables (eg, hematocrit, hemoglobin, lactate, base excess). The trend in human medicine is toward a restrictive strategy (transfuse at hemoglobin level <7 g/dL) compared with a liberal strategy (transfuse at hemoglobin <9–10 g/dL.).[28,29] Recent studies question the restrictive strategy.[30]

PLASMA PRODUCTS

The indications for plasma are controversial in both human and veterinary medicine.[31] Plasma is commonly administered prophylactically in coagulopathic patients with a

Table 1
Blood transfusion guidelines

Product	Composition	Dose	Rate	Notes
Fresh whole blood	RBCs WBCs Platelets All plasma	20 mL/kg	5–10 mL/kg/h <4 h	2 mL/kg may ↑PCV 1% Or transfusion (mL) = [wt (kg) × 90] [desired PCV − recipient PCV]/donor PCV Platelet function begins to decrease within 1 h
Stored whole blood	RBCs ±WBCs All plasma ±Factor V and VIII	20 mL/kg	5–10 mL/kg/h <4 h	2.2 mL/kg may ↑PCV 1% Platelets are nonviable >8 h after collection
Packed red blood cells	RBCs ±WBCs	10–15 mL/kg	5–10 mL/kg/h <4 h	1.5 mL/kg may ↑PCV 1%
FFP	Coagulation factors Antithrombin Albumin Globulins	10–20 mL/kg	5–10 mL/kg/h <4 h	—
Cryoprecipitate	vWF Factor VIII, XIII Fibrinogen Fibronectin	1 unit per 10 kg 1–5 mL/kg	5–10 mL/kg/h <2 h	Start 30 min before surgery Repeat q30 min if highly invasive surgery is anticipated
Cryoprecipitate-poor plasma	Factor II, VII, IX, X Albumin Anticoagulants Fibrinolytic factors	10–30 mL/kg	5–10 mL/kg/h OR 1–2 mL/kg/h <4 h	—
Albumin (canine)	Albumin	Hypotension: 450–800 mg/kg Hypoalbuminemia: Maximum 2 g/kg	≤1 mL/min <6 h	Albumin deficit (g) = 10 × (serum albumin goal − patient's serum albumin) × body weight (kg) × 0.3
Lyophilized platelets	Platelets	1 unit per 5 kg	Slow bolus	Filter not recommended

Abbreviations: PCV, packed cell volume; q, every; RBCs, red blood cells; vWF, von Willebrand factor; WBCs, white blood cells; wt, weight.

potentially higher risk of bleeding. However, studies in human medicine show that abnormal coagulation tests such as prothrombin time and activated partial thrombo-plastin time are not accurate predictors of bleeding.[32–35] Similar findings were found in horses undergoing percutaneous liver biopsies.[36] Viscoelastic testing such as throm-boelastography has shown varying results in human studies but may better predict the risk of bleeding.[37–40] Veterinary studies are needed to determine what tests, if any, can best assess the risk of bleeding and the need for plasma transfusion.

Cryoprecipitate concentrates factors VIII and von Willebrand factor, among others, and is indicated for prevention of bleeding caused by hemophilia A or von Willebrand disease.[41] The smaller volume (compared with FFP) may decrease transfusion reac-tions. Cryoprecipitate-poor plasma (CPP) is the supernatant removed during process-ing and provides factors II, VII, IX, and X and is a suitable treatment in anticoagulant rodenticide toxicosis. In critically ill dogs, albumin levels increased after a constant-rate infusion of CPP, suggesting that CPP may be a treatment option for oncotic sup-port and albumin replacement.[42]

Concentrated albumin products include human serum albumin (HSA) and canine-specific albumin (CSA). Administration of human albumin remains controversial and has been associated with life-threatening hypersensitivity reactions in veterinary pa-tients.[43–45] Repeated transfusions are not recommended.[46] A 5% lyophilized CSA is commercially available. In dogs with septic peritonitis, CSA increased albumin con-centration but was not associated with survival.[47] Canine-specific albumin was well tolerated in healthy dogs, increased albumin level and colloid osmotic pressure, and repeated infusions on days 2 and 14 seemed safe.[48] No feline-specific albumin is currently available and HSA remains the only option for cats. A prospective study in 40 critically ill cats administered HSA reported a significant increase in albumin and no type I or III hypersensitivity reactions.[49] More information regarding the use of albu-min products is provided in Elisa M. Mazzaferro and Thomas Edwards' article, "Update on Albumin Therapy in Critical Illness," elsewhere in this issue.

PLATELET PRODUCTS

Options for platelet transfusion are fresh whole blood, platelet-rich plasma, platelet concentrates, and cryopreserved or lyophilized platelets.[50] The specifics of each platelet product are beyond the scope of this article and it is important to remember that platelets contain erythrocyte antigens and that mismatched platelet transfusions lead to early platelet destruction.[51] The primary indication for platelet transfusion is acute uncontrolled or life-threatening bleeding from severe thrombocytopenia or thrombocytopathia.[50] In patients with platelet destruction, such as idiopathic throm-bocytopenic purpura, the transfused platelets are rapidly destroyed. A study in throm-bocytopenic dogs found that transfusion of cryopreserved platelets increased platelet count but failed to improve clinical bleeding or survival compared with the control group.[52] Lyophilized platelets are commercially available and can be stored at room temperature for 12 months.

COMPATIBILITY TESTING

Commercial kits for dogs test for DEA 1 and include card agglutination assays and an immunochromatographic cartridge method. These kits are useful for initial screening of blood donors and in emergency situations. Confirmation via a gel-based method is recommended when typing blood donors.[53]

All cats should be typed before transfusion, and feline typing kits test for the AB blood group system and provide reliable results. If there is significant autoagglutination or type B or AB results, confirmation of type via a reference laboratory should be considered.[54]

Crossmatching allows the detection of antibodies against erythrocyte antigens. A major crossmatch tests for antibodies in the recipient against donor erythrocytes, whereas a minor crossmatch tests for antibodies in the donor plasma against the recipient's erythrocytes. Compatible crossmatch results do not guarantee compatibility and delayed reactions may occur. Crossmatching can be performed manually, which is time consuming and can be operator dependent, or with commercially available gel crossmatch technology.[55]

Because transfusion of type A blood to a type B cat can be fatal, and cats have naturally occurring alloantibodies, all cats should be crossmatched before transfusion. This crossmatching confirms typing results and evaluates for additional antigens (eg, *MiK*, unrecognized antigens) not detected by typing kits. A retrospective study in 154 transfusion-naive cats had 14.9% incompatible major crossmatches. Febrile transfusion reactions occurred in 10.1% of uncrossmatched cats and 2.5% of crossmatched cats, with no association with survival.[56] Another study in transfusion-naive cats found that major crossmatching did not improve the efficacy of transfusions, nor did it decrease adverse events.[57]

For dogs, crossmatching is often skipped in transfusion-naive dogs because of the lack of clinically important naturally occurring alloantibodies.[58] A retrospective study in transfusion-naive dogs found 17% incompatible crossmatches. Crossmatched dogs had statistically significant higher posttransfusion hematocrits (28.6% ± 7.4%) compared with dogs without crossmatching (25.0% ± 5%). However, no acute hemolytic reactions were documented, and the retrospective nature of the study prevented randomization and introduced bias, making interpretation difficult.[59] Dogs receiving a transfusion more than 4 days after the first transfusion should be crossmatched because of frequent alloimmunization posttransfusion.[58]

BLOOD COLLECTION AND ADMINISTRATION

If using an in-house donor, whole blood can be collected in commercial bags containing an anticoagulant preservative such as citrate-phosphate-dextrose-adenine (CPDA-1). Immediate transfusions of smaller volumes can be collected into syringes with a ratio of 1 mL of anticoagulant (citrate) per 9 mL of blood. Syringes are not appropriate for long-term storage. Donation volumes of 15 to 20 mL/kg from dogs and 10 to 15 mL/kg from cats are considered safe.[60] The optimal technique for administering red blood cells (RBCs) is unknown. For canine blood, a syringe pump using an 18-μm aggregate filter as well as a volumetric peristaltic infusion pump using a standard infusion line with 170 to 260-μm filter significantly shortened RBC survival.[61] In contrast, a similar study in cats showed that a syringe pump and 18-μm aggregate filter did not shorten RBC survival.[62]

MONITORING TRANSFUSIONS

Transfusions should be administered slowly (eg, 0.5–1 mL/kg/h or one-quarter of the final rate) for the first 15 minutes and patients monitored (vital signs, perfusion parameters) closely for an acute reaction. Any vomiting, restlessness, increased respiratory rate or effort, pigmenturia, or urticaria should prompt stopping the transfusion and alerting the clinician. Transfusion reactions can be categorized into nonimmunologic and immunologic as well as acute (<48 hours) or delayed (>48 hours) reactions. Nonimmunologic transfusion reactions include infectious disease transmission, sepsis, citrate toxicity, and transfusion-associated circulatory overload.

Acute immunologic reactions develop when preformed alloantibodies in the recipient bind to erythrocyte antigens in the transfused unit. Acute hemolytic transfusion reactions, a type II hypersensitivity, usually occur within minutes to hours of transfusion and require large enough quantities of preformed alloantibodies to trigger the immune response. Febrile nonhemolytic transfusion reactions (FNHTRs) are the most common reactions in dogs and cats and result in a temperature increase of 1°C or greater within 2 hours of transfusion.[63] If an FNHTR is suspected, the transfusion should be stopped temporarily or the rate decreased. Although common, FNHTRs are usually self-limiting and have minimal clinical significance. Premedication does not prevent FNHTR in human patients and is not routinely recommended.[64]

Transfusion-related acute lung injury (TRALI) is the most common cause of transfusion-related death in humans.[65] Clinical signs include hypoxemia, fever, hypotension, tachycardia, and cyanosis.[66] In humans, TRALI is associated with multiple plasma transfusions, especially from female parturient donors.[67] In dogs, pregnancy does not seem to induce erythrocyte alloantibodies, but other factors, such as leukocyte alloantibodies, have not been investigated.[68] Reports of TRALI in veterinary medicine are limited, with 1 study of possible TRALI reporting a low incidence (3.7%).[66] Transfusion-related immunomodulation has been reported in human patients since the 1970s but remains poorly understood, with both proinflammatory and immunosuppressive effects.[68]

XENOTRANSFUSION

In dire emergencies, transfusion of blood from a different species may be considered if type-matched blood is unavailable. Xenotransfusion of cats with dog blood has been reported and, to date, no severe acute reactions have been described in cats receiving canine blood for the first time.[69] A case report described successful resuscitation of a severely anemic cat with ultrasonography-guided intracardiac canine pRBCs into the left ventricle during CPR.[70] The canine RBCs were short-lived in 2 cats (~4 days) after xenotransfusion, and intravascular hemolysis was common. Both cats survived.[71] Cats seem to have a high prevalence of naturally occurring antibodies against canine erythrocyte antigens, resulting in frequent crossmatch incompatibility.[72] The clinical significance is unclear but a compatible crossmatch or administration of crossmatched species-specific blood products (particularly at 37°C) would be preferred.

AUTOTRANSFUSION

Autotransfusion eliminates infectious disease, immunologic reactions to blood or protein antigens, and hypothermia from cold transfusions. It also offers higher levels of 2,3-DPG and decreased risk of circulatory overload, and provides a convenient supply of compatible blood.[73] Autotransfusion can be performed using cell salvage devices or manually. Ideally, blood is collected sterilely via thoracocentesis, abdominocentesis, or directly from the cavity during surgery and transfused intravenously with an inline filter. Anticoagulants are often unnecessary because cavitary blood quickly defibrinates.[74] Concerns with autotransfusion include contaminated blood (eg, urine, bacteria, fecal matter, or bile) and lack of platelets. Complications include hemolysis, coagulation disorders, microembolism of fat or air, and sepsis.[75]

FUTURE DIRECTIONS

In humans, investigation continues on the association between blood type and specific conditions such as ischemic stroke, pregnancy complications, subarachnoid hemorrhage, acute lymphoblastic leukemia, and venous thromboembolism.[76] It is interesting to speculate whether there are associations with blood type in dogs and cats. Researchers found an enzymatic pathway in the human gut microbiome that removes surface antigens from type A, blood resulting in universal type O blood.[77] This technology has the potential to increase the supply of universal blood and the implications of this research are far-reaching. Interestingly, this comes at a time when experts are questioning the superiority of universal blood types.[6] Type-specific transfusions may be associated with fewer immunologic complications than the use of universal donors. Improving the safety of transfusion may involve washing stored blood and adding scavengers of heme, such as haptoglobin and hemopexin, both of which are being explored in human medicine.[78,79]

DISCLOSURE

None.

REFERENCES

1. Sturgis C. The history of blood transfusion. Burr Med Libr Assoc 1942;30(2): 105–12.
2. Wardrop KJ, Birkenheuer A, Blais MC, et al. Update on canine and feline blood donor screening for blood-borne pathogens. J Vet Intern Med 2016;30(1):15–35.
3. Hayakawa M, Kato S, Matsui T, et al. Blood group antigen A on von Willebrand factor is more protective against ADAMTS 13 cleavage than antigens B and H. J Thromb Haemost 2019;17(6):975–83.
4. Zaremba R, Brooks A, Thomovsky E. Transfusion medicine: An update on antigens, antibodies and serologic testing in dogs and cats. Top Companion Anim Med 2018;34:36–46.
5. Blais M, Berman L, Oakley DA, et al. Canine Dal blood type: a red cell antigen lacking in some dalmatians. J Vet Intern Med 2007;21(2):281–6.
6. Refaai MA, Cahill C, Masel D, et al. Is it time to reconsider the concepts of "universal donor" and "ABO compatible" transfusions? Anesth Analg 2018;126(6): 2135–8.
7. Weinstein NM, Blais M, Harris K, et al. A newly recognized blood group in domestic shorthair cats: the Mik red cell antigen. J Vet Intern Med 2007;21(2):287–92.
8. Nielsen H, Skov F, Dybkjær E, et al. Leucocyte and platelet-derived bioactive substances in stored blood: effect of prestorage leucocyte filtration. Eur J Haematol 1997;58(4):273–8.
9. Sharma R, Marwaha N. Leukoreduced blood components: advantages and strategies for its implementation in developing countries. Asian J Transfus Sci 2010; 4(1):3–8.
10. McMichael MA, Smith SA, Galligan A, et al. Effect of leukoreduction on transfusion-induced inflammation in dogs. J Vet Intern Med 2010;24(5):1131–7.
11. Ekİz E, Arslan M, Akyazi İ, et al. The effects of prestorage leukoreduction and storage duration on the in vitro quality of canine pRBCs. Turk J Vet Anim Sci 2012;36(6):711–7.
12. Corsi R, McMichael MA, Smith SA, et al. Cytokine concentration in stored canine erythrocyte concentrates. J Vet Emerg Crit Care 2014;24(3):259–63.
13. Herring JM, McMichael MA, Smith SA. Microparticles in health and disease. J Vet Intern Med 2013;27(5):1020–33.

14. Smith SA, Ngwenyama TR, O'Brien M, et al. Procoagulant phospholipid concentration in canine erythrocyte concentrates stored with or without prestorage leukoreduction. Am J Vet Res 2015;76(1):35–41.

15. Callan M, Patel R, Rux A, et al. Transfusion of 28-day-old leucoreduced or non-leucoreduced stored red blood cells induces an inflammatory response in healthy dogs. Vox Sang 2013;105(4):319–27.

16. Muro SM, Lee JH, Stokes JV, et al. Effects of leukoreduction and storage on erythrocyte phosphatidylserine expression and eicosanoid concentrations in units of canine packed red blood cells. J Vet Intern Med 2017;31(2):410–8.

17. Lozano L, Blois SL, Wood R, et al. A pilot study evaluating the effects of prestorage leukoreduction on markers of inflammation in critically ill dogs receiving a blood transfusion. J Vet Emerg Crit Care 2019;29(4):385–90.

18. Davidow E, Montgomery H, Mensing M. A Comparison of acute transfusion reactions in 766 dogs receiving either LR or nonLR pRBCs. J Vet Emerg Crit Care 2018;28:S3–4.

19. Blumberg N, Zhao H, Wang H, et al. The intention-to-treat principle in clinical trials and meta-analyses of leukoreduced blood transfusions in surgical patients. Transfusion 2007;47(4):573–81.

20. Schavone J, Rozanski E, Schaeffer J, et al. LR of feline whole blood using a neonatal leukocyte reduction filter: a pilot evaluation. J Vet Intern Med 2012; 26:777.

21. Wurlod VA, Smith SA, McMichael MA, et al. Iron metabolism following intravenous transfusion with stored versus fresh autologous erythrocyte concentrate in healthy dogs. Am J Vet Res 2015;76(11):996–1004.

22. Herring JM, Smith SA, McMichael MA, et al. Microparticles in stored canine RBC concentrates. Vet Clin Pathol 2013;42(2):163–9.

23. Solomon SB, Wang D, Sun J, et al. Mortality increases after massive exchange transfusion with older stored blood in canines with experimental pneumonia. Blood 2013;121(9):1663–72.

24. Hann L, Brown D, King L, et al. Effect of duration of packed red blood cell storage on morbidity and mortality in dogs after transfusion: 3,095 cases (2001–2010). J Vet Intern Med 2014;28(6):1830–7.

25. Maglaras CH, Koenig A, Bedard DL, et al. Retrospective evaluation of the effect of red blood cell product age on occurrence of acute transfusion-related complications in dogs: 210 cases (2010-2012). J Vet Emerg Crit Care 2016;27(1): 108–20.

26. Belpulsi D, Spitalnik SL, Hod EA. The controversy over the age of blood: what do the clinical trials really teach us? Blood Transfus 2017;15(2):112–5.

27. Holowaychuk MK, Musulin SE. The effect of blood usage protocol on the age of packed red blood cell transfusions administered at 2 veterinary teaching hospitals. J Vet Emerg Crit Care 2015;25(5):679–83.

28. Holst LB, Haase N, Wetterslev J, et al. Lower versus higher hemoglobin threshold for transfusion in septic shock. N Engl J Med 2014;371(15):1381–91.

29. Mazer DC, Whitlock RP, Fergusson DA, et al. Restrictive or liberal red-cell transfusion for cardiac surgery. N Engl J Med 2017;377(22):2133–44.

30. Møller A, Nielsen HB, Wetterslev J, et al. Low vs high hemoglobin trigger for transfusion in vascular surgery: a randomized clinical feasibility trial. Blood 2019;133(25):2639–50.

31. Beer K, Silverstein DC. Controversies in the use of fresh frozen plasma in critically ill small animal patients. J Vet Emerg Crit Care 2015;25(1):101–6.

32. Segal JB, Dzik WH, Network1 T. Paucity of studies to support that abnormal coagulation test results predict bleeding in the setting of invasive procedures: an evidence-based review. Transfusion 2005;45(9):1413–25.

33. Caturelli E, Squillante M, Andriulli A, et al. Fine-needle liver biopsy in patients with severely impaired coagulation. Liver 1993;13(5):270–3.

34. Fisher N, Mutimer D. Central venous cannulation in patients with liver disease and coagulopathy – a prospective audit. Intensive Care Med 1999;25(5):481–5.

35. Dzik WH. Predicting hemorrhage using preoperative coagulation screening assays. Curr Hematol Rep 2004;3(5):324–30.

36. Johns I, Sweeney R. Coagulation abnormalities and complications after percutaneous liver biopsy in horses. J Vet Intern Med 2008;22(1):185–9.

37. Spiess BD, Tuman KJ, McCarthy RJ, et al. Thromboelastography as an indicator of post-cardiopulmonary bypass coagulopathies. J Clin Monit 1987;3(1):25–30.

38. Bao H, Du J, Chen B, et al. The role of thromboelastography in predicting hemorrhage risk in patients with leukemia. Medicine 2018;97(13):e0137.

39. Somani V, Amarapurkar D, Shah A. Thromboelastography for assessing the risk of bleeding in patients with cirrhosis—moving closer. J Clin Exp Hepatol 2017; 7(4):284–9.

40. He Y, Xin X, Geng Y, et al. The value of thromboelastography for bleeding risk prediction in hematologic diseases. Am J Med Sci 2016;352(5):502–6.

41. Culler C, Iazbik C, Guillaumin J. Comparison of albumin, colloid osmotic pressure, von Willebrand factor, and coagulation factors in canine cryopoor plasma, cryoprecipitate, and fresh frozen plasma. J Vet Emerg Crit Care 2017;27(6): 638–44.

42. Culler CA, Balakrishnan A, Yaxley PE, et al. Clinical use of cryopoor plasma continuous rate infusion in critically ill, hypoalbuminemic dogs. J Vet Emerg Crit Care 2019;29(3):314–20.

43. Roberts I, Blackhall K, Alderson P, et al. Human albumin solution for resuscitation and volume expansion in critically ill patients. Cochrane Database Syst Rev 2011; 9(11):CD001208.

44. Mathews KA, Barry M. The use of 25% human serum albumin: outcome and efficacy in raising serum albumin and systemic blood pressure in critically ill dogs and cats. J Vet Emerg Crit Care 2005;15:110–8.

45. Trow AV, Rozanski EA, De Laforcade A, et al. Evaluation of use of human albumin in critically ill dogs: 73 cases (2003-2006). J Am Vet Med Assoc 2008;233(4): 607–12.

46. Cohn LA, Kerl ME, Lenox CE, et al. Response of healthy dogs to infusions of human serum albumin. Am J Vet Res 2007;68(6):657–63.

47. Craft EM, Powell LL. The use of canine-specific albumin in dogs with septic peritonitis. J Vet Emerg Crit Care 2012;22(6):631–9.

48. Enders B, Musulin S, Holowaychuk M, et al. Repeated Infusion of lyophilized canine albumin safely and effectively Increases serum albumin and colloid osmotic pressure in healthy dogs. J Vet Emerg Crit Care 2018;28:S5.

49. Vigano F, Blasi C, Carminati N, et al. Prospective review of clinical hypersensitivity reactions after administration of 5% human serum albumin in 40 critically ill cats. Top Companion Anim Med 2019;35:38–41.

50. Hux BD, Martin LG. Platelet transfusions: treatment options for hemorrhage secondary to thrombocytopenia. J Vet Emerg Crit Care 2012;22(1):73–80.

51. Carr R, Hutton JL, Jenkins JA, et al. Transfusion of ABO-mismatched platelets leads to early platelet refractoriness. Br J Haematol 1990;75(3):408–13.

52. Ng ZY, Stokes JE, Alvarez L, et al. Cryopreserved platelet concentrate transfusions in 43 dogs: a retrospective study (2007–2013). J Vet Emerg Crit Care 2016;26(5):720–8.
53. Seth M, Jackson KV, Winzelberg S, et al. Comparison of gel column, card, and cartridge techniques for dog erythrocyte antigen 1.1 blood typing. Am J Vet Res 2012;73(2):213–9.
54. Seth M, Jackson K, Giger U. Comparison of five blood-typing methods for the feline AB blood group system. Am J Vet Res 2011;72(2):203–9.
55. Kessler RJ, Reese J, Chang D, et al. Dog erythrocyte antigens 1.1, 1.2, 3, 4, 7, and Dal blood typing and cross-matching by gel column technique. Vet Clin Pathol 2010;39(5):306–16.
56. McClosky ME, Brown D, Weinstein NM, et al. Prevalence of naturally occurring non-AB blood type incompatibilities in cats and influence of crossmatch on transfusion outcomes. J Vet Intern Med 2018;32(6):1934–42.
57. Sylvane B, Prittie J, Hohenhaus AE, et al. Effect of cross-match on packed cell volume after transfusion of packed red blood cells in transfusion-naïve anemic cats. J Vet Intern Med 2018;32(3):1077–83.
58. Goy-Thollot I, Giger U, Boisvineau C, et al. Pre- and post-transfusion alloimmunization in dogs characterized by 2 antiglobulin-enhanced cross-match tests. J Vet Intern Med 2017;31(5):1420–9.
59. Odunayo A, Garraway K, Rohrbach BW, et al. Incidence of incompatible cross-match results in dogs admitted to a veterinary teaching hospital with no history of prior red blood cell transfusion. J Am Vet Med Assoc 2017;250(3):303–8.
60. Lanevschi A, Wardrop K. Principles of transfusion medicine in small animals. Can Vet J 2001;42(6):447–54.
61. McDevitt RI, Ruaux CG, Baltzer WI. Influence of transfusion technique on survival of autologous red blood cells in the dog. J Vet Emerg Crit Care 2011;21(3):209–16.
62. Heikes BW, Ruaux CG. Effect of syringe and aggregate filter administration on survival of transfused autologous fresh feline red blood cells. J Vet Emerg Crit Care 2014;24(2):162–7.
63. Harrell K, Kristensen A. Canine transfusion reactions and their management. Vet Clin North Am Small Anim Pract 1995;25(6):1333–64.
64. Ning S, Solh Z, Arnold DM, et al. Premedication for the prevention of nonhemolytic transfusion reactions: a systematic review and meta-analysis. Transfusion 2019;59(2):3609–16.
65. Marik PE, Corwin HL. Acute lung injury following blood transfusion: Expanding the definition. Crit Care Med 2008;36(11):3080.
66. Thomovsky EJ, Bach J. Incidence of acute lung injury in dogs receiving transfusions. J Am Vet Med Assoc 2014;244(2):170–4.
67. Pandey S, Vyas GN. Adverse effects of plasma transfusion. Transfusion 2012;52(Suppl 1):65S–79S.
68. Muszynski JA, Spinella PC, Cholette JM, et al. Transfusion-related immunomodulation: review of the literature and implications for pediatric critical illness. Transfusion 2016;57(1):195–206.
69. Bovens C, Gruffydd-Jones T. Xenotransfusion with canine blood in the feline species: review of the literature. J Feline Med Surg 2013;15(2):62–7.
70. Oron L, Bruchim Y, Klainbart S, et al. Ultrasound-guided intracardiac xenotransfusion of canine packed red blood cells and epinephrine to the left ventricle of a severely anemic cat during cardiopulmonary resuscitation. J Vet Emerg Crit Care 2017;27(2):218–23.

71. Euler CC, Raj K, Mizukami K, et al. Xenotransfusion of anemic cats with blood compatibility issues: pre- and posttransfusion laboratory diagnostic and cross-matching studies. Vet Clin Pathol 2016;45(2):244–53.
72. Priolo V, Masucci M, Spada E, et al. Naturally occurring antibodies in cats against dog erythrocyte antigens and vice versa. J Feline Med Surg 2018;20(8):690–5.
73. Robinson DA, Kiefer K, Bassett R, et al. Autotransfusion in dogs using a 2-syringe technique. J Vet Emerg Crit Care 2016;26(6):766–74.
74. Purvis D. Autotransfusion in the emergency patient. Vet Clin North Am Small Anim Pract 1995;25(6):1291–304.
75. Zenoble R, Stone E. Autotransfusion in the dog. J Am Vet Med Assoc 1978; 172(12):1411–4.
76. Pang H, Zong Z, Hao L, et al. ABO blood group influences risk of venous thromboembolism and myocardial infarction. J Thromb Thrombolysis 2020;50:430–8.
77. Rahfeld P, Sim L, Moon H, et al. An enzymatic pathway in the human gut microbiome that converts A to universal O type blood. Nat Microbiol 2019;4(9): 1475–85.
78. Cholette JM, Henrichs KF, Alfieris GM, et al. Washing red blood cells and platelets transfused in cardiac surgery reduces postoperative inflammation and number of transfusions: results of a prospective, randomized, controlled clinical trial. Pediatr Crit Care Med 2012;13(3):290–9.
79. Panch SR, Montemayor-Garcia C, Klein HG. Hemolytic transfusion reactions. N Engl J Med 2019;381(2):150–62.

Extracorporeal Therapies in the Emergency Room and Intensive Care Unit

J.D. Foster, VMD

KEYWORDS

- Intermittent hemodialysis • Plasmapheresis • Continuous renal replacement
- Hemoperfusion • Plasma exchange • Extracorporeal toxin removal

KEY POINTS

- Extracorporeal removal of toxins can prevent complications of organ dysfunction and death.
- Knowledge of the toxin's pharmacokinetic profile can help to guide the selection of the optimal modality of extracorporeal drug removal.
- Severe uremia is refractory to medical management; however, extracorporeal renal replacement therapy can normalize electrolytes, acid–base imbalance, volume status, and remove uremic toxins.
- Immune-mediated diseases may benefit from plasma exchange as an adjunctive treatment to standard immunosuppressive therapy.

EXTRACORPOREAL BLOOD PURIFICATION

Extracorporeal therapies have been performed in experimental animal models for more than 100 years and to treat naturally occurring disease in veterinary patients for more than 50 years. Through manipulation of blood outside of the body, extracorporeal therapies provide opportunities to treat disease and remove toxic substances that cannot be done from within the body. There are a variety of extracorporeal treatments; however, all share the common attributes of removing and returning blood to the patient, need for anticoagulation, and manipulation of the cellular and/or plasma contents of blood. The most commonly performed extracorporeal therapies are intermittent hemodialysis (IHD), continuous renal replacement therapy (CRRT), hemoperfusion (HP), and therapeutic plasma exchange (TPE). Each has their own limitations and characteristics that allow for the development of very targeted therapies. The most common veterinary applications of extracorporeal therapies are used in the treatment

Nephrology/Urology, Internal Medicine, Friendship Hospital for Animals, 4105 Brandywine Street Northwest, Washington, DC 20016, USA
E-mail address: jdfoster@friendshiphospital.com

Vet Clin Small Anim 50 (2020) 1215–1236
https://doi.org/10.1016/j.cvsm.2020.07.014
0195-5616/20/© 2020 Elsevier Inc. All rights reserved.

vetsmall.theclinics.com

of renal failure, acute toxicities, and immune-mediated diseases. An updated list of worldwide hospitals providing extracorporeal therapies can be found at www.asvnu. org.

SOLUTE KINETICS AND OPPORTUNITIES FOR EXTRACORPOREAL MANIPULATION

Nearly all extracorporeal treatments are performed to remove some offending solute(s) from blood. In renal failure, these targets are uremic toxins that accumulate owing to decreased glomerular filtration and renal elimination. Hepatotoxins similarly accumulate in patients with synthetic liver failure. Patients with immune-mediated disease may benefit from the removal of the antigen that triggers disease as well as the offending antibody that is produced in response. Although this concept is easy to comprehend, the significance of such metabolites, toxins, inflammatory mediators, cytokines, and hormones often remains poorly understood.[1–3] Despite this situation, extracorporeal therapies improve the clinical status of patients that are suffering from such conditions. As the role and kinetics of the offending toxic molecules are better understood, extracorporeal therapies can be designed to better improve their removal.

For patients with acute toxicities, the disease-causing substance is often well-known. In dogs with ibuprofen ingestion, it is the ibuprofen itself that is responsible for the adverse effects. Other toxins, such as acetaminophen, are not highly toxic; however, their metabolites are the molecules that cause cell damage. Both the identification of the offending solutes as well as an understanding of its kinetics is crucial to determining which extracorporeal therapy may be used for effective removal. Although not routinely applied to endogenously produced molecules, pharmacokinetics (PK) is the study of exogenous solute absorption, distribution, metabolism, and elimination; a basic understanding of PK is necessary for appropriately prescribing extracorporeal treatment.

Volume of distribution (V_d) is a description of the theoretic distribution of a solute throughout the body. The unit of measure (L/kg) does not reflect an actual volume, but rather provides a relationship of the drug's extravascular and intravascular distribution. Water comprises approximately 60% of total body weight. Solutes with a V_d of 0.6 L/kg typically distribute equally throughout total body water. When the V_d is lower, it indicates restriction of the drug within the intravascular space. A large V_d indicates significant accumulation of the solute in extravascular compartments, such as within the intracellular space or an affinity to accumulate within fat. Lipophilic drugs usually have a large V_d. Extracorporeal techniques are most effective for solutes with a low V_d and are less effective for molecules with a large V_d, because only a small proportion of the drug exists within the intravascular space. A V_d of more than 1 L/kg indicates that less than 5% to 10% of the solute is within the plasma.[4] Prolonged treatment and the processing of numerous blood volumes may be necessary for these treatments to significantly decrease the total body drug concentration. Most drugs exist within the plasma in both a free and protein-bound state. This state is commonly reported as percent protein bound. Drugs with high protein binding are commonly bound to albumin or other plasma proteins, which yields a small V_d.

Clearance is a concept used to describe the rate at which a solute is removed from systemic circulation and reflects the cumulative contribution of all organs participating in the metabolism and excretion of the solute.[5] However, clearance is measured in milliliters per minute per kilogram and reflects the volume of fluid (such as blood or plasma water) that has undergone complete removal of the solute. Hepatic and renal elimination are the 2 main routes of clearance for most drugs. The terminal half-life ($t_{1/2}$)

is the time required for the plasma drug concentration to fall by 50%.[6] Both the V_d and clearance are important contributors to the $t_{1/2}$. Drugs with a large V_d and/or small clearance rate are more likely to have a longer $t_{1/2}$.

Molecular weight is the sum of the weight of all atoms within a given molecule. This value, expressed in Daltons (Da) or grams per mole (typically interchangeable), is helpful to determine if a solute may be too large to pass through the pores within a dialysis membrane. It is important to recognize that protein-bound drugs will have a large molecular weight owing to the size of the bound protein molecule.

PLATFORMS FOR EXTRACORPOREAL BLOOD PURIFICATION

The V_d, molecular weight, and percent protein binding of a solute will help to determine the best method of extracorporeal removal and which platform may most effectively perform this treatment.[7] There are 4 mechanisms of extracorporeal solute removal: diffusion, convection, adsorption, and separation. Both IHD and CRRT rely mostly on diffusion and convection for solute removal. Diffusion occurs when a concentration gradient is created across a permeable membrane such as blood and dialysate across fibers within a hemodialyzer or hemofilter. Molecules move from areas of higher to lower concentration. The permeability of these membranes is mainly determined by the size of pores, thickness of membrane, and surface area.[8] The molecular size of a solute is the main determinant of its ability to be removed via dialysis. Low efficiency (also known as conventional) dialyzers can remove solutes up to 1000 Da, but have higher clearance for solutes less than 500 Da. High efficiency (high-flux) dialyzers can remove solutes up to 11,000 Da.[9]

Convective removal of solutes is performed as a pressure gradient physically moves plasma water and its solutes from one side of the membrane to another. Water is a very small molecule (18 Da) and moves easily across membranes. Solutes are removed via solvent drag as the water crosses the membrane; however, their passage can be restricted by the pore diameter. Because of the physical pressure applied during convection, larger solutes may be removed via convection rather than diffusion for the same dialyzer. Solutes of up to 40,000 Da are easily removed via convection using a high-efficiency dialyzer.

Adsorption is best achieved in HP, where blood or plasma is passed through a sorbent substance that binds and removes solutes from the circulation. Activated charcoal is the most commonly used sorbent molecule in extracorporeal therapies; however, other carbon-, resin-, or polymer-based sorbent columns are also available. Charcoal can irreversibly bind protein- and lipid-bound drugs with great affinity via the van der Waals interaction between the solute and the charcoal.[10] This binding is nonspecific and nontarget solutes may also be bound and removed, including glucose, platelets, coagulation factors, and hormones.[11] To prevent this charcoal is coated to make it more biocompatible, however this decreases its adsorption capability.[12] Charcoal HP can remove solutes well up to 40,000 Da with protein binding of up to 90% to 95%.[13]

Solute separation is performed during plasmapheresis and TPE, where a fraction of whole blood, such as plasma water, is removed along with the molecules that reside within that fraction. This therapy is best for solutes with extensive (>80%) protein binding and a small V_d (ideally <0.5 L/kg).

Although there are several companies that have recently developed veterinary-specific extracorporeal machines, most veterinary practitioners use machines created for adult and pediatric humans. Both IHD and CRRT use hollow fiber semipermeable membranes to remove toxic substances from blood. The main difference between these 2 modalities is the intensity at which this removal is performed. IHD was developed earlier and was the mainstay of treating uremic people. This method can quickly decrease the circulating concentration of most small uremic toxins by more than 80% within 3 hours. However, such rapid shifts in solute and fluid removal may lead to cardiovascular instability. Because most IHD machines do not allow for treatments to extend beyond 8 hours, performing a slow and less intensive treatment was challenging. Thus, CRRT was created as a treatment that could be performed continuously throughout the entire day to be safer for people with hemodynamic instability. By design, it is less efficient to help reduce complications associated with rapid solute removal. However, meta-analyses have shown survival of people with acute kidney injury (AKI) to be similar if they were treated with IHD or CRRT,[13] even those with hemodynamic instability.[14] Such a study has not been performed in veterinary patients. The small size of some veterinary patients creates an opportunity where CRRT machines may be operated to achieve solute clearances similar to IHD treatments. CRRT machines also allow for greater flexibility because most have programmed operational modes to perform purely convective or combination diffusion/convection treatments, whereas IHD clears solutes primarily via diffusion. There are pros and cons to each of these types of machines, which have been discussed elsewhere.[15]

Both IHD and CRRT machines can perform HP with the addition of a sorbent cartridge within the extracorporeal circuit. Some cartridges have been designed to remove specific molecules, such as cytokines, endotoxin, immune complexes, and other mediators of immune response. One sorbent cartridge, CytoSorb, has been used in for the management of critically ill septic people and has shown improvement in inflammatory cytokine concentration and survival rates.[16-18]

Plasmapheresis is the act of separating and removing plasma with return of the cellular component of blood. This term is often incorrectly used to describe TPE, which involves replacing the volume of removed plasma to prevent hypovolemia, decreased colloidal oncotic pressure, or deficiencies in albumin, coagulation factors, and fibrinogen. TPE can be accomplished by filtration and centrifugation methods. Filtration or membrane based TPE can be performed on many CRRT and some IHD machines. It uses a plasma separator—a hemofilter with pores large enough to allow some plasma proteins to cross. Most of these filters have a molecular weight cut-off around 70,000 Da, which is slightly larger than albumin (66,000 Da). Systemic anticoagulation is performed using unfractionated heparin therapy to prevent clotting throughout the extracorporeal circuit. Centrifugal TPE separates whole blood according to density and allows for the removal of any component—namely, plasma, red blood cells, platelets, granulocytes, or mononuclear cells. A major advantage of centrifugal platforms is the ability to use the same machine to perform cytapheresis and cell collection in addition to TPE, something membrane-based systems cannot perform. Most of these treatments are performed using regional citrate anticoagulation; however, systemic heparin therapy can also be administered.

EXTRACORPOREAL TOXIN REMOVAL

A common use of extracorporeal therapies in the emergency setting is an adjunctive therapy for intoxications. Any toxicity that could lead to significant organ dysfunction, serious complications, or death of the patient should be considered for extracorporeal toxin removal (ECTR). An understanding of the toxin's PK is essential for selecting the best type of extracorporeal platform. Many human drugs have undergone preclinical testing in dogs and other species, which may serve as an estimate for PK when species specific data are unavailable. Such information can be obtained via PubMed,

PubChem, and some critical care textbooks. Veterinary drugs that have been approved by the US Food and Drug Administration have undergone some PK evaluation in their target species; this information should be available in the product insert as well as published in drug formularies. It is important to recognize that normal PK parameters may not apply in overdose scenarios. Common drug doses rarely saturate all available enzymes and drug transporters involved in metabolism and elimination. However, saturation may be possible when the amount of drug ingested or administered is markedly increased; in these scenarios it is difficult to anticipate the PK parameters, but the $t_{1/2}$ may be prolonged and total drug exposure may be increased.[4] Unfortunately, most poison control helplines are unfamiliar with ECTR and do not typically recommend it as an effective therapy to remove the offending toxin. These centers may also provide improper recommendations for the timing of extracorporeal therapies, such as recommending hemodialysis only for uremia after ethylene glycol ingestion but not for ECTR. Therefore, emergency clinicians must have a robust understanding of PK and toxicology, as well as having a collegial relationship with the closest providers of ECTR to best identify patients that may benefit from these treatments.

There are several necessary considerations in the decision to use extracorporeal treatment.

The Toxin Is Likely to Cause Significant Organ Dysfunction, Injury, or Death

Drug exposure that results in mild clinical signs or reversible organ injury (eg, a short-term increase in liver enzymes) does not typically benefit from ECTR. In the majority of poisonings occurring within the home, the exact dose of exposure is unknown. People do not commonly have a reliable estimate of the number of pills that were within a bottle before their pet ingesting its contents. Drug exposure must be estimated from the theoretic maximal exposure. The fact that the actual ingestion dose is unknown along with the unavailability of bedside testing for various poisons, ECTR may be considered to be beneficial from the worst case toxin exposure. This amount may be quite higher than actual drug exposure, which can also be decreased by the induction of emesis. In general, the more catastrophic the potential outcome, the stronger the indication for ECTR. For example, the near guarantee of AKI and significant morbidity and mortality after ethylene glycol exposure warrants aggressive treatment with ECTR.

Extracorporeal Clearance Is Likely to Exceed Endogenous Clearance

When evaluating the possible benefit of ECTR for a given toxicity, the $t_{1/2}$ and/or drug clearance should be reviewed. Toxins with a short $t_{1/2}$ are unlikely to be significantly cleared by ECTR, because the time from emergency room presentation to initiation of therapy is rarely immediate. Recommendations for ECTR in people suggest that a poison is dialyzable when more than 30% of the ingested dose can be removed within a 6-hour treatment.[19] Drugs are nondialyzable when less than 3% of the ingested dose is removed during this time. Drugs should have low endogenous clearance rate (<4 mL/kg/min) to be a good candidate for ECTR.[20] After a drug has reached steady-state equilibrium, 97% of the drug is expected to be endogenously eliminated after 5 $t_{1/2}$ intervals. Acetaminophen has been reported to have a $t_{1/2}$ of 23 to 56 minutes in dogs.[21,22] Unless transporter saturation occurs, within 5 hours after acetaminophen exposure, very little of the drug remains. This timing creates a very small window of opportunity for ECTR. In humans, ECTR is indicated for acetaminophen toxicity in people only when they have neurologic complications, a markedly elevated serum acetaminophen concentration, or a marked lactic acidosis.[23] Human guidelines have suggested that, when a poison's V_d exceeds 1 to 2 L/kg, ECTR is unlikely to be effective and should not be pursued.[9,20,24]

Another Antidote or Life-Saving Treatment Is Not Available

Toxicities that may be reversed pharmacologically should have the appropriate antidote administered as quickly as possible. There are few toxicities that provide this therapeutic opportunity. Systemic effects from some organophosphates may be reversed by the administration of atropine, thus decreasing the necessity to increase drug elimination with ECTR.[25] It is important to recognize that as the time from exposure until when an antidote is administered is prolonged, there may already be enough drug exposure to result in significant adverse effects. For example, the conversion of ethylene glycol to glycolic acid may be inhibited by the administration of 4-methylpyrazole (4-MP) or ethanol; however, this conversion begins minutes after ethylene glycol ingestion. At the time of 4-MP or ethanol administration, there may already be a lethal quantity of glycolic acid metabolized. Prevention of death in cats owing to a lethal quantity of ethylene glycol was only prevented by 4-MP when administered within 3 hours after exposure.[26] Studies in dogs shows that 4-MP or ethanol treatment may be effective if administered only within 6 to 8 hours of ingestion.[27–29] If enough time has passed for ethylene glycol to be metabolized to glycolic acid, 4-MP is no longer indicated.[30] Hemodialysis very efficiently removes both ethylene glycol and glycolic acid, suggesting that it is the most effective treatment for ethylene glycol toxicity.[31] Clinicians must be aware of potential antidotes for poisonings, their timeframe of efficacy, and their limitations.

The Benefits of Extracorporeal Toxin Removal Exceed the Risks to Patient Safety

During extracorporeal treatments, a portion of the patient's blood is maintained outside of their body. It is recommended to design an extracorporeal circuit that will contain less than 20% of the patient's blood volume.[32] The red blood cells contained within this volume are unavailable for oxygen delivery; as the percentage of the patient's blood volume within the extracorporeal circuit increases, so does the risk of hypoxia, cardiovascular compromise, and substantial adverse effects. Historically, small patients (<5 kg) may not have been considered candidates for extracorporeal treatments owing to this risk. The increased availability of training opportunities in extracorporeal therapies has provided practitioners with tools to delivery safe and effective extracorporeal treatments. Strategies such as priming the extracorporeal circuit with synthetic colloids or blood have allowed for the delivery of safe ECTR for patients of any size.[33,34] Animals with anemia, cardiac or pulmonary disease, hypovolemia, and hypotension may be at increased risk for complications during ECTR. Astute patient monitoring, preemptive planning, and a well-trained and experienced staff can help to provide safe treatments for nearly all patients. As the risk or magnitude of adverse effect of the toxicity increases, so does the tolerability of potential complications during ECTR. For example, a cat was inadvertently administered a golden retriever's dose of vincristine intravenously, resulting in an exposure of 0.15 mg/kg, exceeding the lethal dose of 0.1 mg/kg. Medical treatment has been ineffective in preventing death in feline vincristine toxicity.[35] For this patient, ECTR is strongly indicated and the risks of this treatment are far overshadowed by the strong likelihood of a fatal outcome. TPE has successfully treated human vincristine toxicity[36] and was safely used to successfully manage feline vincristine toxicity in the author's hospital.

SELECTING THE IDEAL EXTRACORPOREAL TOXIN REMOVAL PLATFORM

Ideally, hospitals providing ECTR will have capabilities to perform IHD, HP, and TPE. Because of the intentional slow rate of solute clearance occurring with CRRT, some have proposed that it is not an appropriate modality to treat toxicities.[20,37,38] For many veterinary patients, their small size may allow for CRRT to deliver more efficient treatments than what can be obtained in humans. In these small patients, CRRT may be an effective means of toxin removal; however, for most toxins, removal will be best with IHD, HP, or TPE. One situation where CRRT may be the ideal treatment is when a toxin has a very large V_d, prolonged clearance, slow intercompartmental transfer rate, and is a molecule with a high sieving coefficient across the hemofilter. CRRT may be able to maintain the plasma drug concentration below toxic a threshold, and prolonged treatment (potentially >24 hours) may be required to enhance total body elimination. By design, many machines performing IHD, HP, and TPE are not capable of treatments beyond 8 hours without starting a new session.

Fig. 1 shows an algorithm to help select the most appropriate method of ECTR based on the limitations as described elsewhere in this article.

Intermittent Hemodialysis

Conventional (low-flux) dialyzers have a small molecular weight cut-off and best remove solutes less than 500 Da, whereas high-efficiency (high-flux) dialyzers may remove solutes easily up to 15,000 Da.[24,39] Solutes from 1000 to 10,000 Da have more efficient clearance with convection compared with diffusion.[40] Purely convective treatment (intermittent hemodiafiltration or HDF) may remove solutes up to 40,000 Da with high-efficiency dialyzers.[9] The removal of toxins via IHD decreases as protein binding increases; however, solutes that are less than 80% protein bound are considered amenable to removal via IHD and HDF.[9,39,40] Increasing treatment time and volume of blood processed during the ECTR treatment allows for more effective removal of solutes with higher degrees of protein binding.[41] Uremia is typically treated with a 4- to 8-hour duration of IHD with variable blood flow rates,[32] where toxicities are treated for 6 to 8 hours using the highest blood flow rate achievable.

Hemoperfusion

Activated charcoal is the most commonly used sorbent substance for ECTR. HP is most effective for solutes with a low to moderate V_d (<1 L/kg).[10] Toxins with a large V_d are less amenable to efficient removal via HP; however, prolonged treatment may allow for a sufficient decrease in total body drug accumulation. Charcoal HP is effective in binding solutes that are less than 95% protein bound.[42] Charcoal HP can remove both lipid- and water-soluble drugs.[43] Solutes up to 40,000 Da can easily bind to charcoal, resulting in effective removal.[44] Saturation of HP columns frequently occurs after 2 to 6 hours of use.[10] Exchanging a second charcoal cartridge may allow for increased solute removal.[45] A typical HP treatment will last 5 to 8 hours and use a blood flow rate of 150 mL/min or less.

Therapeutic Plasma Exchange

Drugs with high (>80%) protein binding and a low V_d (<0.2 L/kg) are ideal for removal with TPE.[46,47] Many of the nonsteroidal anti-inflammatory drugs fit this profile. For a substance that only exists within blood plasma, the exchange of 1 plasma volume would remove 37% of the original concentration. Exchanging 2 plasma volumes produces an 85% decrease, and 3 plasma volumes exchange results in a 95% decrease.[48] Most TPE prescriptions plan to exchange 1.3 to 2.0 plasma volumes;

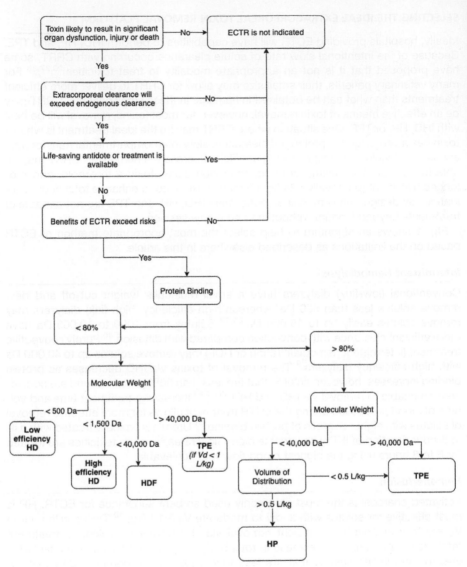

Fig. 1. Algorithm of when to use different methods for ECTR.

however, some have reported success with less volume exchanged.[49,50] Solutes with a larger V_d are less efficiently removed because the drug existing outside of the intravascular space is not immediately available for removal. Molecular weight does not affect the clearance during TPE; solutes of greater than 1,000,000 Da can be removed via TPE.[9]

Other Modalities

Although these platforms are effective in treating most toxicities, other methods may be used where indicated. The following treatments have increasing use in veterinary medicine; however, their exact role in managing disease and intoxications has not been vetted. Anecdotal experience and published case reports exist for several of them.[51] Various resins have been used for HP and may bind targeted solutes differently than activated charcoal. Polymer resins such as CytoSorb and DrugSorb have been designed to remove inflammatory cytokines and aromatic compounds, respectively. Activated carbon sorbents, such as AimaLojic V100s, may have greater affinity and binding capabilities than activated charcoal for some solutes. Albumin and lipid dialysis use sterile dialysate containing albumin or lipid. These techniques can be used for protein- or lipid-bound toxins, allowing the free solute to cross the dialyzer membrane to be entrapped within the dialysate. It is unclear what benefit these have over HP or TPE for veterinary intoxications.

COMMON VETERINARY INTOXICATIONS

Most intoxications require only 1 ECTR session to effectively decrease the serum drug concentration below a toxic threshold. With high drug exposure, the serum concentration may be several folds above a safe threshold. A single ECTR session may result in significant decrease (often >80%) in serum drug concentration; however, the final concentration may still exceed a toxic threshold. For example, AKI has been reported in dogs at a serum ibuprofen concentration of 138 μg/mL.[52] If a dog ingested enough ibuprofen to reach a serum concentration of 800 μg/mL, significant adverse effects would be anticipated and ECTR would be indicated if able to be performed timely. Both TPE and combined HP/HD have been used to treat ibuprofen toxicity in dogs, typically resulting in an 80% to 85% decrease in the serum concentration after treatment.[45,50,53] An 80% decrease in the starting serum concentration of 800 μg/mL would yield a serum ibuprofen concentration of 160 μg/mL, which may still result in AKI and other complications. In this scenario, increasing the dose of ECTR by increasing the amount of blood processed for HP/HD or volumes exchanged for TPE may lead to a greater decrease in the serum concentration. For drugs with a large V_d and slow intercompartmental transfer rates, a second treatment on the following day may be indicated.[47]

Table 1 lists drugs that pose toxic risks for animals as well as which ECTR modalities may be effective. Resources to help determine the best ERCT modality include evaluating published case reports and various chapters in human critical care and nephrology textbooks.

EXTRACORPOREAL MANAGEMENT OF ACUTE KIDNEY INJURY

Both IHD and CRRT used for the treatment of uremia are considered extracorporeal renal replacement therapy (ERRT). The justification for intensive treatment of AKI lies in the possibility of recovery of renal function after an insult. However, a retrospective study of dogs with AKI demonstrated that, of the surviving dogs, only 19% had serum creatinine concentrations return to within the normal reference range.[54] In a study of feline AKI, 25% of cats were discharged with a plasma creatinine concentration within the reference range.[55] Similar to what is observed in humans, AKI in animals is associated with a high mortality rate. Mortality has been reported in several small case series and retrospective studies; however, a meta-analysis of AKI survival was recently published.[56] This article showed a pooled mortality rate of 45% in dogs and 53% in cats. Animals with infectious etiologies of AKI had superior survival to noninfectious causes.

Indications for ERRT in veterinary AKI include anuria or severe oliguria, refractory life-threatening hyperkalemia and academia, hypervolemia, and symptomatic uremia that has failed to respond to conservative management.[15,32,57] Veterinary patients

Table 1
List of common veterinary intoxications grouped by effective ECTR modality

Hemodialysis or Hemofiltration	Charcoal HP (Often Performed in Combination with HD)	TPE
Acetaminophen	Amanita toxins	Amanita toxins
Aspirin	Baclofen[56]	Carprofen[63]
Aluminum[67]	Cannabinoids[57]	Deracoxib[54]
Baclofen	Cyclosporine[58]	Hyperbilirubinemia[64,65]
Bromides	Ibuprofen[43]	Ibuprofen[7,54]
Caffeine	Metaldehyde[59]	Meloxicam[49]
Diethylene glycol	Methotrexate[60]	Naproxen[54,66]
Ethanol[55]	Paraquat[61]	Vincristine
Ethylene glycol[34]	Pentobarbital	
Isopropyl alcohol	Phenobarbital[62]	
Lithium		
Mannitol		
Metaldehyde[49]		
Methanol		
Metformin		
Methyl alcohol		
Theophylline		

Published case reports of effective treatments are noted in citations.
Data from Refs.[7,34,43,49,54-67].

who receive ERRT for AKI typically have more severe disease, more frequent comorbidities, and higher illness scores, which likely give them a poorer prognosis than those with less severe disease who can be managed adequately with conservative therapy. A meta-analysis has shown that dogs and cats treated with hemodialysis as a part of their AKI management had higher mortality rates (53%) compared with those who received conservative care (37%).[56] This finding has also been observed in people with AKI.[58] However, in dogs and cats who survived AKI with the assistance of IHD, the 1-year mortality rates were not markedly different than the 30-day survival rates, suggesting that those patients who survive AKI can do well for some time.[59]

Determining the most appropriate time to initiate ERRT for uric AKI patients who lack life-threatening electrolyte, acid–base, or volume disturbances is not well-established in either human or veterinary medicine.[60–62] There is conflicting evidence in humans; however, some studies have shown that earlier initiation of ERRT is associated with improved mortality rates and a trend toward improved renal recovery in people with AKI.[63–65] Some authors have proposed dialysis should be considered in animals who have a blood urea nitrogen of greater than 80 mg/dL or a serum creatinine concentration of greater than 8 mg/dL.[15] This recommendation suggests starting at a lesser magnitude of uremia than an older recommendation (blood urea nitrogen >100 mg/dL, creatinine >8 mg/dL).[57] In this author's opinion, most dogs and cats with a blood urea nitrogen of less than 120 mg/dL and a creatinine of less than 5 mg/dL can typically be managed well with conservative therapy and the use of enteral feeding tubes. However, this rule is not firm; some patients tolerate uremia better than others. In human medicine, there has been a failure to determine appropriate criteria for the initiation of dialysis for AKI; the heterogeneity of reported studies precludes meta-analyses from determining the optimal time for intervention.[64] Blood urea nitrogen and serum creatinine concentrations may be altered independent of the glomerular filtration rate in critically ill patients, suggesting that functional and structural biomarkers may prove superior in the identification of patients who can benefit from ERRT; however, studies evaluating this claim are needed in both humans and animals. Therefore, the potential benefits and risks of treatment need to be considered, including patient size, associated comorbidities, severity of disease, the local availability of dialysis, and cost. Uremic patients with oligoanuria, hypervolemia, hyperkalemia, and metabolic acidosis may benefit from ERRT.

Both IHD and CRRT can be used for the management of AKI in cats and dogs.[59,66–69] There have been no studies in veterinary patients comparing outcomes between these 2 modalities. There is no obvious advantage of one of these modalities. Because of the small size of veterinary patients, IHD machines can be manipulated to perform treatments with similar clearance rates of what is obtained during CRRT.[15] The blood volume held within the extracorporeal circuit is smaller on some IHD machines (64 mL for Baxter Phoenix neonatal circuit with a Fresenius F3 dialyzer) compared with CRRT (93 mL for Baxter Prismaflex M60 circuit with hemofilter). Most CRRT machines have automated configurations to perform diffusive, convective, or combination therapies.[70] There is no obvious advantage to any of these modalities (continuous hemodialysis, hemofiltration, or hemodiafiltration) in terms of improving morbidity and mortality in AKI. Prolonged IHD involves using either an HD or CRRT platform to deliver a conservative but extended (often 8–12 hours) treatment. Ultimately, the most effective ERRT for AKI is the platform for which the staff (veterinarian and nurses) are most trained, experienced, and comfortable performing. Reviews of the methodology of IHD and CRRT as well as some comparisons has been performed.[15,57,70–72] Because they use prepackaged sterile dialysate and replacement fluid, CRRT machines are quite mobile and may be brought to the patient's cage during treatment. This factor may allow for a critical patient to remain within the intensive care unit, where they can be monitored more closely. However, a downside to performing ERRT within the intensive care unit is the increased foot traffic, distractions, and noise, which can potentially lead to patient restlessness and decreased monitoring acuity. Through the use of prepackaged sterilized fluids, CRRT treatment are generally more expensive than IHD, where dialysate is generated in real time from the hospital's water source. This process requires purification of the water before it can be used for the creation of dialysate; the equipment used for this may hinder the mobility of the IHD machine, depending on the design of the hospital.[73]

ROLE OF THERAPEUTIC PLASMA EXCHANGE IN TREATING IMMUNE-MEDIATED DISEASE

In addition to its role in removing protein-bound toxins, TPE allows for the removal of plasma proteins and other substances involved in the pathophysiology of disease, including antibodies, antigens, paraproteins, and antigen–antibody complexes. TPE has been used as an adjunctive therapy for veterinary immune-mediated disease for decades.[74–76] The most common veterinary diseases treated with TPE are immune-mediated hemolytic anemia and myasthenia gravis.[49,76–80] Many other disorders including immune complex glomerulonephritis, polyradiculoneuritis, hyperviscosity syndrome, and immune-mediated thrombocytopenia have also been treated, although published case reports are sparse.[49,75,76,81–86] Although traditional management of these diseases relies on pharmacologic immunosuppression, the patient is still burdened by the quantity of antibodies that have already been produced before the medical intervention taking effect. This factor may account for the persistent disease that is observed for several days or more after the introduction of immunosuppressive therapy.

As an adjunctive therapy in combination with standard immunosuppressive therapy, TPE has been observed to result in more immediate control of immune-mediated disease. Patients with immune-mediated hemolytic anemia will typically cease autoagglutinating after the first TPE treatment. Myasthenic dogs often improve strength in breathing and walking after TPE. Because immunoglobulins can redistribute from tissue stores the effect is not long lasting; therefore, 3 to 5 TPE treatments may be required before the disease is in remission.

Because of the cost and relative unavailability of apheresis, TPE was often approached as a final effort in refractory cases before euthanasia. This paradigm has been challenged owing to the marked improvement observed in most patients. Some practitioners have advocated for TPE to be considered a first-line therapy for moderate and severe cases of immune-mediated disease. Although randomized prospective studies have not been performed in veterinary medicine, case series have shown improved survival compared with historical controls (unpublished data courtesy of LD Cowgill, 2020). The use of TPE in people has undergone randomized studies, although the strength of evidence is still variable, and has helped to establish consensus guidelines regarding the usefulness of TPE for various diseases.[47] As TPE has gained traction in veterinary medicine, prospective studies are now feasible to better understand which patients can most benefit from treatment and when is the most appropriate time to initiate therapy. Providers of TPE agree that patients should not be referred as a final chance when the patient is moribund; earlier referral allows for the initiation of therapy before a marked decrease in patient stability and tolerance of treatment occurs. Certainly, some patients respond very well to standard treatment and will not show a clear benefit from TPE. TPE should be initiated for patients with more significant disease, who are anticipated to have a prolonged or protracted recovery, preferably as early in the course of the disease as reasonably possible (eg, a patient with immune-mediated hemolytic anemia who has received multiple blood transfusions).

Timing for the initiation of TPE for immune-mediated disease is not well-established. In this author's opinion, TPE could be strongly considered in the following situations.

- In the patient with immune-mediated hemolytic anemia with persistent evidence of ongoing erythrocyte destruction (auto-agglutination, spherocytosis or ghost cells visible on cytology, etc) and requiring 3 or more blood transfusions.
- Patients with severe hyperbilirubinemia with a risk of acute bilirubin encephalopathy and kernicterus.[87,88] The threshold of hyperbilirubinemia associated with adverse neurologic effects has not been well established in dogs in cats, however neurologic decompensation and kernicterus have been reported when the serum total bilirubin concentration was 35.6 to 62.6 mg/dL in dogs[86,89,90] and 17.5 mg/dL in a cat.[91]
- Before adding a third immunosuppressant drug to the patient's current drug regimen.
- Before the administration of human intravenous immunoglobulin, which is associated with risks of hypersensitivity.[92,93]
- In patients with myasthenia gravis or polyradiculoneuritis with progressive respiratory depression, before the requirement of mechanical ventilation.
- Patients with hyperviscosity, resulting in neurologic dysfunction, vascular occlusion, systemic hypertension, or other complications.
- Patients with cutaneous and renal glomerular vasculopathy.[94]
- Patients with confirmed or presumptive immune complex glomerulonephritis, particularly when renal function is rapidly declining.[95]

Based on human recommendations[47] and some shared pathophysiology, the following conditions may benefit from TPE therapy; however, clinical experience may be sparse.

- Meningitis of unknown etiology
- Immune-mediated thrombocytopenia
- Evan's syndrome
- Stabilization before thymectomy in myasthenic patients
- Refractory cases of pemphigus

PRACTICAL CONSIDERATIONS IN PERFORMING EXTRACORPOREAL THERAPIES
Vascular Access

In nearly all circumstances, extracorporeal therapies are best performed through a dedicated dual lumen jugular catheter.[96] Although the author has performed TPE using an arterial catheter placed in the dorsal pedal artery for inlet access and returned blood through a peripheral venous catheter in the cephalic vein, this practice should only be considered in patients who already have an arterial catheter and cannot tolerate sedation or the risks associated with jugular catheter placement (such as hypoxemia owing to pulmonary thromboembolism). People often have TPE performed using 2 peripheral venous catheters (typically 16G); however, this practice is challenging in dogs owing to inability to place such large catheters in many small and medium dogs, an increased tendency for positional occlusion of the vessels, and inadequate blood flow to support the rate of extracorporeal access. Even in large canine patients where it may be possible to use 2 peripheral catheters, it is still preferable to place a jugular catheter because this device provides superior blood flow rates, less occlusion, is unlikely to be removed by the patient, and can be maintained safely over many months.

Catheters should be placed using strict aseptic preparation of the access site and complete barrier protection (cap, mask, sterile gown, gloves, etc) of the operator and assistant. The right jugular vein is the preferred site of vascular access owing to its relatively straight pathway to the cranial vena cava, right atrium, and caudal vena cava. The left jugular vein can be used if the right is inaccessible owing to thrombosis from prior venipuncture, trauma, or other factors that may prevent successful cannulation. A dual lumen catheter should be selected that will be most likely to deliver the blood flow rates needed for therapy. Resistance to blood flow through the catheter is determined through Poiseuille's law, which depends on the catheter width and length. The highest flow rates are obtained by selecting the widest and shortest catheter appropriate for the size of the patient. Hospitals should stock a variety of dialysis and apheresis catheters to fit the diverse sizes and shapes of canine patients, typically ranging from 7Fr × 12 cm through 14Fr × 30 cm. Catheters should be placed using a modified Seldinger technique. Successful placement of the initial peripheral catheter into the jugular vein was found to be successful in only 64% and 77% of cats and dogs, respectively.[97] Ultrasound guidance may be used to aid in the initial cannulation of the jugular vein,[98] which can be challenging in patients with hypervolemia and subcutaneous edema, thrombosis or hematoma from prior venipuncture, or hypovolemic states. A surgical cut-down approach may also be needed in some patients. Fluoroscopy should be used to monitor and guide catheter placement. Blind placement of jugular catheters in critically ill dogs and cats had a 51% complication rate.[97] Fluoroscopy allows the operator to visualize guidewire and catheter placement, helping to prevent incorrect placement and endocardial irritation, and can confirm the final location of the catheter. Catheters used for extracorporeal treatments provide optimal blood flow when the tip is residing within the right atrium. The caudal vena cava is an acceptable option in most patients; however, the distal lumen should be used for inlet (arterial) access to prevent access recirculation.[96]

Blood flow rate necessary to perform aggressive IHD treatment is often greater than 40 mL/min for a cat and greater than 200 mL/min for a dog. Charcoal HP typically uses blood flow rates of less than 150 mL/min to increase the contact time between the blood and the charcoal. Both TPE and CRRT have lower blood flow rates, occasionally less than 10 mL/min. Patients who are to receive only TPE may have a smaller diameter catheter placed than if the patient were to require IHD. For uremic patients, even if the initial few treatments will be performed as CRRT, placing the widest catheter possible is recommended to be able to achieve high blood flow rates needed for IHD or prolonged IHD in the latter sessions.

Patients should not have both jugular veins catheterized; otherwise, cranial venous occlusion and precaval syndrome may occur. In patients who already have a central venous catheter placed in a jugular vein, this catheter should be exchanged over a guidewire for a new catheter dedicated to extracorporeal treatment. A sampling line may be placed in the saphenous or femoral vein. If 1 jugular vein has thrombosed owing to prior venipuncture or catheterization, the placement of a catheter in the contralateral vein may restrict venous drainage and cause precaval syndrome. Subcutaneous edema accumulates within the face and neck and may extend into the thoracic limbs. This phenomenon may resolve after several days, once collateral vessels establish sufficient drainage. Laryngeal edema may create a life-threatening upper airway obstruction, which may require intubation. Removal of the jugular catheter is necessary in this event. Thrombolytics and other intravascular techniques may also be considered to reestablish venous flow. If extracorporeal treatment is still required, access can be obtained through the femoral vein; insertion of the catheter at the most proximal accessible site can accommodate a wide catheter and sufficient blood flow rates. Femoral catheters are more challenging to maintain owing to complications of bandage contamination with urine and feces as well as an increased risk of the patient chewing or dislodging the catheter. An Elizabethan collar should be worn at all times.

Anticoagulation

Most platforms have integrated methods of anticoagulation incorporated into the extracorporeal circuit and operating software. The 2 most often used methods of anticoagulation are systemic heparinization and regional citrate anticoagulation.[99,100] Systemic heparinization is achieved through the delivery of unfractionated heparin into the extracorporeal circuit via an incorporated syringe pump. Enough heparin needs to be administered to prevent coagulation as the blood travels through the extracorporeal circuit. The extracorporeal transit time is one factor that can guide the dose of heparin; transit time (min) = extracorporeal circuit volume (mL) ÷ blood flow rate (mL/min). The effect of heparin is monitored through serial testing of activated clotting time or activated partial thromboplastin time. Generally, the results of these tests should be longer than the extracorporeal transit time; however, individual patient factors need to be considered. Hypocoagulable patients, those with recent trauma or surgery, and those with active bleeding should receive conservative heparinization, but may be more safely managed with regional citrate anticoagulation or a no-heparin treatment.

Regional citrate anticoagulation prevents clotting through induction of hypocalcemia within the extracorporeal circuit. To achieve this state, sodium citrate is added to the extracorporeal circuit as blood is exiting the catheter to decrease the ionized calcium concentration to less than 0.4 mmol. To prevent hypocalcemia in the patient, calcium (either calcium citrate or gluconate) is administered at the return (venous) lumen of the catheter. Serial measurement of the ionized calcium concentration of both the extracorporeal circuit and the patient are required to ensure safety and success. This technique may be safer in hypocoagulable patients, those with active bleeding, and has been used to safely and successfully perform IHD intraoperatively (T Francey, personal communication, 2020).

No-heparin treatments do not result in significant anticoagulation to the patient or the extracorporeal circuit. This technique can be considered in hypocoagulable patients or those with active bleeding when regional citrate anticoagulation is unavailable. This technique uses intermittent saline flushes (30–50 mL every 15–30 minutes) of the extracorporeal circuit to disrupt any forming blood clots.[99] This fluid must be accounted for and removed during treatment via ultrafiltration to prevent a positive fluid balance. The blood flow rate should be maximized to shorten the extracorporeal transit time. Clotting is more likely to occur with this technique, necessitating early discontinuation of therapy; it may not be possible to deliver the entire prescribed dose of ERRT. Administration of a low dose (10–50 U/h) of heparin into the arterial side of the circuit may help to prevent clotting with minimal effects on patient coagulation. In general, no-heparin treatment can be avoided if the staff is trained and experienced with regional citrate anticoagulation, even when the machine does not have this mode incorporated into its operational software.

Patient Monitoring

Patients require continuous monitoring throughout the entire extracorporeal treatment. The treatment should be performed in a location where individualized attention can be given to the patient and all supportive care can be successfully administered. A dedicated room where extracorporeal therapies are performed allows for better control over the environment and prevents the many distractions that can interfere with monitoring. Some critically ill patients, including those who may require mechanical ventilation, vasopressors, and so on, may have optimal monitoring when the treatment is performed within the intensive care unit. The best location depends on both patient status and hospital design. Regardless of location, comfortable bedding, heat support, and supplemental oxygenation should be provided. Only fractious animals require sedation, although patients with status epilepticus or hypoxemia may benefit from injectable anesthesia and/or mechanical ventilation. Patients should wear a harness that can be secured to the treatment table (**Fig. 2**) and also allows the blood lines to be secured to the harness, preventing the patient from pulling out their catheter.

Vital parameters should be assessed before, throughout, and at the completion of treatment. The patient's blood pressure, temperature, heart rate, and respiratory

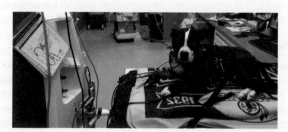

Fig. 2. Patient undergoing hemodialysis. Note the placement of the harness to prevent the patient from dislodging the lines and dialysis catheter.

rate should be measured and recorded. Hypotensive patients should have their blood pressure corrected before the initiation of extracorporeal treatment. Patients with low-normal systolic blood pressure and those where the extracorporeal circuit contains 20% or more of their blood are at risk of intraprocedural hypotension. This condition may be treated with the administration of an intravenous bolus of crystalloid or synthetic colloid or via administration of a vasopressor. The patient's hematocrit should be measured before treatment; priming the circuit with blood may be necessary for anemic patients. Pretreatment coagulation testing should be performed, either activated clotting time or activated partial thromboplastin time when systemic heparinization is used, or serum ionized calcium concentration when performing regional citrate anticoagulation. These tests should be performed every 30 minutes or whenever problems in coagulation are suspected.

Throughout treatment, the patient will have serial monitoring of its vital status and other metrics. Particular attention should be given to the patient at the initiation of treatment and for the first 15 minutes. This time is often when the patient may decompensate and develop hypotension, arrhythmias, hypoxemia, or other life-threatening complications. Vitals should be measured after the patient's blood has completed the initial traverse through the circuit. Any action steps to troubleshoot decompensation should be anticipated and prepared for. Vasopressors should be drawn up and be ready to be administered for patients where hypotension is anticipated. Some patients, particularly cats and small dogs, may benefit from prophylactic administration of vasopressors 5 to 10 minutes before the initiation of extracorporeal therapy. If the patient's cardiovascular status remains stable, these agents may be weaned off during treatment. Blood pressure should be regularly measured at intervals throughout treatment. Cats and small dogs should have a Doppler probe and sphygmomanometer cuff taped in an appropriate place before beginning treatment. This provides an audible pulse signal and allows for immediate measurement in the event of patient instability. Medium and large dogs may have oscillometric blood pressure measurement performed in a similar fashion. Automated measurements can be performed every 5 to 15 minutes according to patient status. Some extracorporeal platforms have an oscillometric blood pressure cuff incorporated into their system; these devices have been validated for correct measurement in humans and may not be accurate in dogs and cats. They should be validated with concurrent blood pressure measurement via dedicated veterinary devices before they are trusted, particularly during hypotensive states when they may be less accurate. A continuous electrocardiogram is monitored throughout treatment for the presence of arrhythmias. Patient heart rate, temperature, respiratory rate, and blood pressure should be recorded every 15 to 30 minutes throughout treatment. Peripheral pulse oxygenation or central venous oxygenation should be measured when possible. Dedicated ancillary devices can measure central venous oxygenation via the extracorporeal circuit and should be used in all treatments.[73] Supplemental oxygenation should be administered to all patients until their cardiopulmonary stability can be assessed during treatment.

Discontinuing Therapy

For most toxicities, a single ECTR session will adequately reduce their serum concentration below a toxic threshold. However, toxins with large V_d, low clearance, or those with particularly high exposure may benefit from 2 or more treatments. Consultation with veterinary toxicologists and clinical pharmacologists is recommended in this scenario because point-of-care testing for most toxicities is unavailable. The length of each ECTR session and volume of blood to be processed should be maximized to achieve the highest extracorporeal treatment. As the V_d of a toxin increases, the volume of blood to be processed should similarly increase. It is common to treat a blood volume of 2 times or less to 10 times in a single session. If troublesome vascular access results in lower than prescribed blood flow rates, the treatment duration should be extended to process an appropriate volume of blood.

The prescription for ERRT in uremic patients is beyond the scope of this article, but thoroughly described elsewhere.[32,70,71] Generally, the initial treatments are more conservative and deliver a smaller dose of dialysis over a longer timeframe. This can help prevent dialysis disequilibrium syndrome and intradialytic hypotension.[101] Performing ERRT too quickly can result in increased complication rate; one study showed 37% of dogs developed neurologic signs when dialyzed for only 60 minutes per session.[102]

After ECTR, the access catheter is typically left in place until it can be determined if the patient will suffer from any adverse complication of the drug exposure. For most nonsteroidal anti-inflammatory drug toxicities, the patient will show azotemia within 48 hours of exposure. If this should occur, the access can then be used for ERRT if warranted by the severity of azotemia. Patients with AKI who are recovering renal function may have ERRT discontinued when their predialysis creatinine is less than 5 mg/dL or their uremia is mild and no longer significantly mitigated with ERRT. The catheter is left in place for 5 to 7 days after the last ERRT treatment to monitor for rebound and to confidently determine if the patient has graduated from requiring ERRT. When not in use, the catheter lumens are locked with an anticoagulant (unfractionated heparin 250–2500 U/mL or 4% citrate) to help prevent thrombosis.

When removing the jugular catheter, direct pressure should be applied for 10 minutes to encourage hemostasis. A temporary bandage should be placed around the neck for 24 hours to protect against contamination. No sutures are typically required, and the skin incision closes by second intention healing.

DISCLOSURE

The authors have nothing to disclose.

REFERENCES

1. Clark WR, Dehghani NL, Narsimhan V, et al. Uremic toxins and their relation to dialysis efficacy. Blood Purif 2019;48(4):299–314.
2. Barreto FC, Barreto DV, Canziani MEF. Uremia retention molecules and clinical outcomes. Contrib Nephrol 2017;191:18–31.
3. Tritto G, Davies N, Jalan R. Liver replacement therapy. Semin Resp Crit Care 2012;33(01):70–9.
4. Roberts DM, Buckley NA. Pharmacokinetic considerations in clinical toxicology. Clin Pharm 2007;46(11):897–939.
5. Toutain PL, Bousquet-Melou A. Plasma clearance. J Vet Pharmacol Ther 2004;27(6):415–25.
6. Toutain PL, Bousquet-Melou A. Plasma terminal half-life. J Vet Pharmacol Ther 2004;27(6):427–39.
7. Monaghan KN, Acierno MJ. Extracorporeal removal of drugs and toxins. Vet Clin North Am Small Anim Pract 2011;41(1):227–38.
8. Haroon S, Davenport A. Choosing a dialyzer: what clinicians need to know. Hemodial Int 2018;22(S2):S65–74.
9. Ghannoum M, Roberts DM, Hoffman RS, et al. A stepwise approach for the management of poisoning with extracorporeal treatments. Semin Dial 2014;27(4):362–70.

10. Ghannoum M, Bouchard J, Nolin TD, et al. Hemoperfusion for the treatment of poisoning: technology, determinants of poison clearance, and application in clinical practice. Semin Dial 2014;27(4):350–61.

11. Winchester JF, MacKay JM, Forbes CD, et al. Hemostatic changes induced in vitro by hemoperfusion over activated charcoal. Artif Organs 1978;2(3):293–300.

12. Denti E, Luboz MP, Tessore V. Adsorption characteristics of cellulose acetate coated charcoals. J Biomed Mater Res 1975;9(2):143–50.

13. Nash DM, Przech S, Wald R, et al. Systematic review and meta-analysis of renal replacement therapy modalities for acute kidney injury in the intensive care unit. J Crit Care 2017;41(JAMA 294 2005):138–44.

14. Schefold JC, Haehling S, Pschowski R, et al. The effect of continuous versus intermittent renal replacement therapy on the outcome of critically ill patients with acute renal failure (CONVINT): a prospective randomized controlled trial. Crit Care 2014;18(1):R11.

15. Cowgill LD, Guillaumin J. Extracorporeal renal replacement therapy and blood purification in critical care. J Vet Emerg Crit Care (San Antonio) 2013;23(2):194–204.

16. Peng Z-Y, Carter MJ, Kellum JA. Effects of hemoadsorption on cytokine removal and short-term survival in septic rats. Crit Care Med 2008;36(5):1573–7.

17. Brouwer WP, Duran S, Kuijper M, et al. Hemoadsorption with CytoSorb shows a decreased observed versus expected 28-day all-cause mortality in ICU patients with septic shock: a propensity-score-weighted retrospective study. Crit Care 2019;23(1):317.

18. Kogelmann K, Jarczak D, Scheller M, et al. Hemoadsorption by CytoSorb in septic patients: a case series. Crit Care 2017;21(1):74.

19. Lavergne V, Nolin TD, Hoffman RS, et al. The EXTRIP (EXtracorporeal TReatments in Poisoning) workgroup: guideline methodology. Clin Toxicol 2012;50(5):403–13.

20. Fertel BS, Nelson LS, Goldfarb DS. Extracorporeal removal techniques for the poisoned patient: a review for the intensivist. J Intensive Care Med 2010;25(3):139–48.

21. KuKanich B. Pharmacokinetics and pharmacodynamics of oral acetaminophen in combination with codeine in healthy Greyhound dogs. J Vet Pharmacol Ther 2016;39(5):514–7.

22. Neirinckx E, Vervaet C, Boever SD, et al. Species comparison of oral bioavailability, first-pass metabolism and pharmacokinetics of acetaminophen. Res Vet Sci 2010;89(1):113–9.

23. Gosselin S, Juurlink DN, Kielstein JT, et al. Extracorporeal treatment for acetaminophen poisoning: recommendations from the EXTRIP workgroup. Clin Toxicol 2014;52(8):856–67.

24. Garlich FM, Goldfarb DS. Have advances in extracorporeal removal techniques changed the indications for their use in poisonings? Adv Chronic Kidney Dis 2011;18(3):172–9.

25. Klainbart S, Grabernik M, Kelmer E, et al. Clinical manifestations, laboratory findings, treatment and outcome of acute organophosphate or carbamate intoxication in 102 dogs: a retrospective study. Vet J 2019;105349.

26. Connally HE, Thrall MA, Hamar DW. Safety and efficacy of high-dose fomepizole compared with ethanol as therapy for ethylene glycol intoxication in cats. J Vet Emerg Crit Care (San Antonio) 2010;20(2):191–206.

27. Grauer GF, Thrall MAH, Henre BA, et al. Comparison of the effects of ethanol and 4-methylpyrazole on the pharmacokinetics and toxicity of ethylene glycol in the dog. Toxicol Lett 1987;35(2–3):307–14.

28. Dial SM, Thrall MA, Hamar DW. 4-Methylpyrazole as treatment for naturally acquired ethylene glycol intoxication in dogs. J Am Vet Med Assoc 1989; 195(1):73–6.

29. Dial SM, Thrall MA, Hamar DW. Efficacy of 4-methylpyrazole for treatment of ethylene glycol intoxication in dogs. Am J Vet Res 1994;55(12):1762–70.

30. Bates N, Rawson-Harris P, Edwards N. Common questions in veterinary toxicology. J Small Anim Pract 2015;56(5):298–306.

31. Schweighauser A, Francey T. Ethylene glycol poisoning in three dogs: importance of early diagnosis and role of hemodialysis as a treatment option. Schweiz Arch Tierheilkd 2016;158(2):109–14.

32. Cowgill LD. Urea kinetics and intermittent dialysis prescription in small animals. Vet Clin North Am Small Anim Pract 2011;41(1):193–225.

33. Posner LP, Willcox JL, Suter SE. Apheresis in three dogs weighing <14 kg. Vet Anaesth Analg 2013;40(4):403–9.

34. Langston C, Cook A, Eatroff A, et al. Blood transfusions in dogs and cats receiving hemodialysis: 230 cases (June 1997–September 2012). J Vet Intern Med 2017;31(2):402–9.

35. Hughes K, Scase TJ, Ward C, et al. Vincristine overdose in a cat: clinical management, use of calcium folinate, and pathological lesions. J Feline Med Surg 2009;11(4):322–5.

36. Pierga J-Y, Beuzeboc P, Dorval T, et al. Favourable outcome after plasmapheresis for vincristine overdose. Lancet 1992;340(8812):185.

37. Kim Z, Goldfarb DS. Continuous renal replacement therapy does not have a clear role in the treatment of poisoning. Nephron Clin Pract 2010; 115(1):c1–6.

38. Ouellet G, Bouchard J, Ghannoum M, et al. Available extracorporeal treatments for poisoning: overview and limitations. Semin Dial 2014;27(4):342–9.

39. King JD, Kern MH, Jaar BG. Extracorporeal removal of poisons and toxins. Clin J Am Soc Nephrol 2019;14(9):1408–15.

40. Bouchard J, Roberts DM, Roy L, et al. Principles and operational parameters to optimize poison removal with extracorporeal treatments. Semin Dial 2014;27(4): 371–80.

41. Eloot S, Schneditz D, Cornelis T, et al. Protein-bound uremic toxin profiling as a tool to optimize hemodialysis. PLoS One 2016;11(1):e0147159.

42. Kawasaki CI, Nishi R, Uekihara S, et al. How tightly can a drug be bound to a protein and still be removable by charcoal hemoperfusion in overdose cases? Clin Toxicol 2005;43(2):95–9.

43. Winchester JF, Harbord NB, Rosen H. Management of poisonings: core curriculum 2010. Am J Kidney Dis 2010;56(4):788–800.

44. Winchester JF. Dialysis and hemoperfusion in poisoning. Adv Ren Replace Ther 2002;9(1):26–30.

45. Tauk BS, Foster JD. Treatment of ibuprofen toxicity with serial charcoal hemoperfusion and hemodialysis in a dog. J Vet Emerg Crit Care (San Antonio) 2016; 26(6):787–92.

46. Schutt RC, Ronco C, Rosner MH. The role of therapeutic plasma exchange in poisonings and intoxications. Semin Dial 2012;25(2):201–6.

47. Padmanabhan A, Connelly-Smith L, Aqui N, et al. Guidelines on the use of therapeutic apheresis in clinical practice – evidence-based approach from the

writing committee of the American society for apheresis: the eighth special issue. J Clin Apher 2019;34(3):171–354.

48. Jones JS, Dougherty J. Current status of plasmapheresis in toxicology. Ann Emerg Med 1986;15(4):474–82.

49. Francey T, Schweighauser A. Membrane-based therapeutic plasma exchange in dogs: prescription, anticoagulation, and metabolic response. J Vet Intern Med 2019;33(4):1635–45.

50. Rosenthal MG, Labato MA. Use of therapeutic plasma exchange to treat nonsteroidal anti-inflammatory drug overdose in dogs. J Vet Intern Med 2019;33(2): 596–602.

51. Londoño LA, Buckley GJ, Bolfer L, et al. Clearance of plasma ivermectin with single pass lipid dialysis in 2 dogs. J Vet Emerg Crit Care (San Antonio) 2017;27(2):232–7.

52. Jackson TW, Costin C, Link K, et al. Correlation of serum ibuprofen concentration with clinical signs of toxicity in three canine exposures. Vet Hum Toxicol 1991;33(5):486–8.

53. Walton S, Ryan KA, Davis JL, et al. Treatment of ibuprofen intoxication in a dog via therapeutic plasma exchange. J Vet Emerg Crit Care (San Antonio) 2017; 27(4):451–7.

54. Vaden SL, Levine J, Breitschwerdt EB. A retrospective case-control of acute renal failure in 99 dogs. J Vet Intern Med 1997;11(2):58–64.

55. Worwag S, Langston CE. Acute intrinsic renal failure in cats: 32 cases (1997-2004). J Am Vet Med Assoc 2008;232(5):728–32.

56. Legatti SAM, Dib RE, Legatti E, et al. Acute kidney injury in cats and dogs: a proportional meta-analysis of case series studies. PLoS One 2018;13(1): e0190772.

57. Cowgill LD, Langston CE. Role of hemodialysis in the management of dogs and cats with renal failure. Vet Clin North Am Small Anim Pract 1996;26(6):1347–78.

58. Elseviers MM, Lins RL, der NPV, et al. Renal replacement therapy is an independent risk factor for mortality in critically ill patients with acute kidney injury. Crit Care 2010;14(6):R221.

59. Eatroff AE, Langston CE, Chalhoub S, et al. Long-term outcome of cats and dogs with acute kidney injury treated with intermittent hemodialysis: 135 cases (1997-2010). J Am Vet Med Assoc 2012;241(11):1471–8.

60. do Nascimento GVR, Gabriel DP, Abrão JMG, et al. When is dialysis indicated in acute kidney injury? Ren Fail 2010;32(3):396–400.

61. Macedo E, Mehta RL. Timing of dialysis initiation in acute kidney injury and acute-on-chronic renal failure. Semin Dial 2013;26(6):675–81.

62. Bagshaw SM, Cruz DN, Gibney RN, et al. A proposed algorithm for initiation of renal replacement therapy in adult critically ill patients. Crit Care 2009; 13(6):317.

63. Liu KD, Himmelfarb J, Paganini E, et al. Timing of initiation of dialysis in critically ill patients with acute kidney injury. Clin J Am Soc Nephrol 2006;1(5):915–9.

64. Karvellas CJ, Farhat MR, Sajjad I, et al. A comparison of early versus late initiation of renal replacement therapy in critically ill patients with acute kidney injury: a systematic review and meta-analysis. Crit Care 2011;15(1):R72.

65. Jamale TE, Hase NK, Kulkarni M, et al. Earlier-start versus usual-start dialysis in patients with community-acquired acute kidney injury: a randomized controlled trial. Am J Kidney Dis 2013;62(6):1116–21.

66. Langston CE, Cowgill LD, Spano JA. Applications and outcome of hemodialysis in cats: a review of 29 cases. J Vet Intern Med 1997;11(6):348–55.

67. Stanley SW, Langston CE. Hemodialysis in a dog with acute renal failure from currant toxicity. Can Vet J La revue vétérinaire canadienne 2008;49(1):63–6.
68. Landerville AJ, Seshadri R. Utilization of continuous renal replacement therapy in a case of feline acute renal failure. J Vet Emerg Crit Car 2004;14(4):278–86.
69. Diehl SH, Seshadri R. Use of continuous renal replacement therapy for treatment of dogs and cats with acute or acute-on-chronic renal failure: 33 cases (2002-2006). J Vet Emerg Crit Car 2008;18(4):370–82.
70. Acierno MJ. Continuous renal replacement therapy in dogs and cats. Vet Clin North Am Small Anim Pract 2011;41(1):135–46.
71. Bloom CA, Labato MA. Intermittent hemodialysis for small animals. Vet Clin North Am Small Anim Pract 2011;41(1):115–33.
72. Fischer JR, Pantaleo V, Francey T, et al. Veterinary hemodialysis: advances in management and technology. Vet Clin North Am Small Anim Pract 2004;34(4): 935–967, vi–vii.
73. Poeppel K, Langston CE, Chalhoub S. Equipment commonly used in veterinary renal replacement therapy. Vet Clin North Am Small Anim Pract 2011;41(1): 177–91.
74. Matus RE, Scott RC, Saal S, et al. Plasmapheresis-immunoadsorption for treatment of systemic lupus erythematosus in a dog. J Am Vet Med Assoc 1983; 182(5):499–502.
75. Matus RE, Gordon BR, Leifer CE, et al. Plasmapheresis in five dogs with systemic immune-mediated disease. J Am Vet Med Assoc 1985;187(6):595–9.
76. Bartges JW. Therapeutic plasmapheresis. Semin Vet Med Surg Animl 1997; 12(3):170–7.
77. Matus RE, Schrader LA, Leifer CE, et al. Plasmapheresis as adjuvant therapy for autoimmune hemolytic anemia in two dogs. J Am Vet Med Assoc 1985;186(7): 691–3.
78. Bartges JW, Klausner JS, Bostwick EF, et al. Clinical remission following plasmapheresis and corticosteroid treatment in a dog with acquired myasthenia gravis. J Am Vet Med Assoc 1990;196(8):1276–8.
79. Crump KL, Seshadri R. Use of therapeutic plasmapheresis in a case of canine immune-mediated hemolytic anemia. J Vet Emerg Crit Care (San Antonio) 2009; 19(4):375–80.
80. Scagnelli AM, Walton SA, Liu C-C, et al. Effects of therapeutic plasma exchange on serum immunoglobulin concentrations in a dog with refractory immune-mediated hemolytic anemia. J Am Vet Med Assoc 2018;252(9):1108–12.
81. Matus RE, Leifer CE, Gordon BR, et al. Plasmapheresis and chemotherapy of hyperviscosity syndrome associated with monoclonal gammopathy in the dog. J Am Vet Med Assoc 1983;183(2):215–8.
82. Forrester SD, Greco DS, Relford RL. Serum hyperviscosity syndrome associated with multiple myeloma in two cats. J Am Vet Med Assoc 1992;200(1):79–82.
83. Boyle TE, Holowaychuk MK, Adams AK, et al. Treatment of three cats with hyperviscosity syndrome and congestive heart failure using plasmapheresis. J Am Anim Hosp Assoc 2011;47(1):50–5.
84. Perondi F, Brovida C, Ceccherini G, et al. Double filtration plasmapheresis in the treatment of hyperproteinemia in dogs affected by Leishmania infantum. J Vet Sci 2018;19(3):472.
85. Lippi I, Perondi F, Ross SJ, et al. Double filtration plasmapheresis in a dog with multiple myeloma and hyperviscosity syndrome. Open Vet J 2015;5(2):108–12.

86. Tovar T, Deitschel S, Guenther C. The use of therapeutic plasma exchange to reduce serum bilirubin in a dog with kernicterus. J Vet Emerg Crit Care (San Antonio) 2017;27(4):458–64.

87. Das S, van Landeghem FKH. Clinicopathological spectrum of bilirubin encephalopathy/kernicterus. Diagnostics (Basel) 2019;9(1):24.

88. Usman F, Diala UM, Shapiro SM, et al. Acute bilirubin encephalopathy and its progression to kernicterus: current perspectives. Res Rep Neonatol 2018;8:33–44.

89. Sangster CR, Stevenson CK, Kidney BA, et al. Kernicterus in an adult dog. Vet Pathol 2007;44(3):383–5.

90. Belz KM, Specht AJ, Johnson VS, et al. MRI findings in a dog with kernicterus. J Am Anim Hosp Assoc 2013;49(4):286–92.

91. Saraiva LH, Andrade MC, Moreira MV, et al. Bilirubin encephalopathy (kernicterus) in an adult cat. JFMS Open Rep 2019;5(1). 205511691983887.

92. Tsuchiya R, Akutsu Y, Ikegami A, et al. Prothrombotic and inflammatory effects of intravenous administration of human immunoglobulin G in dogs. J Vet Intern Med 2009;23(6):1164–9.

93. Spurlock NK, Prittie JE. A review of current indications, adverse effects, and administration recommendations for intravenous immunoglobulin. J Vet Emerg Crit Care (San Antonio) 2011;21(5):471–83.

94. Skulberg R, Cortellini S, Chan DL, et al. Description of the use of plasma exchange in dogs with cutaneous and renal glomerular vasculopathy. Front Vet Sci 2018;5:161.

95. Littman MP. Lyme nephritis. J Vet Emerg Crit Care (San Antonio) 2013;23(2):163–73.

96. Chalhoub S, Langston CE, Poeppel K. Vascular access for extracorporeal renal replacement therapy in veterinary patients. Vet Clin North Am Small Anim Pract 2011;41(1):147–61.

97. Reminga CL, Silverstein DC, Drobatz KJ, et al. Evaluation of the placement and maintenance of central venous jugular catheters in critically ill dogs and cats. J Vet Emerg Crit Care (San Antonio) 2018;28(3):232–43.

98. Hundley DM, Brooks AC, Thomovsky EJ, et al. Comparison of ultrasound-guided and landmark-based techniques for central venous catheterization via the external jugular vein in healthy anesthetized dogs. Am J Vet Res 2018;79(6):628–36.

99. Ross S. Anticoagulation in intermittent hemodialysis: pathways, protocols, and pitfalls. Vet Clin North Am Small Anim Pract 2011;41(1):163–75.

100. Francey T, Schweighauser A. Regional citrate anticoagulation for intermittent hemodialysis in dogs. J Vet Intern Med 2018;32(1):147–56.

101. Zepeda-Orozco D, Quigley R. Dialysis disequilibrium syndrome. Pediatr Nephrol 2012;27(12):2205–11.

102. Melchert A, Barretti P, Ch PT, et al. Intradialytic complications in dogs with acute renal failure submitted to intermittent hemodialysis. Asian J Anim Vet Adv 2017;12(6):288–93.

Respiratory Emergencies

Carissa W. Tong, BVM&S, MRCVS[a], Anthony L. Gonzalez, DVM[b,c],*

KEYWORDS

- Respiratory distress • Hypoxemia • Oxygen • Ventilation

KEY POINTS

- Respiratory distress has a wide spectrum of severity in initial presentation.
- The method of oxygen supplementation selected should provide the highest fraction of inspired oxygen while minimizing patient stress.
- Rapid identification of respiratory distress and localization of respiratory disease play a vital role in stabilization efforts and subsequent diagnostics performed.

INTRODUCTION

Disorders of the respiratory system are a common cause for seeking emergency care in small animals. Presenting clinical signs can have a wide spectrum of severity, with some patients presenting with a mild cough whereas others present in fulminant respiratory distress with imminent fatigue and respiratory or cardiac arrest. Prompt recognition of respiratory distress and the ability to localize upper versus lower respiratory tract dysfunction are important in order to initiate appropriate management in a timely manner. As such, the emergency clinician needs to have an understanding of general respiratory physiology and the pathophysiology and management techniques as they relate to common respiratory diseases seen. This article reviews the basic anatomy of the respiratory tract, physiology relating to gas exchange and development of hypoxemia, and a stepwise approach when faced with a patient in respiratory distress, including localization within the respiratory tract, stabilization and initial diagnostic testing.

ANATOMY OF THE RESPIRATORY SYSTEM

The respiratory system can be divided anatomically into the upper and lower airways, pulmonary parenchyma, pleural space, and thoracic wall. Collectively, the respiratory system functions to move air in and out of the patient (ventilation) and to perform gas

[a] Emergency and Critical Care, Cornell University Veterinary Specialists, 880 Canal Street, Stamford, CT 06902, USA; [b] Cornell University Veterinary Specialists, 880 Canal Street, Stamford, CT 06902, USA; [c] Emergency and Critical Care, Cornell University College of Veterinary Medicine, Ithaca, NY, USA
* Corresponding author. Cornell University Veterinary Specialists, 880 Canal Street, Stamford, CT 06902.
E-mail address: agonzalez@cuvs.org

Vet Clin Small Anim 50 (2020) 1237–1259
https://doi.org/10.1016/j.cvsm.2020.07.002
0195-5616/20/Published by Elsevier Inc.

exchange at the level of the alveoli (oxygenation).[1] Upon inspiration, air enters through the upper airways, which consists of the nasal cavity, nasal sinuses, nasopharynx, larynx, and trachea. This is known as the conducting zone and is where air encounters the most resistance as it is filtered, warmed, and humidified.[1] Air then travels into the lower airways, which consist of bronchi, bronchioles, and the components of the respiratory zone, which includes respiratory bronchioles, alveolar ducts, alveolar sacs, and alveoli.[1] The respiratory zone is where gas exchange occurs in the pulmonary parenchyma via diffusion between the alveoli and capillary blood at the level of the alveoli.[1] Gas exchange occurs along a concentration gradient, allowing oxygen to enter the capillary to then be delivered to tissues and carbon dioxide (CO_2) to enter the alveoli for expiration. The lower airways and pulmonary parenchyma are contained within the pleural space of the chest cavity, which is outlined laterally by the thoracic wall and caudally by the diaphragm. The thoracic wall, diaphragm, and pulmonary parenchyma work together to create negative pressure within the pleural space, ensuring ventilation and oxygenation occur appropriately.[1] The respiratory system is equipped with several built-in defenses against invading pathogens that include nasal hairs, turbinates, the mucociliary apparatus, cough and sneeze reflex, and alveolar macrophages.[1]

CAUSES OF HYPOXEMIA

Hypoxemia is defined as a partial pressure of oxygen in arterial blood (Pa_{O_2}) less than 80 mm Hg, with severe hypoxemia defined as a Pa_{O_2} less than 60 mm Hg. Hypoxemia develops when the process of ventilation or oxygenation does not occur appropriately.[2] The 5 causes of hypoxemia include low fraction of inspired oxygen (Fi_{O_2}), global hypoventilation, right-to-left shunt, diffusion impairment, and ventilation-perfusion (V/Q) mismatch. In clinical practice, V/Q mismatch is the most common cause of hypoxemia, with a variety of diseases as the potential underlying cause, such as moderate to severe pulmonary parenchymal diseases (eg, pneumonia and pulmonary hemorrhage) and pulmonary thromboembolism (PTE).[2]

ANATOMIC LOCALIZATION

Most respiratory diseases can be localized to a specific region of the respiratory system. The ability of the clinician to correctly and rapidly identify the affected region is crucial, because it ensures that the most effective stabilization efforts take place in a timely manner. Numerous studies have shown that a patient's respiratory pattern and breathing sounds can be utilized to identify the source of respiratory distress.[3–5] Localization allows clinicians to create a focused differential diagnosis list and pursue subsequent diagnostics and therapeutics as indicated (**Table 1**). It is equally important for the clinician to be able to recognize patients who are not in true respiratory distress, despite similar appearance. Nonrespiratory look-alikes describe diseases that can result in increased respiratory effort and tachypnea. These can occur secondary to causes unrelated to the respiratory system, such as electrolyte disturbances, metabolic changes, and secondary to pharmacologic interventions.

Upper Airway

Patients with upper airway disease present with increased effort and prolongation during inspiration. Diseases that involve the more rostral portion of the upper airway (eg, nasopharynx) commonly produce stertorous breathing, described as a snoring noise.[4] Diseases in the more caudal portion of upper airway (eg, larynx) tend to produce stridorous breathing, described as a high-pitched whistle.[4] Both stertor and stridor reflect

Table 1
Anatomic localization of the respiratory system with associated diseases and clinical signs

Anatomic Location	Common Diseases	Clinical Signs
Upper airway	• Brachycephalic airway syndrome • Tracheal collapse • Laryngeal paralysis • Nasopharyngeal polyps	• Prolonged inspiration • Stertor • Stridor
Lower airway	• Chronic bronchitis • Feline asthma	• Prolonged expiration • Wheezing • Coughing
Pulmonary parenchyma	• Cardiogenic pulmonary edema • Noncardiogenic pulmonary edema • Pneumonia • Contusions	• Variable thoracic auscultation • May have an impact on both inspiration and exhalation • Signs of systemic illness
Vascular	• PTE	• Acute respiratory distress • Severe respiratory effort with unremarkable parenchymal auscultation
Pleural space	• Pleural effusion • Pneumothorax • Diaphragmatic hernia • Mediastinal/pleural masses	• Restrictive breathing pattern • Decreased heart and lung sounds on auscultation
Thoracic wall	• Flail chest	• Paradoxic breathing pattern • Lack of chest wall movement

increased resistance to airflow encountered in the upper airways. Patients begin to open-mouth breathe as a way to bypass this resistance to air intake and subsequently can become hyperthermic. Obstruction to air movement in the upper airway can be static or dynamic in nature. Static obstructions can be caused by extraluminal or intraluminal masses (eg, neoplasm in dogs and polyps or neoplasms in cats), trauma, or foreign bodies. Dynamic obstructions are seen more commonly in dogs, with the most common underlying diseases including laryngeal paralysis, brachycephalic obstructive airway syndrome, and tracheal collapse.[4] With severe obstruction and increased respiratory effort, airway mucosal edema can develop, which exacerbates the already increased resistance to airflow. A portion of these patients may present as orthopneic, where emergent intubation is necessary to reestablish a patent airway.

Lower Airway

With lower airway disease, increased effort and prolongation are seen during exhalation, because there is an increased resistance secondary to airway narrowing or collapse. An expiratory push can be seen in patients in attempts to overcome this resistance. Patients often have a chronic history of a combination of coughing, wheezing, and respiratory distress.[4,6] The most common lower airway disease seen in cats is feline asthma.[6] Recently, potassium bromide has been reported to cause neutrophilic-eosinophilic lower airway disease in cats.[7] In dogs, lower airway disease may include chronic bronchitis, eosinophilic bronchopneumopathy, or neoplasia.

Pulmonary Parenchyma

Patients with pulmonary parenchymal disease can have increases in both inspiratory and expiratory effort, with accompanying increases in chest and abdominal wall excursions.[5] Abnormalities in lung sounds, such as crackles, wheezes, or absence of lung sounds, can be noted on auscultation.[5] These patients also can exhibit signs of systemic illness. The pulmonary parenchyma can be affected by a variety of diseases, including pulmonary edema (cardiogenic or noncardiogenic), bronchopneumonia, contusions, hemorrhage, and interstitial diseases.

Cardiogenic pulmonary edema should be suspected in patients presenting in respiratory distress with pulmonary crackles and a concurrent heart murmur. In cats, the concurrent presence of a gallop rhythm, hypothermia, tachycardia, and tachypnea is strongly suggestive of underlying cardiac disease causing distress.[3] The absence of a heart murmur does not rule out a cardiac cause for respiratory cause of respiratory distress in cats. In addition to murmurs, dysrhythmias also should be made note of because dogs with arrhythmogenic right ventricular cardiomyopathy and dilated cardiomyopathy do not often develop a murmur but may have dysrhythmias present.

Noncardiogenic pulmonary edema can be caused by head trauma, prolonged seizures, and acute upper airway obstruction, such as strangulation or sharp pull of a neck lead.[8] The edema formation is thought to occur secondary to massive sympathetic activity that leads to increased hydrostatic pressure and permeability in the lungs.[9]

Numerous types of pneumonia exist in dogs and cats, including aspiration, lipid, hematogenous, infectious, and parasitic pneumonia.[10] Clinical signs may be mild earlier in the disease, with patients exhibiting an intermittent soft cough.[10] As the disease progresses, patients can develop a productive, moist cough with development of increased respiratory effort, exercise intolerance, fever, and often systemic signs, such as anorexia and severe lethargy.[10]

Vascular

PTE is a potentially life-threatening condition where an obstruction of a pulmonary vessel or vessels by a thrombus occurs secondary to an underlying disease that causes hypercoagulability.[11] The pulmonary artery is affected most commonly. An acute PTE can cause significant hypoxemia such that the patient can develop respiratory distress in the face of unremarkable thoracic auscultation or radiographs.[11]

Pleural Space

Abnormal accumulation of fluid, air, or soft tissue (eg, mediastinal mass or diaphragmatic hernia) can occupy the pleural space and result in a reduction of functional residual capacity,[12] the volume of gas that is left behind in the lungs at the end of expiration after a normal tidal breath.[1] This volume maintains a gas reserve between breaths and prevents small airways from collapsing.[1] As such, patients classically present with a rapid, shallow restrictive breathing pattern. A dyssynchronous (or paradoxic) breathing pattern also has been shown to be associated with pleural space disease.[4] On auscultation, patients with pleural effusion or soft tissue accumulation often have decreased lung sounds ventrally, whereas patients with air accumulation tend to have decreased lung sounds dorsally.

Fluid accumulation in the pleural space (pleural effusion) can occur secondary to various disease processes, including right-sided heart failure, neoplasia, infection (pyothorax), hemorrhage (hemothorax), and chylothorax.[12] Dogs presenting with hemothorax should be evaluated for concurrent pericardial effusion and pulmonary hemorrhage, because anticoagulant rodenticide toxicity can lead to diffuse hemorrhage. A pneumothorax can develop secondary to blunt or penetrating trauma, esophageal perforation, rupture of pulmonary lesions (eg, neoplasia or bullae), lung lobe torsion,[12] and has been reported to occur spontaneously in cats with chronic lower airway disease.[13]

Thoracic Wall

Thoracic wall diseases include congenital malformation, trauma-induced injury, cervical spinal disease, and neuromuscular disease.[14] Disease of the thoracic wall can be identified by decreased outward movements of the thoracic wall during inspiration, which leads to hypoventilation. Patients with thoracic wall disease often have short and shallow breaths with decreased chest expansion, increased abdominal effort and may exhibit cheek puffing. They do not respond to oxygen because their primary problem is ventilation, not oxygenation, and as such, may require mechanical ventilation.

Look-Alikes

Acid-base and metabolic disturbances

Patients with metabolic acidosis may develop tachypnea as a compensatory mechanism to normalize systemic pH by blowing off CO_2.[15] Kussmaul breathing, which is described as a deep, slow, labored breathing pattern, can develop in patients with profound metabolic acidosis.[15] Electrolyte disturbances (hypokalemia and hypocalcemia) and hypoglycemia also can have an impact on respiratory muscle function.[16,17] Cats with hyperthyroidism can exhibit signs such as tacyhpnea, including tachypnea, and in chronic unregulated cats exhibit respiratory weakness and, and reduced respiratory muscle contractions.[18]

Decreased oxyhemoglobin content

A decrease in oxyhemoglobin content adversely affects the ability of oxygen to carry and deliver oxygen, resulting in tissue hypoxia. This can be seen in patients with anemia or dyshemoglobinemias (eg, carboxyhemoglobin and methemoglobinemia).[19,20] Tachypnea develops as a compensatory mechanism for the tissue hypoxia.

Pain/distress

Patients can become severely tachypneic due to sympathetic stimulation secondary to pain or stress causing alteration in their respiratory pattern.[21] Pain caused by thoracic wall injuries also can limit expansion of the thoracic wall, leading to shallow breathing and hypoventilation.[14]

Pharmacologic

Various medications also may create abnormalities in the respiratory pattern of a patient. Some opioids can cause central respiratory depression (eg, fentanyl), whereas others (eg, hydromorphone and methadone) cause tachypnea and panting. Agents that induce neuromuscular blockade (eg, atracurium) may cause respiratory paralysis. Propofol is a drug used for induction of anesthesia in small animal patients and frequently causes respiratory depression or apnea. Slow administration of propofol can reduce apneic events. Pretreatment with flow-by oxygen is recommended to avoid propofol-induced hypoventilation and hypoxemia during anesthesia induction.

PATIENT HISTORY

Obtaining an accurate and detailed history can be extremely informative. A patient's history prior to the onset of distress can provide either a clear cause for the respiratory clinical signs (eg, traumatic injury) or valuable information for the clinician to pair with the signalment and examination findings when beginning to formulate a list of differential diagnoses. For example, a young dog that presents for increased respiratory effort may lead the clinician to consider infectious pneumonia as the top differential diagnosis, whereas the same presentation in an older dog with a history of voice change may lead the clinician to consider laryngeal paralysis with secondary aspiration pneumonia. It also is prudent to ask questions about relevant preexisting medical conditions (eg, cardiac disease, neoplasia, and endocrinopathies) and any current medications the patient is receiving. Depending on the presenting signs, potential exposure to various toxins, such as smoke inhalation or anticoagulant rodenticide, should be asked about. The speed of progression of respiratory distress also should be ascertained as it helps clinicians prioritize diseases on their differential lists. In cats, signs of lethargy and abnormal behavior may precede respiratory distress. Lastly, depending on the region, the patient's travel history also may help rule in or out other infectious causes of respiratory illness, such as fungal disease.

INITIAL STABILIZATION

Patients presenting in respiratory distress should be considered critical because many can be on the verge of decompensation and respiratory arrest. Their tolerance of stress from handling and restraint is minimal, creating a very narrow window for evaluation, which requires an organized and strategic approach to an initial assessment. The plan should be shared with the support team to ensure everyone moves in unison with any needed equipment or instruments made readily available and to avoid unnecessary stressors that can further exacerbate respiratory compromise.

Oxygen Therapy

Oxygen therapy should be provided immediately upon triage for patients presenting in respiratory distress. There are various ways to provide supplemental oxygen in small animals (**Table 2**). Ideally, the method selected would provide the highest Fio_2 with the

Table 2 Methods of oxygen supplementation	
Method of Oxygenation	**Mean Fraction of Inspired Oxygen Achieved (%)**
Flow-by oxygen	24–45
Face mask	35–55
Unilateral nasal catheter	30–50
Bilateral nasal catheter	30–70
Oxygen hood	21–60
Oxygen cage	21–60
HFOT	21–100
Positive-pressure ventilation	21–100
Hyperbaric oxygen	100

Adapted from Sumner C, Rozanski E. Management of respiratory emergencies in small animals. Vet Clin North Am Small Anim Pract. 2013;43(4):799-815; with permission.

least amount of stress imposed on the patient. This ultimately is determined on an individual basis, taking into account patient characteristics, severity of hypoxemia, and clinic resources.

Flow-by oxygen
Flow-by oxygen is the simplest method to provide supplemental oxygen, is generally well tolerated, and can reach Fio_2 levels of 0.25 to 0.4 with flow rates of 2 L/min.[22] Drawbacks to this method are that it achieves a low Fio_2, requires a handler to hold the oxygen tubing to the patient, and ultimately is a short-term strategy. Oxygenation has been shown to be significantly improved if oxygen is provided with a face mask compared with conventional flow-by techniques, where the oxygen tubing is held near the patient's nares.[23] Flow-by and face mask techniques allow short-term provision of oxygen and are well suited during initial patient assessment for immobilized patients or those recovering from anesthesia.

Oxygen hoods
Oxygen hoods can be better tolerated than face masks, especially with patients who are mobile. Although available for purchase, an oxygen hood can be made easily by fitting an Elizabethan (E)-collar on the patient with a clear plastic wrap that covers two-thirds of the hood, allowing the remaining space open for ventilation and elimination of heat and CO_2. An oxygen tube is secured to the inner aspect of the E-collar.[24] An oxygen hood has been shown to achieve an oxygen concentration of 70% within 90 seconds.[25] Patients should be closely monitored as the use of an oxygen hood does carry a risk for accumulation of CO_2 and condensation with subsequent overheating.[24]

Oxygen cage
Oxygen cages often are utilized to provide a constant rate of oxygen supplementation. Commercially available cages are designed to regulate Fio_2, temperature, and humidity with a scavenger system for CO_2.[24] Cages are a minimally invasive way to provide oxygen supplementation up to a concentration of 60% and allow for continuous visual monitoring of the patient. Use of an oxygen cage is limited by a patient's size, as larger dogs either do not fit in the cage or tend to overheat. A caretaker's ability to hear respiratory sounds is muted by the door. In addition, whenever the door or window is opened for monitoring or therapy, there is rapid loss of oxygen concentration within the cage.[24]

Nasal oxygen
Nasal oxygen is a more invasive modality compared with the options discussed previously. This can be provided via placement of a nasal catheter or use of commercially available nasal prongs. Nasopharyngeal catheters can be made from a red rubber atheter or infant feeding tube and generally are easily placed and well tolerated by most patients.[24] The placement of nasopharyngeal catheters is outlined in **Box 1**. Nasal prongs are limited in use as the prongs do not fit every patient, whereas with nasal catheters, the size of the catheter used can be adjusted based on the size of a patient's nares. Placement of bilateral nasal catheters allows for higher oxygen concentrations, of up to 50% to 60%, to be reached, versus a unilateral nasal catheter, achieving oxygen concentrations of 27% to 40%.[26] Both nasal prongs and nasal catheters should be connected to a humidified oxygen source to minimize desiccation of the nasal mucosa.[24] Nasal oxygen may prove less effective in patients that are panting excessively.

> **Box 1**
> **Nasopharyngeal oxygen catheter placement**
>
> *Equipment required*
>
> 1. Oxygen flowmeter with attached bubble humidifier
> 2. Red rubber catheter
>   A. 3.5F to 5F for small dogs and cats
>   B. 5F to 8F for medium dogs
>   C. 8F to 10F for large dogs
> 3. Sterile lubricating jelly
> 4. Proparacaine ophthalmic drops or 2% lidocaine gel
> 5. Nonabsorbable suture material and suturing instruments
> 6. E-collar
> 7. With or without Christmas tree adapter
>
> *Procedure*
>
> 1. Apply 2 drops of proparacaine ophthalmic drops or topical lidocaine gel into the desired nares.
> 2. Premeasure the tube from the nose to the lateral canthus of the eye and mark the tube accordingly. This places the tip of the tube into the nasopharynx.
> 3. Apply a small amount of lubricating jelly onto the distal end of the tube.
> 4. Insert the tube into the nose and advance until the premarked point.
>   A. Cats: insert the tube in a ventromedial direction.
>   B. Dogs: insert the tube in a dorsomedial direction, then ventromedially.
> 5. Once the tube is in place, secure the tube as close to the nasal planum as possible using the Chinese finger trap suturing method. A second suture should be placed either on the side of the face or on the forehead.
> 6. Connect the catheter to the oxygen tubing and turn on flowmeter.
> 7. Place E-collar to prevent the patient from removing the catheter.
>
> *Adapted from* Boyle J. Oxygen Therapy. In: Burkitt Creedon JM, Davis H eds. Advanced Monitoring and Procedures for Small Animal Emergency and Critical Care. 1st ed. Chichester, UK: Wiley-Blackwell; 2012:263-273; with permission.

High-flow oxygen therapy

High-flow oxygen therapy (HFOT) has gained use as a noninvasive method to support the hypoxemic patient when conventional oxygen therapy is not sufficient.[27–29] It involves the use of specialized nasal cannulas that allow the administration of heated and humidified oxygen at concentrations up to 100% with flow rates as high as 60 L/min. It is speculated that HFOT provides patients with some degree of positive end-expiratory pressure/continuous positive airway pressure.[27] HFOT has been shown to be a successful therapeutic option with minimal complications in a population of dogs with moderate to severe hypoxemia.[27]

Hyperbaric oxygen therapy

Hyperbaric oxygen therapy involves the delivery of 100% oxygen that is pressurized to a value above atmospheric pressure, allowing more oxygen to be made available for diffusion into the pulmonary capillaries.[30] It has been reported to be beneficial in patients with carbon monoxide poisoning, severe burns, wounds, and thromboembolic diease, as well as post-cardiopulmonary resuscitation.[30] Hyperbaric oxygen therapy is not a widely available treatment modality in veterinary medicine and thus its use in acute hypoxemia has not been fully validated.

Complications of Oxygen Therapy

- Oxygen toxicity: prolonged exposure to high oxygen concentrations (eg, 100% oxygen for more than 12 hours) can predispose patients to oxygen toxicity. It is believed that the toxic effects are due to the formation of oxygen-derived free radical species, which induce endothelial and epithelial cell damage, increase endothelial permeability, and ultimately cause inflammation and alveolar damage.[22]
- Absorption atelectasis: high concentrations of oxygen being delivered to the alveoli result in a washout of the nitrogen support skeleton, resulting in alveolar collapse.[22]
- Hypoventilation: hypoventilation is seen in patients where oxygen has replaced CO_2 as the main respiratory stimulus, such as patients with chronic obstructive pulmonary disease. Under normal conditions, CO_2 is a primary stimulus for breathing. In animals with chronic obstructive pulmonary disease or in some brachycephalic breeds, oxygen replaces CO_2 as the stimulus for breathing. Supplementation with oxygen can decrease respiratory drive and result in significant hypoventilation.[22]

Establishing Intravascular Access

Obtaining vascular access is a key component of emergency stabilization of the patient with respiratory distress. It gives the clinician the ability to intravenously (IV) administer rapidly acting drugs for bronchodilation, sedation, or induction of anesthesia if emergent endotracheal intubation is needed (**Table 3**). A peripheral IV catheter should be placed once the patient is deemed stable enough to endure restraint. Over-the-needle peripheral catheters are used routinely and can be placed readily in the cephalic, accessory cephalic, or lateral saphenous vein.

Sedation

Sedation and anxiolytics often are used in the emergency setting to reduce the stress associated with respiratory difficulty. This is useful particularly with patients in an upper respiratory crisis. In patients in whom an underlying cardiac cause has not been fully ruled out, the decision to use sedation should be made cautiously as some sedative agents have a degree of cardiovascular depressant effects.[31] For a majority of patients, low-dose butorphanol (00.1–0.3 mg/kg; IV, intramuscularly [IM], or subcutaneously [SQ]) and/or acepromazine (0.005–0.02 mg/kg; IV, IM, or orally) can be considered because they have a rapid onset of action and can be administered IM. A disadvantage of butorphanol and acepromazine is that neither of them has direct reversal agents. Benzodiazepines, such as midazolam or diazepam, could be considered as adjunct sedatives, with a 0.1 mg/kg to 0.3 mg/kg dose, IV, IM (midazolam only), or PO. The benzodiazepines may cause excitement, particularly in cats.[31] Appropriate monitoring should take place with any use of sedatives, such that any adverse effects can be acted on and immediately reversed, when necessary.

Other Pharmacologic Agents

Bronchodilators could be considered in patients presenting with lower airway disease, such as feline asthma or bronchitis. Both aminophylline (8–10 mg/kg, IV) and terbutaline (0.01 mg/kg, SQ or IM) are injectable bronchodilators, which should be considered

Table 3
Common pharmacologic agents used in respiratory emergencies

Drug	Dose	Route	Comments
Acepromazine	0.005–0.02 mg/kg	IV, IM, PO	• May cause hypotension
Aminophylline	8–10 mg/kg	IV	• May cause tachycardia, central nervous system stimulation
Butorphanol	0.05–0.3 mg/kg	IV, IM	• May cause respiratory depression
Dexamethasone sodium phosphate	0.1–0.15 mg/kg	IV, IM, SQ	• Anti-inflammatory dose
Dexmedetomidine	2–5 µg/kg	IV, IM	• Reversible • Minimal respiratory depression
Diazepam	0.2–0.4 mg/kg	IV	• PO may cause fulminant hepatic failure in cats • Reversible • May cause excitement or myoclonus if given alone
Furosemide	1–4 mg/kg	IV, IM, SQ	• May cause prerenal azotemia, worsen preexisting nephropathies
Midazolam	0.2–0.4 mg/kg	IV, IM	• Reversible • May cause excitement or myoclonus if given alone
Terbutaline	0.01 mg/kg	IM, SQ	• May cause tachyarrhythmias

Data from Plumb DC. Plumb's Veterinary Drugs. https://www.plumbsveterinarydrugs.com. Updated September 2017. Accessed December 10, 2019.

initially due to the ease of administration. Aminophylline causes direct bronchial smooth muscle relaxation, increases the strength of diaphragmatic contraction, has weak chronotropic and inotropic effects, and can lead to centrally mediated respiratory stimulation in some patients.[31]

Injectable glucocorticoids can be a valuable tool to reduce swelling in patients presenting with an upper airway obstruction, such as in laryngeal paralysis or brachycephalic airway syndrome. Dexamethasone sodium phosphate (0.1–0.15 mg/kg, IV, SQ, or IM) is commonly utilized as it has a quick onset (1–2 h) and an intermediate duration of action (24–36 h).[31] Long-acting steroids (eg, methylprednisolone acetate) have mineralocorticoid effects that can lead to acute plasma volume expansion. As such, they are not recommended in the acute setting because they may precipitate congestive heart failure, particularly in cats.[32] It also is important that clinicians establish whether a patient recently has been given nonsteroidal anti-inflammatories prior to presentation, because coadministration with glucocorticoids may precipitate adverse gastrointestinal effects, such as ulceration and perforation.

In patients where congestive heart failure is suspected or not able to be completely ruled out, a trial dose of injectable furosemide (1–4 mg/kg; IV, IM, or SQ) can be considered. Improvement of clinical signs after furosemide administration may help clinicians further narrow down their differential diagnoses to cardiac causes.

Control of Hyperthermia

Patients presenting with respiratory distress, in particular brachycephalic breeds or dogs with laryngeal paralysis, often are unable to thermoregulate.[33] Active cooling measures should be started immediately when hyperthermia is noted in order to minimize the development of deleterious systemic effects (eg, disseminated intravascular coagulation).[34] Active cooling via a fan, wetting the fur, or even shaving down the fur may be considered to reduce the core body temperature. Cooling efforts should be discontinued once the core body temperature reaches 103.5°F to 104°F (39.7°–40°C) to prevent rebound hypothermia and shivering.[34] Often, sedation and oxygen supplementation prove sufficient.

EMERGENCY PROCEDURES
Thoracocentesis

Thoracocentesis involves entering the thoracic cavity, most commonly to remove fluid or air from the pleural space. A thoracocentesis generally is performed between the seventh and ninth intercostal spaces, with the needle directed dorsally for air and ventrally for fluid. The site of needle insertion can be guided by use of a cage-side ultrasound to visualize accessible pockets of fluid or an area where there is an absent glide sign indicating a pneumothorax.[35] Based on patient size, the pleural space can be entered with a butterfly catheter such as in cats and small dogs, or with a needle or over-the-needle IV catheter of various gauges in medium to large dogs. A thoracocentesis can be either of diagnostic value, where the goal is to collect a sample to confirm the presence and/or evaluate the cause of air or fluid accumulation, or of therapeutic value, where the volume removed is sufficient to alleviate clinical signs. Development of respiratory signs in cats and dogs due to pleural effusion occurs once a volume of 20 mL/kg and 30-60 mL/kg is reached within the pleural space, respectively.[36] In patients with moderate to severe distress, a thoracocentesis should be performed prior to any additional testing, such as venipuncture or thoracic radiographs. Risks associated with thoracocentesis include hemorrhage, infection, iatrogenic lung or cardiac puncture, and pneumothorax.[35] As a rule of thumb, any pleural fluid collected should be analyzed as it may help reveal the causative etiology (**Table 4**).

Thoracostomy Tube

In some patients, air can continue to accumulate within the pleural space until a tension pneumothorax forms, which can be seen when thoracic or pulmonary injury acts as a 1-way valve, allowing air into the pleural space during inspiration but prevents expulsion during expiration. In these cases, when negative pressure cannot be obtained in the pleural space following repeat thoracocentesis due to the reaccumulation of air, unilateral or bilateral placement of a thoracostomy tube should be considered.[35] The most common type of thoracostomy tube used is an Argyle tube, which utilizes a trocar for entry into the thoracic cavity. Use of the trocarized tube is advantageous in that the tubes come in various lengths and sizes (8–32 French [F]); however, placement generally requires general anesthesia. As an alternative, commercially available over-the-wire thoracic drainage catheters[a] are now available, that utilize the modified Seldinger technique for placement (**Box 2**). These are usually well tolerated by most patients with use of sedation or local anesthesia, and have been shown to be effective with minimal complications.[35] Despite being available in only 12-gauge and 14-gauge sizes, the over-the-wire thoracic drainage catheters have demonstrated comparable efficacy to large-bore catheters when aspirating thick fluid, such has that observed in cases of pyothorax.[37]

Temporary Tracheostomy

A temporary tracheostomy may be required to alleviate a life-threatening upper airway obstruction, which can be secondary to severe laryngeal swelling or hemorrhage, foreign body, or neoplasia.[38] Ideally, a tracheostomy is performed under controlled

Table 4
In-house evaluation of pleural effusion

Gross examination and physical characteristics	Includes transparency or turbidity, color, odor, clots, and fibrin
TP	Transudate: TP <2.5 g/dL, TNCC <3000/uL
TNC	Modified transudate: TP >2.5 g/dL, TNCC <3000/uL Exudate: TNCC >3000/uL
PCV	Evaluate for hemorrhagic effusion
Triglyceride and cholesterol	Evaluates for chylous effusion • Fluid cholesterol-triglyceride ratio <1 • Fluid triglyceride, >100 mg/dL
Cytologic examination	Performed on spun-down sample Evaluates for bacteria, fungal, or plant materials

Abbreviations: PCV, packed cell volume, TNCC, total nucleated cell count; TP, total protein concentration.
Adapted from Bohn AA. Analysis of canine peritoneal fluid analysis. Vet Clin North Am Small Anim Pract. 2017;47(1):123-133; with permission.

settings with the patient under general anesthesia with a cuffed endotracheal tube in place. If endotracheal intubation is unsuccessful or a complete occlusion cannot be relieved, an emergent slash tracheostomy may be required.[39] Contraindications to performing a tracheostomy include coagulopathies, obstruction (eg, mass, foreign body, and tracheal collapse) distal to the site of tracheostomy, and previous tracheal stent placement.[38] Readers are referred to additional sources regarding the details of tracheostomy tube placement.[38]

Mechanical Ventilation

Mechanical ventilation is indicated when a patient is failing conventional oxygen therapy or has impending signs of respiratory fatigue. Generally speaking, the rule of 60s can be applied as criteria for when to consider mechanical ventilation:

- Severe hypoxemia (Pao_2 <60 mm Hg) on Fio_2 0.6
- Hypoventilation with severe hypercapnia ($Paco_2$ >60 mm Hg)
- Excessive respiratory effort with impending fatigue or failure

Mechanical ventilation relieves the patient's work of breathing and provides relief from distress. Prognosis for a patient's ability to be weaned from the ventilator highly depends on the underlying disease process. Dogs and cats that require mechanical ventilation due to traumatic pulmonary contusions and congestive heart failure have 30% and 62.5% survival rates, respectively.[40,41] Those requiring ventilation due to acute lung injury (ALI) or acute respiratory distress syndrome (ARDS), however, have a poor prognosis, with one-twelfth of dogs and one-quarter cats surviving to discharge.[42]

DIAGNOSTICS

Once anatomic localization of the cause of respiratory difficulty is complete and stabilization efforts are under way, the clinician can be begin formulating a differential list and diagnostic plan. The importance of having a systematic and strategic diagnostic plan cannot be underplayed, because it allows the clinician to perform diagnostics in a stepwise fashion that provides the greatest amount of information without further jeopardizing a patient's stability.

| **Box 2** |
| **Thoracostomy tube placement** |

Equipment required

1. Clippers
2. Surgical scrub (eg, chlorhexidine gluconate, 4%)
3. Sterile gloves
4. Sterile drape and supplies
5. Sterile instruments: needle holder, nonabsorbable suture, #11 blade
6. MILA guide wire style thoracostomy tube set (includes 18-g over-the-needle, guide wire, dilator, and thoracostomy tube)
7. Local anesthetic

Procedure

1. Depending on stability, patients can be placed into either sternal or lateral recumbency for placement.
2. Shave the thoracic wall between rib spaces 5 to 11 and surgically prepare the site using chlorhexidine scrub and alcohol.
3. Don sterile gloves and drape the site.
4. Local anesthetic (lidocaine, bupivacaine) can be injected into the SQ space and the intercostal muscles at the planned site of insertion. Intercostal nerve block also can be performed.
5. The skin is pulled cranially and a small full thickness stab incision is made into the skin at the insertion site, usually over seventh–eighth intercostal space.
6. An 18-g over-the-needle catheter is inserted through the stab incision into the thoracic cavity.
7. Thoracostomy tube is placed via the modified Seldinger technique.
   A. The needle stylet of the catheter is removed and the guide wire is fed through the catheter cranially until two-thirds of the wire is passed into the thoracic cavity.
   B. The catheter is withdrawn over the guide wire, leaving the guide wire in the thoracic cavity. It is prudent that the clinician does not let go of the guide wire at any time.
   C. The small-bore thoracostomy tube is fed into the thorax over the guide wire.
   D. The guide wire is removed from the distal end of the thoracostomy tube and the tube is clamped as soon as the guide wire is removed.
   E. A luer lock cap is placed onto the proximal end of the thoracostomy tube.
8. Once the tracheostomy tube is inserted into the thorax, the skin is released, creating an SQ tunnel for the thoracostomy tube.
9. The tube is secured to the patient at the 2 wings and base with sutures.
10. A sterile adherent dressing is placed over the insertion site.
11. A radiograph should be taken to confirm appropriate placement in the pleural space.

Adapted from Lombardi R, Savino E, Waddell LS. Pleural Space Drainage. In: Burkitt Creedon JM, Davis H eds, Advanced Monitoring and Procedures for Small Animal Emergency and Critical Care. 1st ed. Chichester, UK: Wiley-Blackwell; 2012:378-392; with permission.

Pulse Oximetry

Pulse oximetry is a noninvasive measurement that provides a crude estimate of Pao_2, utilizing spectrophotometric technology to estimate the oxygen saturation of hemoglobin in arterial blood.[43] Oxygen saturation, as measured by pulse oximetry (Spo_2) measurements are correlated to Pao_2 via the oxygen-hemoglobin dissociation curve.[2,43] An Spo_2 of greater than 97% is considered normal as it correlates to a Pao_2 of 80 mm Hg to 100 mm Hg, while $SpO2$ readings of 95% and 90% are considered abnormal, as they correlate to Pao_2 of 80 mm Hg and 60 mm Hg, respectively.[2] The accuracy of each measurement should be verified by matching the patient's heart rate to the calculated heart rate displayed and by the signal strength of the reading. Spo_2 readings should also be evaluated in conjunction with a patient's respiratory effort and any interference (eg, supplemental oxygen). Limitations with use of pulse oximetry include the inability to differentiate oxyhemoglobin from dyshemoglobinemia and numerous factors that could produce erroneous results, including severe anemia, hypoperfusion, excessive fluorescent light, and motion artifact.[43]

Arterial Blood Gas

An arterial blood gas (ABG) is considered the gold standard for evaluating oxygenation. The ABG also concurrently evaluates a patient's overall acid-base status, with some panels containing additional parameters (eg, blood glucose, lactate, and electrolytes). Normal parameters of ABG samples and expected acid-base compensations are outlined in **Table 5**. Arterial samples can be drawn from the dorsal metatarsal, coccygeal, sublingual, femoral, or aural arteries into preheparinized syringes and then analyzed by benchtop machines.[44]

A Pao_2 of less than 80 mm Hg indicates hypoxemia, with less than 60 mm Hg indicative of severe hypoxemia. The Pao_2, along with calculation of the maximal expected partial pressure of oxygen within the alveolus (Pao_2), is used in calculating the alveolar to arterial (A-a) gradient. The Pao_2 is obtained from the blood gas and the Pao_2 is derived from the alveolar gas equation: $Pao_2 = [(P_B - P_{H2O}) \times Fio_2] - [Paco_2/RQ]$, where P_B is barometric pressure (mm Hg), P_{H2O} is water vapor pressure (mm Hg), and RQ is respiratory quotient, commonly 0.8.[44] Assuming atmospheric pressure of 760 mm Hg, a water vapor of 47 mm Hg, and Fio_2 0.21, the equation can be rearranged as $Pao_2 = 150 - Paco_2/0.8$. Once the Pao_2 is calculated, the A-a gradient is calculated by subtracting Pao_2 from Pao_2. Normally, the A-a gradient is approximately less than 10 mm Hg and indicates normal pulmonary function.[44] Values greater than 15 to 20 are considered abnormal and indicate some form of diffusion impairment.[44]

Older dogs are more likely to have a higher $Paco_2$ and a lower Pao_2, which could imply their A-a gradient is higher. One exception to this rule is that brachycephalic breeds tend to have a higher A-a gradient than mesocephalic or dolichocephalic breeds.[45] At higher altitudes, where the barometric pressure is considerably lower than that of sea level, the actual barometric pressure obtained at the time of blood sample collection should be used for calculation. The A-a gradient can be calculated only when the ABG is obtained from a patient breathing room air with no oxygen supplementation. A normal Pao_2 is generally 5 times the Fio_2. For patients on supplemental oxygen, a Pao_2/Fio_2 (PF) ratio can be calculated. In veterinary patients, a PF ratio of greater than or equal to 450 to 500 is considered normal, whereas a PF ratio less than 300 indicates ALI and a PF ratio less than 200 indicates ARDS.[46] An Spo_2/Fio_2 ratio has been investigated as a surrogate for PF ratio, showing good correlation in healthy dogs.[47] No current studies are available investigating correlation and its use in patients with respiratory disease.

Table 5
Normal arterial blood gas parameters and guidelines for compensation

Value	Dog	Cat
pH	7.31–7.46	7.21–7.41
Pao$_2$	92 mm Hg (80–105)	105 mm Hg (95–115)
Paco$_2$	37 mm Hg (32–43)	31 mm Hg (26–36)
Sao$_2$	>95%	>95%

Disturbances	Guideline for Compensation
Metabolic acidosis	Each 1 mEq/L decrease in HCo$_3$ decreases PCo$_2$ by 0.7 mm Hg
Metabolic alkalosis	Each 1 mEq/L decrease in HCo$_3$ increases PCo$_2$ by 0.7 mm Hg
Respiratory acidosis	
Acute	Each 1 mm Hg increase in PCo$_2$ increases HCo$_3$ by 0.15 mEq/L
Chronic	Each 1 mm Hg increase in PCo$_2$ increases HCo$_3$ by 0.35 mEq/L
Respiratory alkalosis	
Acute	Each 1 mm Hg decrease in PCo$_2$ increases HCo$_3$ by 0.25 mEq/L
Chronic	Each 1 mm Hg decrease in PCo$_2$ increases HCo$_3$ by 0.55 mEq/L

Abbreviations: HCO3, bicarbonate; SaO2, oxygen saturation
Adapted from de Morais HSA, DiBartola, SP. Ventilatory and metabolic compensation in dogs with acid-base disturbances. J Vet Emerg Crit Care. 1991;1(2):39–49; with permission.

Ventilation also can be assessed by measuring Paco$_2$. Aside from a true airway obstruction, it is rare for small animal patients to present with hypercarbia. A venous blood gas also can be used to evaluate ventilation in a patient and tends to require less technical expertise than obtaining an arterial sample. In patients with normal perfusion, the venous partial pressure of carbon dioxide usually is 5 mm Hg higher than the Paco$_2$.[44] A low Pco$_2$ is reflective of hyperventilation and the patient's increased breathing effort. In intubated patients, capnometry/capnography also can be used to determine the efficiency of ventilation.

Radiographs

Radiographs are one of the most commonly utilized diagnostic imaging techniques. They are readily available and allow assessment of the airways and cardiopulmonary structures.[48] Radiographs should not be attempted until a patient is deemed stable, as the stress of positioning may result in respiratory or cardiac arrest. This is important particularly in feline patients that have a high sympathetic drive. Sedation often is required and can provide great relief.

Although common practice is to take 2 orthogonal views, it is recommended to perform 3-view studies when possible, to maximize detection of lesions and minimize superimposition of structures.[48] Imaging the cervical region also may be of use in certain patients, such as those with a cough, or if an upper airway obstruction is suspected. Any opacities in the pulmonary parenchyma and pattern of distribution, cardiac and pulmonary vessel size, and mainstem airways all should be evaluated. A vertebral heart scale (VHS) can be calculated from a right lateral thoracic radiograph to assess cardiac size. To do this, a long axis measurement of the heart is taken from the ventral aspect of the mainstem bronchus to the apex of the heart, and a short axis measurement is taken perpendicular to the long axis, at the level of the caudal vena cava. These measurements then are aligned with the vertebral column at the cranial edge of the fourth vertebrae, and vertebral bodies wtihin each measurement are quantified to give the VHS.[49] A VHS of greater than 9.3 was found to be highly specific for the presence of heart disease in cats presenting with acute respiratory distress.[49] In dogs and cats, noncardiogenic pulmonary edema is most likely to have a bilaterally symmetric distribution in the caudodorsal lung field.[50] When caused by airway obstruction, it often is asymmetric and unilateral (right-sided) with dorsal distribution.[50]

Dynamic diseases, such as tracheal collapse and mainstem bronchial collapse, may not be seen or may be underestimated on radiography. Macready and colleagues[51] showed that even with paired inspiratory and expiratory thoracic radiographs, radiography misdiagnosed the location of tracheal collapse and failed to diagnose tracheal collapse entirely in 44% and 8% of dogs, respectively. In patients with dynamic disease, fluoroscopy and/or bronchoscopy may be necessary to determine diagnosis.

Lung Ultrasonography

Point-of-care lung ultrasonography (LUS) has gained use as a diagnostic tool and is more commonly used in the emergency setting due to its ease in performance and requirement of minimal equipment.[52] The 2 widely used techniques to evaluate the thoracic cavity include the focused assessment with sonography for trauma scan and the veterinary bedside lung ultrasound examination protocol.[52,53] Although serving as a quick way to detect the presence of fluid, both can also be used to detect pulmonary edema via the presence of ultrasound artifacts, known as B lines (commonly referred to as lung rockets).[52,53] B lines have been shown to be diagnostic for alveolar-interstitial diseases and can be a sensitive test for differentiating cardiac versus noncardiac causes of pulmonary edema.[54–56] Compared with traditional radiography, LUS is able to detect a higher incidence of alveolar-interstitial syndrome.[55] Besides evaluating for the presence of B-lines, ultrasonographic measurement of the left atrium (LA) compared to the measurement of the aortic root (Ao), known as the LA:Ao ratio, may aid clinicians in distinguishing between cardiac versus noncardiac causes of respiratory abnormalities. The LA:Ao ratio normally is 1:1. LA enlargement resulting in an La:Ao ratio >1.5 was found to be 97% sensitive and 100% specific for detecting congestive heart failure in cats.[56]

Several other artifacts can be noted on LUS that have diagnostic value. The absence of a glide sign, created by the parietal and visceral pleural surfaces gliding over each other during respiration, indicates the presence of a pneumothorax.[57] Recent evaluation of pneumothorax in dogs revealed that an abnormal subpleural sign, known as a curtain sign, also may indicate a pneumothorax.[58] Several other subpleural signs, including the shred sign, tissue sign, and nodule sign, have also been described.[54,59] For additional information, readers are referred to the Gregory R. Lisciandro's article, "Cageside Ultrasound in the ER and ICU," elsewhere in this issue.

Advanced Imaging

Use of advanced imaging, such as fluoroscopy, tracheobronchoscopy, and computed tomography (CT), may be indicated in certain cases. Awake fluoroscopy allows dynamic assessment of the larger airways (trachea and mainstem bronchi) during both phases of respiration, providing a more global assessment of airway collapse.[51] Tracheobronchoscopy is the best modality to evaluate upper and lower airway collapse, allowing visualization of any macroscopic changes to the airways and for the presence of foreign bodies or masses in the airway that may be contributing to the patient's clinical signs.[60] CT has shown superior sensitivity in detecting pulmonary parenchymal changes in both veterinary and human medicine.[61–64] The use of CT is limited by the need for sedation or anesthesia; imaging capabilities also are restricted largely to veterinary referral centers. CT pulmonary angiography is the gold standard for the diagnosis of PTE in humans and has been shown to be a reliable modality in dogs.[65,66] A CT pulmonary angiography can be performed under sedation whilst simultaneously administering a bolus of contrast media. The thorax is scanned for complete or partial intraluminal arterial filling defects, which are diagnostic for a PTE.[66]

Airway Sampling

Airway samples can be obtained via a transtracheal wash (TTW), endotracheal wash (ETW), or bronchoalveolar lavage (BAL). The samples collected can be submitted for cytologic evaluation, fluid analysis, and aerobic, anerobic, or fungal cultures, where indicated. The TTW is a minimally invasive procedure that can be performed with/without mild sedation and is usually reserved for medium to large dogs. For small dogs (<10 kg) and cats, an ETW is recommended. ETW is more invasive than TTW because it requires placement of a sterile endotracheal tube under brief general anesthesia.[67] A guide to performing an ETW is outlined in **Box 3**. A BAL, performed under general anesthesia, allows for visualization of airways and sampling via fluid collection and brush cytology, using specialized equipment.[60] As such, BAL is not a modality routinely used on an emergency basis despite its increased sensitivity compared with TTW and BAL.[59] The main complication seen with airway sampling is oxygen desaturation or cyanosis, with other potential complications to include pneumothorax, and tracheal laceration with subsequent SQ emphysema.[67]

Oropharyngeal swabs are often utilized for respiratory polymerase chain reaction (PCR) panels, showing high sensitivity and specificity for the detection of canine adenovirus type 2, canine distemper virus, and *Bordetella bronchiseptica* in dogs.[68–70] The diagnostic use of deep oropharyngeal swabs was shown not to be useful for culture samples in a population of puppies with community-acquired pneumonia.[68] Ultrasound-guided fine needle aspirates can be considered in consolidated lung lobes or masses that are on the periphery of the lung field. Although rare, complications include pneumothorax, pulmonary hemorrhage, and death.[71]

Clinicopathologic Evaluation

Comprehensive bloodwork, such as a complete blood cell count and biochemistry, often is performed to systemically evaluate the metabolic status of a patient but tends to not be diagnostic for any specific underlying respiratory disease. Certain findings with corresponding clinical signs, however, may lead a clinician to consider specific disorders, such as peripheral eosinophilia in a dog with eosinophilic bronchopneumopathy.

The SNAP prohormone brain natriuretic peptide (proBNP) test measures N-terminal fragment of the proBNP (NT-proBNP), which is released during increased myocardial wall stretch. Its use in differentiating cardiac and noncardiac causes of respiratory distress has been demonstrated in both dogs and cats.[56,72] The NT-proBNP levels in pleural fluid may differentiate cardiac versus noncardiac cause of pleural effusion in cats.[73] The NT-proBNP levels can be increased in other conditions, such as pulmonary hypertension, dysrhythmias, renal disease, and systemic hypertension, where secondary myocardial stretch may occur.[74] Serologic testing for fungal, viral, and protozoal pathogens, in addition to PCR and virus isolation assays, should be considered when deemed appropriate.

Viscoelastic testing may serve the most use when evaluating for hypercoagulability as support for a suspected PTE. Thromboelastography is a well-established modality for in-hospital viscoelastic testing.[75] Its use is limited, however, by need for specialized equipment and delicate sample collection in order to minimize erroneous results.

Box 3
Endotracheal wash procedure

Equipment required

1. IV catheter

2. Short-acting anesthetic agents (eg, propofol and alfaxalone)

3. Laryngoscope

4. Sterile gloves

5. 3 to 5 syringes with sterile 0.9% saline
   A. 3-mL to 5 mL-aliquots for cats and small dogs
   B. 10-mL to 20-mL aliquots for larger dogs

6. Sterile endotracheal tubes

7. Sterile red rubber catheter (5–8F)

8. Sterile specimen container

9. A suction catheter and wall-mount mechanical suction unit

10. Aerobic culture transport medium

11. Ethylenediamine tetraacetic acid (EDTA) and nonserum separator tubes

Procedure

1. The patient is positioned into sternal recumbency.

2. An injection of short-acting anesthetic agents is given IV and titrated to effect to allow endotracheal intubation.

3. A laryngoscope is used to assist intubation with a sterile endotracheal tube, taking care to avoid contamination of the tube with oropharyngeal secretions.

4. Once the patient is intubated, a sterile red rubber catheter is introduced through the endotracheal tube.

5. An aliquot of sterile saline is instilled through the catheter and flushed into the airways.

6. Retrieval of fluid
   A. The syringe used to flush the saline into the airway can be used to manually aspirate the fluid instilled.
   B. Alternatively, a suction catheter is inserted into the endotracheal tube. The suction catheter can be connected to a suction unit through a sterile specimen container, where fluid can be aspirated into the container. Gentle, intermittent suction is applied to retrieve fluid sample.

7. If insufficient sample is obtained, instillation of saline aliquots can be repeated.

8. The fluid retrieved is placed into aerobic culture transport medium, EDTA, and nonserum separator tubes to be submitted for laboratory analysis.

9. Once the procedure is performed, patients should be monitored until they are awake and can be extubated.

10. Patients may need additional suction if excessive fluid is suspected in the airway via auscultation.

Adapted from Syring RS. Tracheal Washes. In: King LG, ed. Textbook of Respiratory Disease in Dogs and Cats. 1st ed. St. Louis, MO: Saunders; 2004: 128-134; with permission.

The recent availability of point-of-care viscoelastic devices have allowed rapid cage-side in vitro assessment of global coagulation. Readers are referred to evidence-based guidelines on viscoelastic testing in veterinary medicine created by the Partnership on Rotational ViscoElastic Test Standardization initiative.[76]

Heartworm testing can be performed utilizing bedside rapid SNAP tests, which are widely available and have a high sensitivity and specificity.[77] Canine SNAP tests detect the adult worm antigen, whereas the feline tests detect the antibody.[77,78] Clinicians also are encouraged to evaluate a blood smear for evidence of circulating microfilaria.

A Baermann fecal test is traditionally used for evaluation of lung worms (Angiostrongylus vasorum); however, its accuracy is variable due to intermittent shedding of the parasite.[79] Alternatively, an ELISA SNAP test is available for cage-side use with a high sensitivity and specificity in detecting lungworm antigens.[80]

SUMMARY

Respiratory distress is a common emergency in dogs and cats and can have a wide spectrum of clinical signs that range from mild to severe at the time of initial presentation, often in patients that are critical. As such, it is crucial for clinicians to feel confident in the recognition of respiratory distress and subsequent localization of the disease. Care must be exercised when evaluating patients in respiratory distress and a strategic diagnostic plan should be created that minimizes the risk of further respiratory compromise to the patient. Clear communication and planning with support staff will help alleviate any unnecessary stress and uncertainties, allowing the most effective handling of these patients while in hospital and ultimately optimizing outcome.

DISCLOSURE

The authors have nothing to disclose.

REFERENCES

1. West JB. Chapter 1 Structure and function. In: Respiratory physiology: the essentials. 9th edition. Baltimore (MD): Lippincott Williams & Wilkins; 2012. p. 1–11.
2. Haskins SC. Hypoxemia. In: Silverstein DC, Hopper K, editors. Small Animal Critical Care Medicine. 2nd edition. St. Louis: Saunders; 2015. p. 81–6.
3. Sigrist NE, Adamik KN, Doherr MG, et al. Evaluation of respiratory parameters at presentation as clinical indicators of the respiratory localization in dogs and cats with respiratory distress. J Vet Emerg Crit Care 2001;21(1):13–23.
4. Holt DE. Upper Airway Obstruction, Stertor, and Stridor. In: King L, editor. Textbook of Respiratory Disease in Dogs and Cats. 1st edition. St Louis: Saunders; 2004. p. 34–42.
5. Fonfara S, de la Heras Alegret L, German AJ, et al. Underlying diseases in dogs referred to a veterinary teaching hospital because of dyspnea: 229 cases (2003-2007). J Am Vet Med Assoc 2011;239(9):1219–24.
6. Johnson LR, Vernau W. Bronchoscopic findings in 48 cats with spontaneous lower respiratory tract disease (2002-2009). J Vet Intern Med 2011;25(2):236–43.
7. Bertolani C, Hernandez J, Gomes E, et al. Bromide-associated lower airway disease: A retrospective study of seven cats. J Feline Med Surg 2012;14(8):591–7.
8. Mandell DC. Respiratory Distress in Cats. In: King L, editor. Textbook of Respiratory Disease in Dogs and Cats. 1st edition. St Louis: Saunders; 2004. p. 12–7.

9. Adamantos S, Hughes D. Pulmonary Edema. In: Silverstein DC, Hopper K, editors. Small Animal Critical Care Medicine. 2nd edition. St. Louis: Saunders; 2015. p. 116–9.

10. Brady CA. Bacterial Pneumonia in Dogs and Cats. In: King L, editor. Textbook of Respiratory Disease in Dogs and Cats. 1st edition. St. Louis: Saunders; 2004. p. 412–21.

11. Goggs R, Benigni L, Fuentes VL, et al. Pulmonary thromboembolism. J Vet Emerg Crit Care 2009;19(1):30–52.

12. Silverstein D. Pleural space disease. In: Textbook of respiratory disease in dogs and cats. 1st edition. St Louis (MO): Saunders; 2004. p. 49–53.

13. White HL, Rozanski EA, Tidwell AS, et al. Spontaneous pneumothorax in two cats with small airway disease. J Am Vet Med Assoc 2003;222(11):1573–5.

14. Donahue S, Silverstein DC. Chest Wall Disease. In: Silverstein DC, Hopper K, editors. Small Animal Critical Care Medicine. 2nd edition. St. Louis: Saunders; 2015. p. 148–50.

15. Gallo de Moraes A, Surani S. Effects of diabetic ketoacidosis in the respiratory system. World J Diabetes 2019;10(1):16–22.

16. Lee JA. Nonrespiratory Look-alikes. In: Silverstein DC, Hopper K, editors. Small Animal Critical Care Medicine. 2nd edition. St. Louis: Saunders; 2015. p. 157–60.

17. de Brito Galvão JF, Schenck PA, Chew DJ. A Quick Reference on Hypocalcemia. Vet Clin North Am Small Anim Pract 2017;47(2):249–56.

18. Scott-Moncrieff JC. Feline Hyperthyroidism. In: Feldman E, Nelson R, Reusch C, Scott-Moncrieff JC, editors. Canine and Feline Endocrinology. 4th edition. St Louis: Saunders; 2015. p. 136–95.

19. Sobhakumari A, Poppenga RH, Pesavento JB, et al. Pathology of carbon monoxide poisoning in two cats. BMC Vet Res 2018;14(1):67.

20. Rumbeiha WK, Lin YS, Oehme FW. Comparison of N-acetylcysteine and methylene blue, alone or in combination, for treatment of acetaminophen toxicosis in cats. Am J Vet Res 1995;56(11):1529–33.

21. Hernandez-Avalos I, Mota-Rojas D, Mora-Medina P, et al. Review of different methods used for clinical recognition and assessment of pain in dogs and cats. Int J Vet Sci Med 2019;7(1):43–54.

22. Tseng LW, Drobatz KJ. Oxygen supplementation and humidification. In: King L, editor. Textbook of Respiratory Disease in Dogs and Cats. 1st edition. St Louis: Saunders; 2004. p. 205–13.

23. Wong AM, Uquillas E, Hall E, et al. Comparison of the effect of oxygen supplementation using flow-by or a face mask on the partial pressure of arterial oxygen in sedated dogs. N Z Vet J 2019;67(1):36–9.

24. Boyle J. Oxygen Therapy. In: Burkitt Creedon J, Davis H, editors. Advanced monitoring and procedures for small animal emergency and critical care. 1st edition. Ames (IA): Wiley-Blackwell; 2012. p. 263–73.

25. Engelhardt MH, Crowe DT. Comparison of six non-invasive supplemental oxygen techniques in dogs and cats. J Vet Emerg Crit Care 2004;14(S1):S1–17.

26. Dunphy ED, Mann FA, Dodam JR, et al. Comparison of unilateral versus bilateral nasal catheters for oxygen administration in dogs. J Vet Emerg Crit Care 2002; 12(4):245–51.

27. Keir I, Daly J, Haggerty J, et al. Retrospective evaluation of the effect of high flow oxygen therapy delivered by nasal cannula on PaO2 in dogs with moderate-to-severe hypoxemia. J Vet Emerg Crit Care 2016;26(4):598–602.

28. Daly JL, Guenther CL, Haggerty JM, et al. Evaluation of oxygen administration with a high-flow nasal cannula to clinically normal dogs. Am J Vet Res 2017; 78(5):624–30.

29. Jagodich TA, Bersenas AME, Bateman SW, et al. Comparison of high flow nasal cannula oxygen administration to traditional nasal cannula oxygen therapy in healthy dogs. J Vet Emerg Crit Care 2019;29(3):246–55.

30. Birnie GL, Fry DR, Best MP. Safety and tolerability of hyperbaric oxygen therapy in cats and dogs. J Am Anim Hosp Assoc 2018;54(4):188–94.

31. Plumb DC. Plumb's Veterinary Drugs. 2017. Availble at: https://www.plumbsveterinarydrugs.com. Accessed December 10, 2019.

32. Smith SA, Tobias AH, Fine DM, et al. Corticosteroid-associated congestive heart failure in 12 cats. Intern J Appl Res Vet Med 2004;2:159–70.

33. Davis MS, Cummings SL, Payton ME. Effect of brachycephaly and body condition score on respiratory thermoregulation of healthy dogs. J Am Vet Med Assoc 2017;251(10):1160–5.

34. Johnson SI, McMichael M, White G. Heatstroke in small animal medicine: a clinical practice review. J Vet Emerg Crit Care 2006;16(2):112–9.

35. Lombardi R, Savino E, Waddell LS. Pleural Space Drainage. In: Burkitt Creedon J, Davis H, editors. Advanced monitoring and procedures for small animal emergency and critical care. 1st edition. Ames (IA): Wiley-Blackwell; 2012. p. 378–92.

36. Cockshutt JR. Management of fracture-associated thoracic trauma. Vet Clin North Am Small Anim Pract 1995;25(5):1031–46.

37. Fetzer TJ, Walker JM, Bach JF. Comparison of the efficacy of small and large-bore thoracostomy tubes for pleural space evacuation in canine cadavers. J Vet Emerg Crit Care 2017;27(3):301–6.

38. Mazzaferro EM. Temporary tracheostomy. Top Companion Anim Med 2013; 28(3):74–8.

39. Mann FA, Flanders MM. Temporary tracheostomy. In: Burkitt Creedon J, Davis H, editors. Advanced monitoring and procedures for small animal emergency and critical care. 1st edition. Ames (IA): Wiley-Blackwell; 2012. p. 306–17.

40. Campbell VL, King LG. Pulmonary function, ventilator management, and outcome of dogs with thoracic trauma and pulmonary contusions: 10 cases (1994-1998). J Am Vet Med Assoc 2000;217(10):1505–9.

41. Edwards TH, Erickson Coleman A, Brainard BM, et al. Outcome of positive-pressure ventilation in dogs and cats with congestive heart failure: 16 cases (1992-2012). J Vet Emerg Crit Care 2014;24(5):586–93.

42. Balakrishnan A, Drobatz KJ, Silverstein DC. Retrospective evaluation of the prevalence, risk factors, management, outcome, and necropsy findings of acute lung injury and acute respiratory distress syndrome in dogs and cats: 29 cases (2011-2013). J Vet Emerg Crit Care 2017;27(6):662–73.

43. Jubran A. Pulse oximetry. Crit Care 2015;19(1):272.

44. Rieser TM. Arterial and venous blood gas analyses. Top Companion Anim Med 2013;28(3):86–90.

45. Hoareau GL, Jourdan G, Mellema M, et al. Evaluation of arterial blood gases and arterial blood pressures in brachycephalic dogs. J Vet Intern Med 2012;26(4): 897–904.

46. Wilkins PA, Otto CM, Baumgardner JE. Acute lung injury and acute respiratory distress syndromes in veterinary medicine: Consensus definitions: The Dorothy Russell Havemeyer Working Group on ALI and ARDS in Veterinary Medicine. J Vet Emerg Crit Care 2007;17(4):333–9.

47. Calabro JM, Prittie JE, Palma DA. Preliminary evaluation of the utility of comparing SpO2/FiO2 and PaO2/FiO2 ratios in dogs. J Vet Emerg Crit Care 2013;23(3): 280–5.

48. Ober CP, Barbe D. Comparison of two- vs. three-view thoracic radiographic studies on conspicuity of structured interstitial patterns in dogs. Vet Radiol Ultrasound 2006;47(6):542–5.

49. Sleeper MM, Roland R, Drobatz KJ. Use of the vertebral heart scale for differentiation of cardiac and noncardiac causes of respiratory distress in cats: 67 cases (2002-2003). J Am Vet Med Assoc 2013;242(3):366–71.

50. Bouyssou S, Specchi S, Desquilbet L, et al. Radiographic appearance of presumed noncardiogenic pulmonary edema and correlation with the underlying cause in dogs and cats. Vet Radiol Ultrasound 2017;58(3):259–65.

51. Macready DM, Johnson LR, Pollard RE. Fluoroscopic and radiographic evaluation of tracheal collapse in dogs: 62 cases (2001–2006). J Am Vet Med Assoc 2007;230(12):1870–6.

52. Lisciandro GR. Abdominal and thoracic focused assessment with sonography for trauma, triage, and monitoring in small animals. J Vet Emerg Crit Care 2011;21(2): 104–22.

53. Lisciandro GR, Fosgate GT, Fulton RM. Frequency and number of ultrasound lung rockets (B-lines) using a regionally based lung ultrasound examination named vet BLUE (veterinary bedside lung ultrasound exam) in dogs with radiographically normal lung findings. Vet Radiol Ultrasound 2014;55(3):315–22.

54. Ward JL, Lisciandro GR, Ware WA, et al. Lung ultrasonography findings in dogs with various underlying causes of cough. J Am Vet Med Assoc 2019;255(5): 574–83.

55. Ward JL, Lisciandro GR, DeFrancesco TC. Distribution of alveolar-interstitial syndrome in dogs and cats with respiratory distress as assessed by lung ultrasound versus thoracic radiographs. J Vet Emerg Crit Care 2018;28(5):415–28.

56. Ward JL, Lisciandro GR, Ware WA, et al. Evaluation of point-of-care thoracic ultrasound and NT-proBNP for the diagnosis of congestive heart failure in cats with respiratory distress. J Vet Intern Med 2018;32(5):1530–40.

57. Lisciandro GR, Lagutchik MS, Mann KA, et al. Evaluation of a thoracic focused assessment with sonography for trauma (TFAST) protocol to detect pneumothorax and concurrent thoracic injury in 145 traumatized dogs. J Vet Emerg Crit Care 2008;18(3):258–69.

58. Boysen S, McMurray J, Gommeren K. Abnormal curtain signs identified with a novel lung ultrasound protocol in six dogs with pneumothorax. Front Vet Sci 2019;6:291.

59. Simonetta C, Valentina D, Tommaso M. Thoracic ultrasound: a method for the work-up in dogs and cats with acute dyspnea. J Anim Sci Res 2017;1(1):1–6.

60. Johnson L. Small Animal Bronchoscopy. Vet Clin North Am Small Anim Pract 2001;31(4):691–705.

61. Nemanic S, London CA, Wisner ER. Comparison of thoracic radiographs and single breath-hold helical CT for detection of pulmonary nodules in dogs with metastatic neoplasia. J Vet Intern Med 2006;20(3):508–15.

62. Self WH, Courtney DM, McNaughton CD, et al. High discordance of chest x-ray and computed tomography for detection of pulmonary opacities in ED patients: Implications for diagnosing pneumonia. Am J Emerg Med 2013;31(2):401–5.

63. Reetz JA, Caceres AV, Suran JN, et al. Sensitivity, positive predictive value, and interobserver variability of computed tomography in the diagnosis of bullae

associated with spontaneous pneumothorax in dogs: 19 cases (2003-2012). J Am Vet Med Assoc 2013;243(2):244–51.

64. Traub M, Stevenson M, McEvoy S, et al. The use of chest computed tomography versus chest x-ray in patients with major blunt trauma. Injury 2007;38(1):43–7.

65. Goggs R, Chan DL, Benigni L, et al. Comparison of computed tomography pulmonary angiography and point-of-care tests for pulmonary thromboembolism diagnosis in dogs. J Small Anim Pract 2014;55(4):190–7.

66. Marschner CB, Kristensen AT, Rozanski EA, et al. Diagnosis of canine pulmonary thromboembolism by computed tomography and mathematical modelling using haemostatic and inflammatory variables. Vet J 2017;229:6–12.

67. Finke MD. Transtracheal wash and bronchoalveolar lavage. Top Companion Anim Med 2013;28(3):97–102.

68. Piewbang C, Rungsipipa A, Poovorawan Y, et al. Development and application of multiplex PCR assays for detection of virus-induced respiratory disease complex in dogs. J Vet Med Sci 2017;78(12):1847–54.

69. Canonne AM, Billen F, Tual C, et al. Quantitative PCR and cytology of bronchoalveolar lavage fluid in dogs with Bordetella bronchiseptica infection. J Vet Intern Med 2016;30(4):1204–9.

70. Sumner CM, Rozanski EA, Sharp CR, et al. The use of deep oral swabs as a surrogate for transoral tracheal wash to obtain bacterial cultures in dogs with pneumonia. J Vet Emerg Crit Care 2011;21(5):515–20.

71. Zekas LJ, Crawford JT, O'Brien RT. Computed tomography-guided fine-needle aspirate and tissue-core biopsy of intrathoracic lesions in thirty dogs and cats. Vet Radiol Ultrasound 2005;46(3):200–4.

72. Fox PR, Oyama MA, Reynolds C, et al. Utility of plasma N-terminal pro-brain natriuretic peptide (NT-proBNP) to distinguish between congestive heart failure and non-cardiac causes of acute dyspnea in cats. J Vet Cardiol 2009;11(Suppl 1): S51–61.

73. Wurtinger G, Henrich E, Hildebrandt N, et al. Assessment of a bedside test for N-terminal pro B-type natriuretic peptide (NT-proBNP) to differentiate cardiac from non-cardiac causes of pleural effusion in cats. BMC Vet Res 2017;13(1):394.

74. de Lima GV, Ferreira F da S. N-terminal-pro brain natriuretic peptides in dogs and cats: A technical and clinical review. Vet World 2017;10(9):1072–82.

75. Donahue SM, Otto CM. Thromboelastography: A tool for measuring hypercoagulability, hypocoagulability, and fibrinolysis. J Vet Emerg Crit Care 2005; 15(1):9–16.

76. Goggs R, Brainard B, deLaforcade AM, et al. Partnership on Rotational Visco-Elastic Test Standardization (PROVETS): Evidence-based guidelines on rotational viscoelastic assays in veterinary medicine. J Vet Emerg Crit Care 2014; 24(1):1–22.

77. Stillman BA, Monn M, Liu J, et al. Performance of a commercially available in-clinic ELISA for detection of antibodies against Anaplasma phagocytophilum, Anaplasma platys, Borrelia burgdorferi, Ehrlichia canis, and Ehrlichia ewingii and Dirofilaria immitis antigen in dogs. J Am Vet Med Assoc 2014;245(1):80–6.

78. Venco L, Marchesotti F, Manzocchi S. Feline heartworm disease: A'Rubik's-cube-like' diagnostic and therapeutic challenge. J Vet Cardiol 2015;17(Suppl 1):S190–201.

79. Canonne AM, Billen F, Losson B, et al. Angiostrongylosis in dogs with negative fecal and in-clinic rapid serological tests: 7 Cases (2013-2017). J Vet Intern Med 2018;32(3):951–5.

80. Schnyder M, Stebler K, Naucke TJ, et al. Evaluation of a rapid device for serological in-clinic diagnosis of canine angiostrongylosis. Parasite Vectors 2014;7:72.

Ocular Emergencies in Small Animal Patients

Rachel Matusow Wynne, DVM, MS[a,b]

KEYWORDS

- Canine • Feline • Ophthalmic • Examination • Emergency • Glaucoma • Uveitis
- Cornea

KEY POINTS

- Ocular emergencies vary from relatively benign to vision or life threatening, with significant overlap in clinical signs.
- Careful ophthalmic examination in dim light conditions with a bright light source and competent head restraint are crucial to diagnosing ocular disease.
- Adjunctive ophthalmic diagnostic testing should be performed to rule out corneal ulceration, glaucoma, and dry eye before empiric topical antibiotic or steroid medications are prescribed.
- Most emergency conditions present with ocular redness, cloudiness, discomfort, apparent bulging, or vision loss. Differential diagnoses can be considered on this basis.

INTRODUCTION

Diverse emergent ophthalmic conditions present with similar or overlapping clinical signs, but underlying ophthalmic diseases range from the relatively benign to those with the potential to cause permanent blindness if not promptly addressed. Ophthalmic emergencies may represent primary ocular conditions or ocular manifestations of potentially life-threatening systemic disease. Emergency practitioners must become familiar with differential diagnoses, develop strong ophthalmic examination skills, and understand when to apply ancillary diagnostic testing to rule out conditions that threaten vision, comfort, globe, or life. This article reviews practical tips for small animal ophthalmic examination, differential diagnoses by presenting clinical signs, and basic treatment strategies for a selection of ophthalmologic emergencies.

EMERGENCY OPHTHALMIC EXAMINATION

An effective ophthalmologic examination requires adequate patient restraint, a dimly lit room, a bright light source, methodical inspection of periocular and ocular structures, and appropriate ancillary testing.[1–3] Staff should be instructed to immobilize

a Cornell University Veterinary Specialists, 880 Canal Street, Stamford, CT 06902, USA; b Cornell University College of Veterinary Medicine, Ithaca, NY, USA
E-mail address: rwynne@cuvs.org

Vet Clin Small Anim 50 (2020) 1261–1276
https://doi.org/10.1016/j.cvsm.2020.07.003
0195-5616/20/© 2020 Elsevier Inc. All rights reserved.

the patient's head with both hands while holding the patient's body with their own trunk, arms, and an assistant if necessary (**Fig. 1**). Care should be taken to avoid compression of the jugular veins or excessive eyelid manipulation, because both have a significant impact on intraocular pressure.[4,5] Lights should remain bright during initial examination of the head, adnexa, and menace response but should be dimmed before attempting detailed corneal or intraocular examination. Dim lighting is particularly important for patients with corneal opacification (pigment, edema), because bright room light dramatically reduces corneal transparency in these conditions. The ophthalmic examination should be performed in a consistent order regardless of presenting clinical signs, typically moving from extraocular structures to ocular surface to anterior segment to posterior segment or fundic examination.

Assessment of intraocular pressure, fluorescein staining, and Schirmer tear values should be considered in every ophthalmic emergency case. Patients eventually diagnosed with glaucoma commonly have a history of treatment with topical antibiotic or steroid medications prescribed for a red eye. Performing tonometry at the initial visit could prevent ongoing pressure-related discomfort and have a significant positive impact on prognosis for vision. Similarly, fluorescein staining is important for the detection of unsuspected ulcerations before administration of topical steroids. Early detection and treatment of dry eye can improve prognosis for response to other therapies (for conjunctivitis, corneal ulceration) and reduces the risk of disease progression over time.

DIAGNOSIS AND TREATMENT OF EMERGENT OPHTHALMIC CONDITIONS

Common presenting signs for ophthalmic emergencies in small animals include ocular redness, cloudiness, discomfort (squinting, third eyelid elevation, rubbing/scratching at the eye, increased tearing), perceived globe enlargement, and vision loss. The challenge for emergency clinicians is to determine the specific underlying cause and initiate appropriate medical or surgical management.

The Red Eye

Ocular redness is present in most ophthalmic emergencies. Identifying the precise anatomic location of this redness narrows the differential list for underlying conditions.

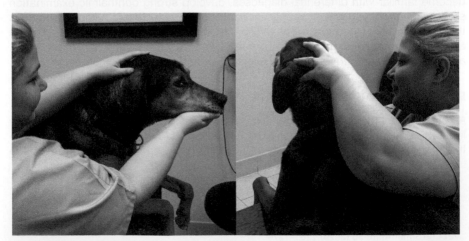

Fig. 1. Complete, three-dimensional immobilization of the head is critical to performing an effective ophthalmic examination in small animals.

Common sources of increased ocular redness include conjunctival hyperemia, episcleral injection, corneal neovascularization, and hemorrhage (conjunctival, subconjunctival, anterior chamber [hyphema], iridal, vitreal, or retinal).

Conjunctival hyperemia is the least specific finding and should be differentiated from episcleral injection, because the latter typically indicates intraocular disease (uveitis or glaucoma). Conjunctival vessels are mobile, branching, smaller in diameter, and more likely to cause a diffuse redness, whereas episcleral vessels are relatively immobile, branch minimally, and run in an anterior-posterior direction over the perilimbal sclera.[2,6–8] Subconjunctival hemorrhage results in focal or multifocal regions of redness that obscure conjunctival vasculature and underlying sclera; underlying causes include trauma, strangulation, vasculitis, and coagulopathy (**Fig. 2**).

Corneal neovascularization patterns can also provide clues to the underlying disease process: superficial vessels tend to be long and branching, whereas deep stromal vessels form straighter/denser hedgelike configurations. Superficial corneal neovascularization indicates ocular surface disease (eg, superficial ulceration, frictional irritation, keratoconjunctivitis sicca), stromal vessels indicate stromal inflammation (ulcers, immune mediated), or intraocular disease if circumferential (glaucoma, uveitis)[7] (**Fig. 3**). Dense corneal neovascularization is frequently mistaken for hyphema. Care should be taken to differentiate redness (blood vessels) in the cornea from extravasated blood in the anterior chamber.

Hyphema and vitreal or retinal hemorrhages typically arise secondary to uveitis/chorioretinitis (infectious disease, neoplasia), coagulopathies/clotting disorders, ocular trauma, systemic hypertension,[9,10] or chronic rhegmatogenous retinal detachment. Patients with poor choroidal pigmentation naturally have a red appearance to their fundus, which can be differentiated from retinal or vitreal hemorrhage by the vascular pattern of the redness (the blood being contained within the choroidal vessels radiating from the region of the optic nerve head).[10]

The Cloudy Eye

A clear visual axis is maintained by highly specialized anatomic and physiologic properties of the cornea, anterior chamber, lens, and vitreous.[11,12] Ophthalmic disease often permanently or temporarily disrupts these mechanisms, leading to loss of transparency and reduced vision. Cloudy eyes are best evaluated in dim light with a bright light source. A front-to-back, stepwise approach facilitates localization of cloudiness: look for loss of transparency in the cornea first, followed by the anterior chamber, lens, and vitreous. To accomplish this, establish whether structures posterior to the area in

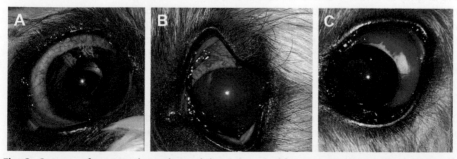

Fig. 2. Sources of extraocular redness. (*A*) Conjunctival hyperemia, (*B*) episcleral injection, (*C*) conjunctival and subconjunctival hemorrhage.

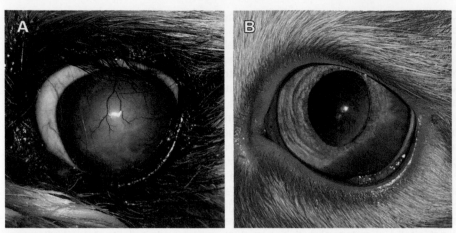

Fig. 3. Superficial corneal vessels are long and branching (*A*), whereas stromal neovascularization tends to be hedgelike in appearance (*B*).

question are easily visible: for example, if the iris detail is easily visible, the cornea and anterior chamber are likely transparent and ocular cloudiness is more likely a result of lens or vitreal opacity (**Fig. 4**).

Primary differentials for corneal cloudiness with concurrent discomfort include corneal edema secondary to ulceration, anterior uveitis, or glaucoma; comfortable eyes with corneal cloudiness should be evaluated for scars, lipid or mineral deposits, or chronic corneal edema secondary to corneal endothelial disease. Diffuse cloudiness of the anterior chamber is most likely caused by aqueous flare, whereas hypopyon, fibrin, and anteriorly prolapsed vitreous form discrete opacities within the aqueous humor. Lenticular (nuclear) sclerosis appears cloudy from afar but causes no significant obstruction of the tapetal reflection or fundic examination, whereas significant cataract blocks passage of light and prevents visualization of the posterior segment. Clinically relevant vitreal opacities are rare in dogs and cats, although retinal elevation into the vitreal space can appear cloudy and obscure visualization of the optic nerve and choroid/tapetum lucidum.

The Acutely Blind Eye

Detailed ophthalmic evaluation including fundus examination and maze testing in dim and brightly lit environments is indicated for patients with acute-onset vision loss. The most urgent conditions to be ruled out are glaucoma, anterior lens luxation, uveitis, hyphema, and retinal detachment secondary to systemic hypertension. To narrow a differential diagnosis list, it is helpful to determine whether (1) vision loss is affecting 1 or both eyes and (2) whether there is concurrent discomfort. See **Table 1** for differential diagnoses.

The Uncomfortable Eye

Ocular discomfort typically manifests with some combination of rubbing, scratching, blepharospasm, enophthalmia, third eyelid elevation, or reduced appetite/lethargy. Trauma, ocular surface irritation (eg, trichiasis, foreign material, dry eye), corneal ulceration, corneal laceration, corneal foreign body, uveitis, glaucoma, anterior lens luxation, and orbital cellulitis/abscess are common causes of ocular discomfort.

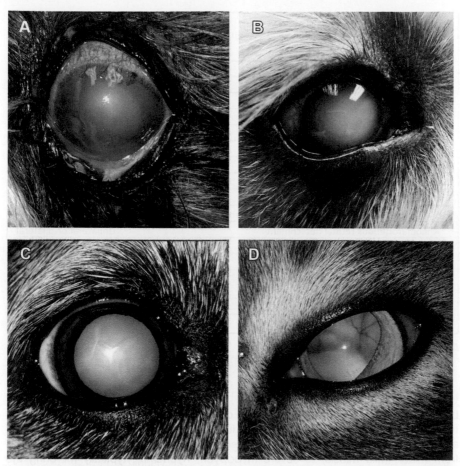

Fig. 4. Ocular cloudiness can be localized by determining which structures lie anterior and posterior to the opacity. (*A*) Corneal edema impairs visualization of the anterior chamber, iris, lens, and posterior segment. (*B*) The cornea is transparent but lipemic aqueous flare obscures the iris, lens, and posterior segment. (*C*) Lenticular opacity (mature cataract) prevents visualization of the posterior segment, whereas corneal, anterior chamber, and iris details remain crisp. (*D*) Retinal detachment creates a veil within the vitreous space that is seen here through the transparent cornea, anterior chamber, and lens.

Application of a topical anesthetic agent such as proparacaine hydrochloride 0.5% ophthalmic solution facilitates examination, reduces risk of falsely increased intraocular pressure measurements caused by blepharospasm, and minimizes the risk of further trauma (such as rupture of a deep corneal ulcer) during examination. Application of a second drop 1 minute after the first has been shown to extend the duration topical anesthesia,[13] and corneal culture is not significantly affected by proparacaine application.[14] If planned, Schirmer tear testing should be performed before administration of topical anesthetic agents.

Corneal ulceration
Fluorescein staining should be performed in every uncomfortable eye. Corneal ulcers frequently cause acute-onset conjunctival hyperemia, corneal edema,

Table 1	
Differential diagnoses for acutely blind eyes in small animals	
Causes	**Eyes Affected**
Painful Causes	
Glaucoma (primary, secondary)	Unilateral or bilateral
Anterior lens luxation	Typically unilateral
Uveitis	Unilateral or bilateral
Trauma	Typically unilateral
Hyphema	Unilateral or bilateral
Non–overtly Painful Causes	
Glaucoma	Unilateral or bilateral
Progressive cataract	Unilateral or bilateral
Sudden acquired retinal degeneration syndrome	Bilateral
Rhegmatogenous retinal detachment	Unilateral or bilateral
Exudative/serous retinal detachment	Unilateral or bilateral
End-stage progressive retinal atrophy	Bilateral
Retinal toxicity (fluoroquinolone (cat), ivermectin, and so forth)	Bilateral
Optic neuritis	Unilateral or bilateral
Central nervous system lesion	Unilateral or bilateral

Data from Refs.[4,15-18]

blepharospasm, and epiphora or purulent ocular discharge. Corneal neovascularization develops over days to weeks after initial development of the corneal wound and varies from superficial to stromal depending on ulcer depth. Reflex uveitis varies from minor (mild miosis) to severe (hypopyon, hyphema), typically mirroring the severity of corneal ulceration. If a visible corneal defect (divot) is present, the ulcer should be considered deep[12] and likely infected (**Fig. 5**). However, fluorescein stain can pool in a healed stromal ulcer (corneal facet), so thorough rinsing is important. If active ulceration is present (fluorescein positive), the emergency clinician should rule out ongoing underlying causes (conjunctival foreign body, trichiasis, keratoconjunctivitis sicca, lagophthalmos, infection), establish depth (superficial vs stromal), and tailor topical and oral therapy to severity of ulceration[7]: an uncomplicated superficial ulcer may heal on 3 times daily prophylactic topical antibiotic alone, whereas a septic stromal ulcer should be addressed with topical antibiotic and antiproteolytic (serum, plasma, ethylenediaminetetraacetic acid [EDTA], acetylcysteine) drops every 2 to 6 hours, topical cycloplegic medication (atropine, cyclopentolate) every 12 to 24 hours, and oral analgesics. Referral should be offered for any patient with a stromal ulcer or potential corneal perforation; surgical stabilization is often recommended for ulcers with greater than or equal to 50% stromal loss.[7,12] Drops are preferable to ointments for deep ulcers to minimize risk of ointment entering the anterior chamber in the case of perforation. If corneal perforation is suspected, broad-spectrum oral antibiotic therapy should be initiated. Only superficial, nonhealing ulcers with loose epithelial edges and without ongoing underlying disease are candidates for cotton-swab debridement; if a deep ulcer is not healing, ongoing infection is likely and debridement is contraindicated.[7,12]

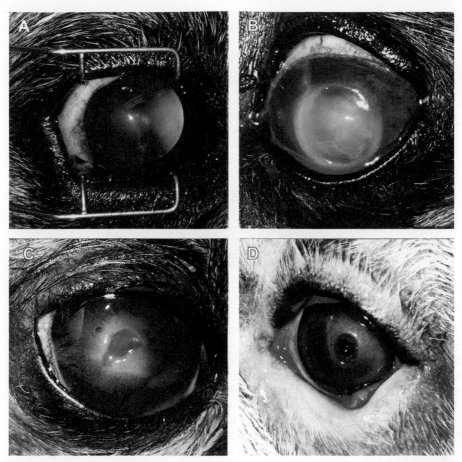

Fig. 5. Corneal ulcers vary in depth and diameter. (*A*) A superficial ulcer does not alter corneal curvature. (*B*) A wide, flat-appearing stromal (deep) ulcer. (*C*) A narrow-diameter but deep stromal ulcer. (*D*) A deep stromal ulcer with central progression to descemetocele.

Corneal foreign body

Patients presenting with corneal foreign bodies typically have a history of contact with brush, leaves, or thorny plants. Superficial to full-thickness foreign material (typically brown plant matter) will be visible in the cornea, with accompanying discomfort, discharge, and anterior uveitis. Superficially embedded (flat-appearing, nonpenetrating) corneal foreign bodies can often be removed via hydropulsion with eyewash in a syringe fitted with a 25-gauge needle with the needle tip removed.[7,19] Penetrating corneal foreign bodies (**Fig. 6**) should be referred to a veterinary ophthalmologist for slit-lamp biomicroscopy; partial-thickness objects may be removed with topical anesthesia alone, whereas perforating foreign bodies require microsurgical intervention with primary wound closure. Medical treatment is similar to that for corneal ulceration.

Corneal laceration

Corneal lacerations in dogs and cats are frequently caused by a fellow cat in the household, broken glass, or projectile objects thrown from landscaping equipment. Cat-claw injuries are particularly common in young puppies that have not yet

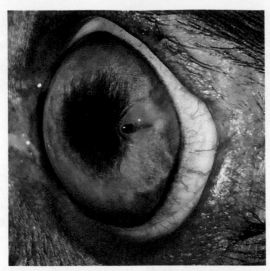

Fig. 6. Perforating corneal foreign body (thorn) in a young hunting dog after a day in the woods.

developed a strong menace response. Ophthalmic examination reveals a linear, partial-thickness to full-thickness corneal wound, variable degree of corneal edema, blepharospasm, ocular discharge, and reflex uveitis (**Fig. 7**). Referral to a veterinary ophthalmologist should be considered for all corneal lacerations. Full-thickness corneal lacerations are commonly associated with concurrent lens capsule rupture, requiring aggressive medical and/or surgical treatment to prevent severe intraocular inflammation or septic endophthalmitis. Corneal lacerations may require primary microsurgical repair, particularly in the face of ongoing aqueous humor leakage or

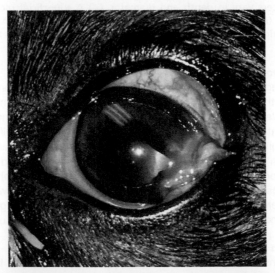

Fig. 7. Perforating corneal laceration with fibrin plug and iris prolapse causing secondary dyscoria in a dog after unwitnessed trauma.

poor apposition of wound edges.[20] Concurrent phacoemulsification may be indicated when lens trauma is present. Inadequate treatment of phacoclastic uveitis or septic implantation into the lens can result in an eye that heals well initially but becomes painful and blind within several weeks of injury.[7] If the laceration is superficial or referral is not available, treat as for a similar-depth corneal ulceration; therapy should include oral antibiotic therapy if corneal perforation is suspected.

Glaucoma

Significant intraocular pressure increase typically results in vision loss, corneal edema, and episcleral injection. Once increased intraocular pressure has been diagnosed, examination should focus on differentiating primary from secondary glaucoma in dogs: primary glaucoma is hereditary in certain breeds; typically presents in middle-aged dogs; often affects one eye before the other; and causes episcleral injection, conjunctival hyperemia, pupil dilatation, and corneal edema without other significant anterior segment changes.[4] Glaucoma is typically secondary in cats. Evidence of secondary glaucoma includes visible anterior lens luxation; hyphema; miosis despite increased intraocular pressure; diffuse or focal iris thickening (infiltrative lesion); and other signs of trauma, inflammation, or systemic disease. Specific risk factors for secondary glaucoma in dogs include cataract surgery, anterior lens luxation, uveitis (lens induced, immune mediated, infectious disease related), primary or metastatic intraocular neoplasia, trauma, and hyphema.[21,22] Patients with secondary glaucoma associated with suspected systemic disease should undergo thorough physical examination and appropriate diagnostic testing.

Dorzolamide 2% hydrochloride ophthalmic solution can be safely applied to canine or feline eyes with primary or secondary glaucoma every 8 hours, making this a good first-line medication[23]; fixed-combination dorzolamide 2%/timolol maleate 0.5% ophthalmic solution is slightly more potent and can be used every 12 hours,[24] although timolol is contraindicated in patients with respiratory or cardiac disease.[23] For primary glaucoma in dogs, twice-daily latanoprost 0.005% ophthalmic solution is an extremely effective treatment[25] that can be used in conjunction with dorzolamide or dorzolamide/timolol. However, efficacy of latanoprost is limited in feline patients with glaucoma, and use is contraindicated in dogs until anterior lens luxation can be definitively ruled out.[1,3]

Diagnosis of acute-onset primary glaucoma should be followed by prompt administration of appropriate antiglaucoma medications and in-hospital monitoring for a response to treatment, because persistent pressure increase leads to permanent vision loss. Target pressure is less than 20 mm Hg to minimize risk of ongoing vision loss in dogs.[4] Prompt referral should be considered if possible. If pressure is unresponsive to topical medications within a matter of hours, aqueous paracentesis or intravenous (IV) treatment with mannitol should be considered to prevent progressive permanent vision loss (1 g/kg IV over 20–30 minutes, withhold water for 1–2 hours, avoid in patients with renal or cardiac disease).[26,27] Maximal topical medical therapy must be continued concurrently, because pressure reduction secondary to IV mannitol or aqueous paracentesis is short lived at approximately 1 hour.[28]

Anterior lens luxation

Anterior lens luxation is a common cause of secondary glaucoma and emergency presentation in dogs.[22] However, severe corneal edema frequently makes diagnosis challenging for emergency veterinarians. Dark room lighting and a bright light source held at an angle to the observer are important for examination,[28] and degree of suspicion should be increased if the pupillary margin of the iris cannot be identified (**Fig. 8**). Any

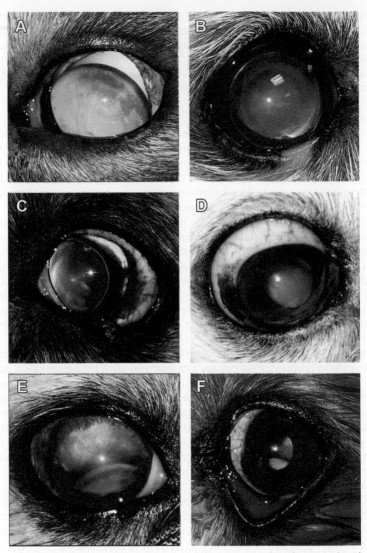

Fig. 8. A visible lens equator indicates lens instability. Anterior lens luxation (*A, B*), lens sub-luxation with aphakic crescent (*C, D*), and posterior lens luxation (*E, F*). Image B courtesy of J. Disney, DVM, MS, DACVO, Midvale, UT.

terrier breed dog with acute-onset intraocular pressure increase should be thoroughly evaluated for anterior lens luxation because of their hereditary predisposition to lens instability,[4] although other breeds are affected as well.[1] Dorzolamide 2% ophthalmic solution can be administered safely to eyes with anterior lens luxation, but latanoprost is contraindicated because of exacerbation of pupillary block glaucoma.[23,29] Referral to a veterinary ophthalmologist is recommended, because surgical lens extraction is typically the treatment of choice.[16] Transcorneal reduction of anterior lens luxation is a nonsurgical intervention for acute anterior lens luxation with a similar long-term success rate to intracapsular lens extraction. Pharmacologic mydriasis is induced and the lens is encouraged to move posterior to the iris via application of transcorneal pressure with a cotton-tipped applicator under topical anesthetic and lubricant, with or without sedation or general anesthesia. If the anterior lens luxation is successfully reduced, immediate-term and then long-term topical miotic therapy (twice-daily latanoprost 0.005% ophthalmic solution) is necessary to attempt to prevent recurrence.[30]

Anterior lens luxation it typically secondary to chronic uveitis in cats and is less likely to cause acute increase in intraocular pressure and emergency presentation.[28] Posterior lens luxation is not an emergent condition in dogs or cats, although concurrent glaucoma or retinal detachment should be ruled out.

Uveitis

Canine and feline patients with anterior uveitis often present because of secondary ocular discomfort. Examination may reveal ocular redness (episcleral injection, conjunctival hyperemia, circumlimbal stromal corneal neovascularization, rubeosis iridis), cloudiness (corneal edema, keratic precipitates, aqueous flare, hypopyon, cataract), excessive tearing, reduced intraocular pressure, miosis, and discomfort affecting 1 or both eyes. Uveitis can result from primary ocular disease (corneal ulceration, cataract, trauma, intraocular neoplasia) or as an ocular manifestation of neoplastic (eg, lymphoma), immune-mediated (vasculitis, uveodermatologic syndrome), or infectious (bacterial, fungal, parasitic, viral, protozoal) disease.[15] Thorough physical examination is important, and laboratory work and thoracic and abdominal imaging should be considered if systemic disease is suspected. Infectious-disease testing must be tailored to the patient and geographic area. A high percentage of cases remain idiopathic in both dogs and cats.[31] In some geographic regions, empiric therapy with doxycycline may be appropriate while infectious-disease testing is pending. Symptomatic therapy should include topical and/or oral antiinflammatories and atropine (contraindicated in secondary glaucoma)[15] (**Fig. 9**).

Horner's syndrome

Ocular signs of Horner's syndrome (enophthalmia, third eyelid elevation, ptosis, miosis) can mimic ocular discomfort and uveitis in dogs and cats (**Fig. 10**). Fluorescein staining and tonometry should be used to rule out corneal ulceration, uveitis, and glaucoma. Application of topical anesthetic may be used to rule out ocular surface

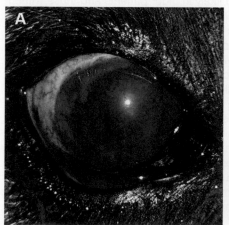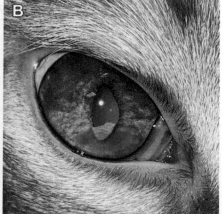

Fig. 9. (A) Canine eye with anterior uveitis and low intraocular pressure. (B) Feline eye with anterior uveitis (lymphoma) and secondary glaucoma.

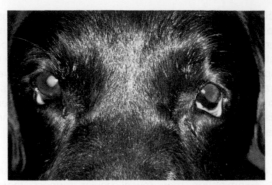

Fig. 10. Horner syndrome in the left eye of a dog with concurrent bilateral mature cataract.

discomfort by lack of response. Resolution of clinical signs in response to topical application of 1 drop of 1% phenylephrine ophthalmic solution within 20 to 60 minutes is consistent with a diagnosis of Horner's syndrome.[17]

The Apparently Enlarged Eye

Bulging eye is a common presenting complaint for canine and feline patients, requiring the clinician to distinguish between buphthalmos, exophthalmos, proptosis, and optical illusion (**Fig. 11**). Truly enlarged eyes are typically blind, because buphthalmia is the result of chronic pressure increase.[4,6] Corneal edema and exophthalmia often create an illusion of globe enlargement; if intraocular pressure is normal and the eye is visual, buphthalmia is unlikely and exophthalmia or optical illusion should be considered.

Exophthalmia describes anterior displacement of the globe. Although blinking may be impaired by exophthalmia, the eyelids remain anterior to the globe equator (differentiating this condition from proptosis). Exophthalmia can be conformational (breed related) or secondary to space-occupying orbital disease. An exophthalmic eye has palpably reduced retropulsion compared with the contralateral side.[2] The most common underlying causes of acquired exophthalmia are orbital cellulitis/abscess (dogs) and orbital neoplasia (dogs and cats). Orbital cellulitis should be prioritized in young or painful patients, whereas neoplasia is more likely in older patients and those without discomfort. Less common differential diagnoses for acquired exophthalmia include salivary mucoceles/sialoceles, zygomatic sialoadenitis, acute-stage masticatory myositis (bilateral, with third eyelid elevation), and extraocular polymyositis (bilateral, without third eyelid elevation).[32] Imaging via orbital ultrasonography, computed tomography, or MRI with sample collection for cytology and culture may be indicated, although initial empiric treatment with antiinflammatories and broad-spectrum systemic antibiotic therapy such as cephalosporins or potentiated penicillins is appropriate for cases of suspected orbital abscess in dogs and cats.[33]

Brachycephalic dogs are predisposed to traumatic proptosis, and more significant trauma is required to precipitate proptosis in cats and nonbrachycephalic dogs.[32] Dog fight and vehicular trauma common causes.[34] By definition, the eyelid margins are entrapped posterior to the globe equator (unable to blink), with a variable degree of anterior globe displacement, strabismus, miosis, hyphema, and ulcerative keratitis. Patients should be screened for concurrent nonophthalmic trauma. The eye should be lubricated immediately. Positive direct and consensual (from injured to normal eye) pupillary light responses are favorable prognostic indicators for vision after globe replacement/tarsorrhaphy procedure.[34] Enucleation should be recommended in

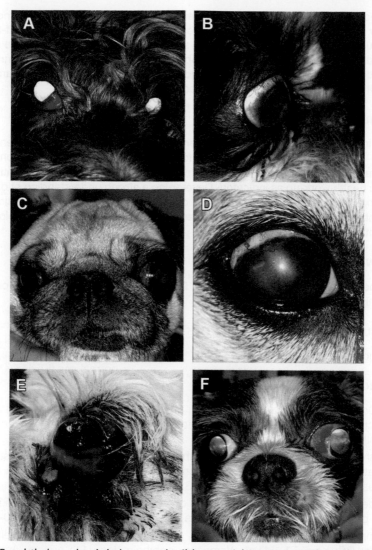

Fig. 11. Exophthalmos, buphthalmos, and mild or partial proptosis can be difficult to diagnose correctly. (*A*) Exophthalmos secondary to orbital neoplasia. (*B*) Breed-related exophthalmos. (*C*) Marked buphthalmos of the left eye is a sign of chronic glaucoma. (*D*) Haab striae (*asterisks*) are breaks in the Descemet membrane that indicate buphthalmia and end-stage glaucoma. (*E*) Traumatic proptosis requiring enucleation. (*F*) Traumatic proptosis-like injury without posterior entrapment of eyelid margins; temporary tarsorrhaphy is indicated.

cases with more than 2 suspected rectus muscle avulsions, complete hyphema, other severe globe trauma/rupture, or owner inability to provide future enucleation or treatment of dry eye if needed.[32,35] Long-term complications after correction include permanent vision loss, keratoconjunctivitis sicca, phthisis bulbi, and strabismus. In 1 study, 28% of surgically replaced eyes retained vision at last follow-up and most blind eyes remained comfortable.[34] Once prognosis and owner preference are established, emergency enucleation or globe replacement with temporary tarsorrhaphy should be promptly performed under general anesthesia. It is important to prevent self-trauma before surgery, because the optic chiasm and vision in the contralateral eye can be damaged by traction on the proptosed globe. Postoperatively, oral antiinflammatory, analgesic, and antibiotic medications should be prescribed; consider topical antibiotic therapy if leaving a medial gap in the temporary tarsorrhaphy.

SUMMARY

Small animal clinicians can successfully identify ocular conditions that threaten vision, comfort, or life by establishing a routine for careful ophthalmic examination, using appropriate diagnostic testing, and performing a thorough physical examination and systemic health work-up as indicated. Developing a strong understanding of differential diagnoses based on presenting signs can help guide examination, testing, and treatment. When indicated, prompt referral to a veterinary ophthalmologist is important.

ACKNOWLEDGMENTS

The author thanks Julia Disney, DVM, MS, DACVO for her assistance in the preparation of this article.

DISCLOSURE

The author has nothing to disclose.

REFERENCES

1. McDonald JE, Kiland JA, Kaufman PL, et al. Effect of topical latanoprost 0.005% on intraocular pressure and pupil diameter in normal and glaucomatous cats. Vet Ophthalmol 2015;19:13–23.
2. Featherstone HJ, Heinrich CL. Ophthalmic examination and diagnostics. In: Gelatt KN, Gilger BC, Kern TJ, editors. Veterinary ophthalmology. 5th edition. Ames (IA): John Wiley and Sons; 2013. p. 533–613.
3. Studer ME, Martin CL, Stiles J. Effects of 0.005% latanoprost solution on intraocular pressure in healthy dogs and cats. Am J Vet Res 2000;61(10):1220–4.
4. Plummer CE, Regnier A, Gelatt KN. The canine glaucomas. In: Gelatt KN, Gilger BC, Kern TJ, editors. Veterinary ophthalmology. 5th edition. Ames (IA): John Wiley and Sons; 2013. p. 1050–145.
5. Klein HE, Krohne SG, Moore GE, et al. Effect of eyelid manipulation and manual jugular compression on intraocular pressure measurement in dogs. J Am Vet Med Assoc 2011;238(10):1292–5.
6. Miller PE. The Glaucomas. In: Maggs DJ, Miller PE, Ofri R, editors. Slatter's fundamentals of veterinary ophthalmology. 4th edition. St. Louis (MO): Elsevier Inc; 2008. p. 230–57.
7. Maggs DJ. Cornea and Sclera. In: Maggs DJ, Miller PE, Ofri R, editors. Slatter's fundamentals of veterinary ophthalmology. 4th edition. St. Louis (MO): Elsevier Inc; 2008. p. 175–202.
8. Maggs DJ. Conjunctiva. In: Maggs DJ, Miller PE, Ofri R, editors. Slatter's fundamentals of veterinary ophthalmology. 4th edition. St. Louis (MO): Elsevier Inc; 2008. p. 135–50.

9. Ofri R. Vitreous. In: Maggs DJ, Miller PE, Ofri R, editors. Slatter's fundamentals of veterinary ophthalmology. 5th edition. St. Louis (MO): Elsevier Inc; 2012. p. 277–84.

10. Ofri R. Retina. In: Maggs DJ, Miller PE, Ofri R, editors. Slatter's fundamentals of veterinary ophthalmology. 5th edition. St. Louis (MO): Elsevier Inc; 2012. p. 285–317. https://doi.org/10.1016/B978-0-7216-0561-6.50018-6.

11. Samuelson DA. Ophthalmic anatomy. In: Gelatt KN, Kern TJ, Gilger BC, editors. Veterinary ophthalmology. 5th edition. Ames (IA): John Wiley and Sons; 2013. p. 39–170.

12. Ledbetter EC, Gilger BC. Diseases and surgery of the canine cornea and sclera. In: Gilger BC, Gelatt KN, Kern TJ, editors. Veterinary ophthalmology. 5th edition. Ames (IA): John Wiley and Sons; 2013. p. 976–1049.

13. Herring IP, Bobofchak MA, Landry MP, et al. Duration of effect and effect of multiple doses of topical ophthalmic 0.5% proparacaine hydrochloride in clinically normal dogs. Am J Vet Res 2005;66(1):77–80.

14. Edwards SG, Maggs DJ, Byrne BA, et al. Effect of topical application of 0.5% proparacaine on corneal culture results from 33 dogs, 12 cats, and 19 horses with spontaneously arising ulcerative keratitis. Vet Ophthalmol 2019;22(4): 415–22.

15. Hendrix DV. Diseases and surgery of the canine anterior uvea. In: Gilger BC, Gelatt KN, Kern TJ, editors. Veterinary ophthalmology. 5th edition. Ames (IA): John Wiley and Sons; 2013. p. 1146–98.

16. Davidson MG, Nelms SR. Diseases of the lens and cataract formation. In: Gelatt KN, Gilger BC, Kern TJ, editors. Veterinary ophthalmology. 5th edition. Ames (IA): John Wiley and Sons; 2013. p. 1199–233.

17. Webb AA, Cullen CL. Neuro-ophthalmology. In: Gelatt KN, Gilger BC, Kern TJ, editors. Veterinary ophthalmology. 5th edition. Ames (IA): John Wiley and Sons; 2013. p. 1820–96.

18. Narfstrom K, Petersen-Jones SM. Diseases of the canine ocular fundus. In: Gelatt KN, Gilger BC, Kern TJ, editors. Veterinary ophthalmology. 5th edition. Ames (IA): John Wiley and Sons; 2013. p. 1303–92.

19. Labelle AL, Psutka K, Collins SP, et al. Use of hydropulsion for the treatment of superficial corneal foreign bodies: 15 cases (1999–2013). J Am Vet Med Assoc 2014;244(4):476–9.

20. Paulsen ME, Kass PH. Traumatic corneal laceration with associated lens capsule disruption: a retrospective study of 77 clinical cases from 1999 to 2009. Vet Ophthalmol 2012;15(6):355–68.

21. Johnsen DAJ, Maggs DJ, Kass PH. Evaluation of risk factors for development of secondary glaucoma in dogs: 156 cases (1999-2004). J Am Vet Med Assoc 2006;229(8):1270–4.

22. Gelatt KN, MacKay EO. Secondary glaucomas in the dog in North America. Vet Ophthalmol 2004;7(4):245–59.

23. Maggio F. Glaucomas. Top Companion Anim Med 2015;30(3):86–96.

24. Plummer CE, MacKay EO, Gelatt KN. Comparison of the effects of topical administration of a fixed combination of dorzolamide–timolol to monotherapy with timolol or dorzolamide on IOP, pupil size, and heart rate in glaucomatous dogs. Vet Ophthalmol 2006;9(4):245–9.

25. Gelatt KN, MacKay EO. Effect of different dose schedules of latanoprost on intraocular pressure and pupil size in the glaucomatous Beagle. Vet Ophthalmol 2001;4(4):283–8.

26. Alario AF, strong TD, Pizzirani S. Medical Treatment of Primary Canine Glaucoma. Vet Clin North Am Small Anim Pract 2015;45(6):1235–59.

27. Volopich S, Mosing M, Auer U, et al. Comparison of the effect of hypertonic hydroxyethyl starch and mannitol on the intraocular pressure in healthy normotensive dogs and the effect of hypertonic hydroxyethyl starch on the intraocular pressure in dogs with primary glaucoma. Vet Ophthalmol 2006;9(4):239–44.

28. Sapienza JS. Feline Lens Disorders. Clin Tech Small Anim Pract 2005;20(2): 102–7.

29. Willis AM. Ocular hypotensive drugs. Vet Clin North Am Small Anim Pract 2004; 34(3):755–76.

30. Montgomery KW, Labelle AL, Gemensky-Metzler AJ. Trans-corneal reduction of anterior lens luxation in dogs with lens instability: a retrospective study of 19 dogs (2010-2013). Vet Ophthalmol 2014;17(4):275–9.

31. Wiggans KT, Vernau W, Lappin MR, et al. Diagnostic utility of aqueocentesis and aqueous humor analysis in dogs and cats with anterior uveitis. Vet Ophthalmol 2013;17(3):212–20.

32. Spiess BM, Pot SA. Diseases and surgery of the canine orbit. In: Gelatt KN, Gilger BC, Kern TJ, editors. Veterinary ophthalmology. 5th edition. Ames (IA): John Wiley and Sons; 2013. p. 793–831.

33. Wang AL, Ledbetter EC, Kern TJ. Orbital abscess bacterial isolates and in vitro antimicrobial susceptibility patterns in dogs and cats. Vet Ophthalmol 2009; 12(2):91–6.

34. Pe'er O, Oron L, Ofri R. Prognostic indicators and outcome in dogs undergoing temporary tarsorrhaphy following traumatic proptosis. Vet Ophthalmol 2019; 206:1186.

35. Miller PE. Ocular emergencies. In: Maggs DJ, Miller PE, Ofri R, editors. Slatter's fundamentals of veterinary ophthalmology. 4th edition. St. Louis (MO): Elsevier Inc; 2008. p. 419–26.

Biosecurity Measures in Clinical Practice

Christopher G. Byers, DVM, CVJ

KEYWORDS

- Hospital-acquired infection • Nosocomial infection • Zoonotic disease • Biosecurity
- Fomite • Infection control • Disinfection • Hand hygiene

KEY POINTS

- Veterinary teams should develop biosecurity programs to help prevent spread of infection to other animals and people in a hospital environment.
- Essential components of effective veterinary biosecurity programs include elimination and substitution of pathogens and hazards, engineering controls, administrative controls, and the use of personal protective equipment.
- Hand hygiene is the most effective step for preventing transmission of infectious agents.

INTRODUCTION

Hospitalized companion animals have increased susceptibility for hospital-acquired/nosocomial infections. Such patients typically have compromised immune systems due to a variety of health conditions, and they are potentially exposed to shedding of infectious agents from other animals. Veterinarians have a responsibility to help reduce unintentional disease transmission and to protect both patients and hospital personnel from common biosecurity hazards, including zoonotic infections potentially found in hospital environments. Veterinarians should proactively manage biosecurity risks in hospital, because these threats have an impact on health of veterinary patients and personnel, hospital operations, and client confidence.

ROUTES OF DISEASE TRANSMISSION

In order to persist over long periods of time, pathogens require reservoirs in which they normally reside. Reservoirs can be living organisms or nonliving sites. Regardless of the reservoir, transmission must occur for infection to spread. Transmission from reservoir to patient occurs first. Then, a patient transmits the infectious agent to other susceptible patients or to inanimate objects. Infectious microorganisms are transmitted in veterinary hospitals via 5 main routes[1]:

4321 North 136th Street, Omaha, NE 68164, USA
E-mail address: criticalcaredvm@gmail.com
Website: http://www.CriticalCareDVM.com

Vet Clin Small Anim 50 (2020) 1277–1287
https://doi.org/10.1016/j.cvsm.2020.07.004
0195-5616/20/© 2020 Elsevier Inc. All rights reserved.

vetsmall.theclinics.com

1. Direct contact
2. Indirect contact (also known as fomite transmission)
3. Vector transmission
4. Droplet/airborne
5. Common vehicle

Direct contact transmission occurs when an animal or person comes in direct contact with an infected animal or person. Indirect contact transmission occurs when a susceptible host touches a contaminated, inanimate object, called a fomite, and transfers the contaminated material to a susceptible portal of entry, most commonly mucous membranes, without specific animal-to-human or animal-to-animal contact. Pathogens transmitted indirectly via fomites are a major cause of hospital-acquired infections. Many hospitalized patients are infected with contagious pathogens; as such, surfaces throughout a hospital are more likely to be contaminated with infectious agents. Furthermore, portable items can be contaminated near one patient and then become a source of transmission to patients or personnel in other areas of a hospital.

Transmission also may occur via vectors. Vector transmission occurs when a biological vector (eg, arthropod) acquires a pathogen from 1 animal and transmits it to another. Heartworm disease is a common example of a disease transmitted by a vector (mosquito). Fleas, ticks, and flies are other common biological vectors of disease.

When patients sneeze, cough, bark, and so forth, small droplets containing microorganisms may be propelled through the air, leading to droplet transmission. This form of transmission involves the movement of a pathogen to a new host over a distance of less than 1 m. When the transmitted distance is greater than 1 m, the preferred term is airborne transmission. Dust and fine particles, known as aerosols, can carry pathogens and facilitate airborne transmission. Many droplet exposures are best characterized as medium to large particle aerosols (ie, >100 μm). These aerosols are too large to be inhaled but may cause disease after contact with mucosal or conjunctival surfaces.

Common vehicle transmission applies to microorganisms transmitted by contaminated items, such as food, water, intravenous fluids, medications, blood products used during transfusions, and medical equipment.

Veterinary team members should remember that many diseases affecting dogs and cats are zoonotic in nature, thus posing potential risks to personnel and owners alike. Zoonotic agents may be transmitted via all of the routes discussed previously.[2]

HIERARCHY OF INFECTION CONTROL

A common tactic for addressing infection control in veterinary hospitals is the use of a 5-tier hierarchy pyramid (**Fig. 1**).[3] Top tiers generally are considered more effective than lower ones, and not all tiers are applicable to every situation.

The elimination and substitution tiers describe practices that may be implemented to prevent pathogens from entering hospitals and/or to physically remove them from facilities.[3] For example, pest management practices—including ectoparasite control and prompt disposal of food waste and other materials—are imperative for infection control. Unfortunately, both elimination and substitution—although most effective— also tend to be the most difficult to implement in veterinary hospitals.

Engineering controls are facility constructs designed to help remove pathogens from a veterinary facility and/or enhance adherence to biosecurity protocols.[3] An important consideration should be given to heating, ventilation, and air conditioning.

Administrative controls are hospital policies and procedures designed to address both team member and patient traffic flow when pathogens are suspected or known.[3] Policies to address medical waste disposal are of paramount importance. Another

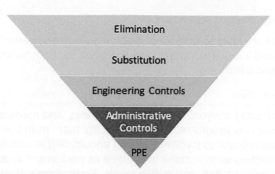

Fig. 1. Five-tier hierarchy of infection control. (*Courtesy of* Centers of Disease Control and Prevention. The National Institute for Occupational Safety and Health (NIOSH). National Institute for Occupational Safety and Health. Hierarchy of controls. Available at https://www.cdc.gov/niosh/topics/hierarchy/default.html. Accessed 6 October 2019.)

essential administrative control is appropriate antimicrobial stewardship.[4] The drafting of policies that promote the judicious use of antimicrobials is necessary to help prevent the development of drug-resistant pathogens. Similarly, protocols to identify high-risk patients (eg, immunocompromised patients) and perform necropsies, use of isolation units, and placement and maintenance of intravenous and urinary catheters all are vital administrative controls in effective biosecurity programs.[4]

Personal protective equipment (PPE) is unique clothing and equipment to protect team members and patients that may be exposed to suspected or known pathogens.[5] The use of PPE helps prevent pathogen exposure and spread.

PRINCIPLES OF INFECTION CONTROL

Every veterinary hospital should develop a comprehensive program for biosecurity control. Management should identify enthusiastic and capable team member(s) to develop and implement specific biosecurity protocols. These individuals should be empowered to recruit other individuals to cultivate staff training programs, create checklists, and generate biosecurity surveillance protocols. Critical components of such programs include the following.

Hand Hygiene

Hand hygiene is the number 1 weapon in preventing the spread of microorganisms and refers to washing with soap and water or using alcohol-based hand rubs containing 60% to 95% alcohol.[6,7] Proper hand hygiene unequivocally removes and kills myriad pathogens without compromising the integrity of the skin. Hand hygiene should be performed[7]

- Before and after contact with a patient and/or animal owner
- Immediately after contact with blood, body fluids, nonintact skin, mucous membranes, or contaminated items (even when gloves are worn during contact)
- Immediately after removing gloves, when moving from contaminated body sites to clean body sites during client care
- After touching objects and medical equipment in the immediate patient care vicinity
- Before eating
- After using the restroom

- After coughing/sneezing into a tissue

When hands are not visibly soiled, use of alcohol gel is the preferred method of hand hygiene. **Boxes 1** and **2** detail recommended protocols for both handwashing and the use of alcohol-based gels.[6,7]

Cleaning and Disinfection

Cleaning and disinfecting environment surfaces, fomites, and medical devices are integral parts of biosecurity programs.[8,9] Every hospital team member needs to understand protocols and processes involved. Teams should define who is responsible for cleaning and disinfecting each surface and piece of equipment in all patient rooms, treatment areas, surgical suites, and public areas. Furthermore, they should develop a schedule for achieving cleaning and disinfection goals.

Different areas of veterinary hospitals pose different levels of biosecurity risk. Human work areas that do not get much animal traffic should be cleaned thoroughly and routinely on a daily basis. Daily disinfection of every surface in these areas of the hospital, however, typically is not needed. In contrast, areas where sick or potentially sick animals are examined and/or treated require more stringent disinfection. Isolation units, intensive care units, and surgical suites require the strictest cleaning and disinfection protocols. Hospital teams are encouraged to develop systems to designate areas of different risk.

Cleaning and disinfecting are 2 distinct processes.[10] Cleaning is the removal of visible foreign material on objects or surfaces and is the first step in environmental sanitation. Disinfection of the inanimate environment decreases the bioburden and limits cross-transmission of pathogens in hospital environments. Most disinfectants are ineffective in the presence of dirt and organic matter.[11] As such, cleaning must occur first before disinfection to effectively remove feces, urine, blood, respiratory secretions, and/or dirt. Proper cleaning/disinfecting is a 4-step process, and gloves and appropriate attire should be worn (**Box 3**).[12]

An ideal disinfectant is one that is broad spectrum, works in any environment, and is nontoxic, nonirritating, noncorrosive, and relatively inexpensive. Unfortunately, no disinfectant is ideal. Therefore, careful consideration of the characteristics of a

---

Box 1
Recommended handwashing protocol

1. Remove all hand and arm jewelry.

2. Wet hands and forearms with warm water.

3. Add at least 3 mL to 5 mL (1–2 full pumps) of soap to palm of hand.

4. Lather all hand surfaces—pay particular attention to the areas between fingers, backs of hands, underneath fingernails, and thumbs.

5. Rinse under warm water until all soap residue is removed.

6. Dry hands with paper towel or warm air dryer.

Data from Boyce JM, Pittet D. Guideline for Hand Hygiene in Health-Care Settings; recommendations for the Healthcare Infection Control Practices Advisory Committee and the HICPAC/SHEA/APIC/IDSA Hand Hygiene Task Force. Infect Control Hosp Epidemiol 2002;23(12 Suppl):S3-S40 and Pittet D, Allegranzi B, Boyce K, et al. The World Health Organization Guidelines on Hand Hygiene in Health Care and their consensus recommendations. Infection Control Hosp Epidemiol 2009;30(7):611-622.

> **Box 2**
> **Recommended protocol for use of alcohol-based hand rub**
>
> 1. Remove all hand and arm jewelry.
> 2. Ensure hands are visibly clean.
> 3. Apply 1 to 2 full pumps (or 2–3 cm diameter pool of product) onto 1 palm.
> 4. Spread product over all surfaces of hands—pay particular attention to the areas between fingers, backs of hands, underneath fingernails, and thumbs.
> 5. Rub hands until product is dry (minimum of 15–20 seconds).
>
> *Data from* Boyce JM, Pittet D. Guideline for Hand Hygiene in Health-Care Settings; recommendations for the Healthcare Infection Control Practices Advisory Committee and the HICPAC/SHEA/APIC/IDSA Hand Hygiene Task Force. Infect Control Hosp Epidemiol 2002;23(12 Suppl):S3-S40 and Pittet D, Allegranzi B, Boyce K, et al. The World Health Organization Guidelines on Hand Hygiene in Health Care and their consensus recommendations. Infection Control Hosp Epidemiol 2009;30(7):611-622.

disinfectant is essential to select the most useful, effective, and cost-efficient product (**Table 1**).[13,14] Use of the proper concentration of a disinfectant is important to achieve the best results for each situation. Some products have different dilutions depending on the desired use of the product. The product label lists the best concentration to use for each situation.

There are a variety of ways to apply disinfectants.[13] Object surfaces or walls may be treated with a disinfectant solution by wiping, brushing, spraying, or misting. Portable items should be soaked in a container of disinfectant. Appropriate contact times are essential.[14] Disinfectants may vary in the contact time needed to kill versus inactivate microorganisms. Areas being disinfected should be well soaked with the disinfectant selected to avoid drying before the end of the optimum contact time. Some chemicals may have residual activity whereas others may evaporate quickly.

Heat, light, and radiation also may be appropriately used to reduce or eliminate microorganisms in a hospital environment.[15] The use of heat is a one of the oldest physical controls against microorganisms. Although both moist heat (autoclave and steam) and dry heat (flame and baking) can be used to inactivate microorganisms, moist heat is more effective and requires less time than dry heat. Sunlight and UV light can have a detrimental effect on several microorganisms and may be practical methods for inactivating viruses, mycoplasma, bacteria, and fungi, in particular those that are airborne.

> **Box 3**
> **Four-step process for cleaning and disinfecting**
>
> Step 1: mechanical removal of organic material
>
> Step 2: cleaning with soap or general cleaner with subsequent rinsing and drying
>
> Step3: applying disinfectant and allow to sit for the required contact time
>
> Step 4: rinsing disinfectant and drying area well
>
> *Data from* Quinn PJ, Markey BK. Disinfection and disease prevention in veterinary medicine. In: Block SS, editor. Disinfection, sterilization and preservation. 5th edition. Philadelphia: Lippincott, Williams & Wilkins. 2001; pp1069-1103.

Table 1
Characteristics of selected disinfectants

	Alcohols	Alkalis	Aldehydes	Chlorine	Iodine	Peroxygen Compounds	Phenols	Quaternary Ammonium Compounds	Biguanides
Bactericidal	Y	Y	Y	Y	Y	Y	Y	Y	Y
Viricidal	±	Y	±	Y	Y	Y	Y	Y enveloped	±
Fungicidal	Y	Y	Y	Y	Y	±	Y	Y	N
Sporicidal	N	Y	Y	Y	±	Y	N	Y	N

Abbreviations: ±, variable/limited activity; N, not effective; Y, effective.
Data from Fraise AP, Lambert PA, et al. (eds) Russel, Hugo, & Ayliffe's Principles and Practice of Disinfection, Preservation and Steriliztion, 5th ed. 2013. Ames, IA: Wiley-Blackwell and McDonnell GE. Antisepsis, Disinfection, and Sterilization: Types, Action, and Resistance. 2007. ASM Press, Washington DC.

UV light sterilizing capabilities are limited on surfaces because of its lack of penetrating power. Other forms of radiation are used less frequently but may include the use of microwaves or gamma radiation. Freezing is not a reliable method of sterilization but may help reduce heavy numbers of bacteria.

Performing routine follow-up evaluations of hospital areas is essential to verify pathogens have been destroyed. Visual inspection of cleanliness is important, but bacteriologic samples also should be obtained to determine the efficacy of the cleaning and disinfecting protocols. Failure of these programs may be due to an ineffective disinfectant, careless use of an effective disinfectant, and/or a variety of environmental factors (eg, temperature, relative humidity). The timing of sample collection is important, and the best time to sample is 2 days to 3 days after disinfection. Samples for microbiological testing should not be taken from a wet surface because the disinfectant still may be acting, and disinfectant residues may prevent growth of microorganisms in culture media.

Personal Protective Equipment

PPE includes items, such as gloves, gowns, masks, respirators, goggles, and face shields, used to create barriers that protect skin, clothing, mucous membranes, and the respiratory tract from infectious agents.[16] The items selected for use depend on the infectious agent, type of interaction, and the method of microorganism transmission.

PPE should be donned in the following order[16]:

1. Gown
2. Mask or respirator
3. Goggles or face shield
4. Gloves

The Occupational Safety and Health Administration (OSHA) standards require employers to provide PPE for employees with hazard exposure in the workplace, train employees on the proper use of PPE, and properly maintain, store, and dispose of PPE.

Gowns should be donned if skin or clothing is likely to be exposed to blood or body fluids. Properly fitted gowns should cover the torso fully from neck to knee, arms to the end of wrists, and wrap around the back. They should fasten in back of the neck and waist. Veterinary team members should wear surgical masks/respirators and goggles/face shields if there is a reasonable chance a spray of blood or body fluids may occur to the mouth or nose. A properly fitted mask should have secured ties or elastic bands at the middle of the head and neck. The flexible band should be manipulated to fit the nose bridge, and the mask should fit snugly to the face and below the chin. Googles/face shields should be adjusted to fit over the eyes/face. Gloves should be worn when touching blood, body fluids, nonintact skin, mucous membranes, and contaminated items. Gloves also always should be worn during activities involving vascular and urinary access. They should extend to cover the wrist of an isolation gown.

PPE should be removed immediately after use and should be doffed in proper order to prevent contamination of skin or clothing. The recommended order for doffing PPE is gown first, then shoe covers, followed by gloves, and lastly mask/respirator and goggles/face shield.[16] Any PPE or other disposable items saturated with blood or body fluids, such that fluid may be poured, squeezed, or dripped from the item, should be discarded into a biohazard bag. Any PPE not saturated may be placed directly in the trash.

Needlestick and Sharps Injury Prevention

Literature shows as many as one-third of all sharps injuries occur during disposal.[17] Veterinary medical team members, especially credentialed veterinary technicians, are particularly at risk, because they sustain the most needlestick injuries. The Centers for Disease Control and Prevention estimates 62% to 88% of sharps injuries can be prevented simply by using safer medical devices.[18] Safe handling of needles and other sharp devices are components of standard precautions that are implemented to prevent health care worker exposure to bloodborne pathogens. The Needlestick Safety and Prevention Act mandates the use of sharps with engineered safety devices when suitable devices exit.[19]

Recalling the hierarchy of infection control, a common sense approach for needlestick and sharps injury prevention (from most effective to least effective) is

- Elimination and substitution—whenever applicable and appropriate for patient care, substitute injections by administering medications via another route. Furthermore, jet injectors may be substituted for syringes and needles.
- Engineering controls—use of needles that retract, sheathe, or blunt immediately after use can reduce the incidence of needle/sharp injuries.
- Administrative controls—develop hospital policies that enhance team member knowledge of needle/sharps safety and limit exposure to needle/sharps hazards. Other effective policies include activating safety devices on needles and other sharps immediately after use; discarding used needles immediately after use; eliminating the practices of recapping, bending, and cutting; placing used needles, lancets, or other contaminated sharps in a leak-proof, puncture-resistant sharps container that either is red in color or labeled with a biohazard label; and not overfilling sharps containers.
- PPE—proper use of PPE like goggles, face shields, gloves, masks, and gowns may provide an effective barrier from needle/sharps injuries.

Laundry

Properly laundering reusable blankets, towels, and scrubs is an essential component of effective biosecurity protocols.[20] Veterinary hospitals should have the appropriate equipment to facilitate effective washing and hot air drying of laundry.[20] Special consideration should be given to laundry generated in isolation units, by suspected and known infected animals, and in surgical suites. Ideally, single-use items should be used in isolation units and for patients with suspected or known infectious diseases. Soiled items should be disposed properly in appropriate medical waste receptacles according to local, state, and federal regulations. An alternative approach is to presoak laundry from isolation units and infected animals in diluted bleach (ie, 9 parts water and 1 part bleach) for 10 minutes prior to routine washing and hot air drying.[20] Surgical laundry, including towels and wraps, ideally should be washed and hot air dried separately from other hospital laundry.

Waste Disposal

The Environmental Protection Agency regulates the disposal of products with environmental impact. The OSHA regulates issues associated with potential employee exposure to hazardous substances. Guidance pertaining to products used in the workplace that have an impact on human health is provided by the National Institute for Occupational Safety and Health. The Drug Enforcement Administration regulates the disposal of controlled substances. Veterinary practices that ship hazardous materials are subject to regulation by the Department of Transportation, whereas those that ship materials via air are subject to regulation by the Federal Aviation Administration. In general, state regulations supersede federal regulations in that they may be more stringent.

Medical waste refers to waste products that are not considered general waste. It is produced from health care premises, such as hospitals, clinics, doctors'/ dentists' offices, veterinary hospitals, and laboratories. Regulated medical waste, also known as biohazardous waste, is a subset of medical waste that poses a significant risk of transmitting infection to people. Regulated medical waste generated from veterinary facilities includes sharps waste, animal carcasses, body parts, bedding, and related wastes when animals are intentionally infected with organisms likely to be pathogenic to healthy humans for the purposes of research.

Sharp items should be disposed of in containers that are puncture resistant, leak-proof, closable, and labeled with the biohazard symbol or red in color. Sharps containers should be replaced when filled up to the indicated full line. Items that should be discarded into sharps containers include contaminated items that may easily cause cuts or punctures in the skin, including needles, lancets, broken glass, and rigid plastic vials. Syringes or blood collection tube holders attached to needles also must be discarded still attached to the needles. Similarly, non-sharp disposable items saturated with blood or body fluids should be discarded into biohazard bags that are puncture-resistant, leak-proof, and labeled with a biohazard symbol or red in color. Such items may include used PPE and disposable rags or cloths.

The American Veterinary Medical Association has established best management practices for pharmaceutical disposal.[21] It urges members to

- Follow all applicable federal, state, local, and tribal regulations and guidelines for disposal of all pharmaceutical waste.
- Be knowledgeable of regulations that apply to controlled substances or hazardous, chemotherapeutic, trace chemotherapeutic, mixed, or radiologic waste.
- Maintain close inventory control.
- Avoid pouring/flushing pharmaceuticals down drains or toilets as well as burning pharmaceutical waste, unless permitted by authorities of oversight.
- Segregate waste and utilize appropriate waste brokers, including reverse distributors, whenever possible.
- Train employees on proper disposal of pharmaceutical waste.

SUMMARY

Infection control, biosecurity, and biosafety are essential functions of all veterinary hospitals. Veterinary facilities have a responsibility to protect personnel and clients from exposure to zoonotic disease agents. Hospital teams should develop biosecurity protocols that optimize patient care while concurrently minimizing the risk of hospital-acquired infection. Good biosecurity practices are not the only feature defining excellence in veterinary care, but it is impossible to achieve excellent patient care without employing logical infection control procedures.

DISCLOSURE

Dr C.G. Byers serves as a consultant for Dechra Pharmaceuticals and is a member of the Scientific Advisory Board for Veterinary Recommended Solutions.

REFERENCES

1. Morley PS. Biosecurity of veterinary practices. Vet Clin North Am Food Anim Pract 2002;18(1):133–55.
2. Wright JG, Jung S, Holman RC, et al. Infection control practices and zoonotic disease risks among veterinarians in United States. J Am Vet Med Assoc 2008; 232(12):1863–72.
3. National Institute for Occupational Safety and Health. Hierarchy of controls. Available at: https://www.cdc.gov/niosh/topics/hierarchy/default.html. Accessed October 6, 2019.
4. Gibbons JD, MacMahon K. Workplace safety and health for the veterinary health care team. Vet Clin North Am Small Anim Pract 2015;45(2):409–26.
5. Williams CJ, Scheftel JM, ELchos BL, et al. Compendium of Veterinary Standard Precautions for Zoonotic Disease Prevention in Veterinary Personnel: National Association of State Public Health Veterinarians: Veterinary Infection Control Committee 2015. J Am Vet Med Assoc 2015;247(11):1252–77.
6. Boyce JM, Pittet D. Guideline for Hand Hygiene in Health-Care Settings; recommendations for the Healthcare Infection Control Practices Advisory Committee and the HICPAC/SHEA/APIC/IDSA Hand Hygiene Task Force. Infect Control Hosp Epidemiol 2002;23(12 Suppl):S3–40.
7. Pittet D, Allegranzi B, Boyce K, et al. The World Health Organization Guidelines on Hand Hygiene in Health Care and their consensus recommendations. Infect Control Hosp Epidemiol 2009;30(7):611–22.
8. Murphy CP, Reid-Smith RJ, Boerlin P, et al. *Escherichia coli* and selected veterinary and zoonotic pathogens isolated from environmental sites in companion animal veterinary hospitals in southern Ontario. Can Vet J 2010;51(9):963–72.
9. Cherry B, Burns A, Johnson GS, et al. *Salmonella typhimurium* outbreak associated with veterinary clinic. Emerg Infect Dis 2004;10(12):2249–51.
10. Ewart SL. Disinfectants and control of environmental contamination. In: Smith BL, editor. Large Animal Internal Medicine: diseases of horses, cattle, sheep and goats. 3rd edition. St. Louis (MO): Mosby; 2001. p. 1371–80.
11. Willett HP. Ch. 10. Sterilization and disinfection. In: Joklik WK, editor. Zinsser microbiology. East Norwalk (CT): Appleton and Lange; 1992. p. 188–200.
12. Quinn PJ, Markey BK. Disinfection and disease prevention in veterinary medicine. In: Block SS, editor. Disinfection, sterilization and preservation. 5th edition. Philadelphia: Lippincott, Williams & Wilkins; 2001. p. 1069–103.
13. Fraise AP, Maillard J-Y, Sattar S, et al, editors. Russel, Hugo, & Ayliffe's principles and practice of disinfection, preservation and steriliztion. 5th edition. Ames (IA): Wiley-Blackwell; 2013.
14. McDonnell GE. Antisepsis, disinfection, and sterilization: types, action, and resistance. Washington (DC): ASM Press; 2007.
15. Rutala WA, Weber DJ. Healthcare Infection Control Practices Advisory Committee (HICPAC). 2008. Guideline for disinfection and sterilization in healthcare facilities. Available at: http://www.cbc.gov/hicpac/Disinfection_Sterilization/toc.html. Accessed October 6, 2019.
16. Honda H, Iwata K. Personal protective equipment and improving compliance among healthcare workers in high-risk settings. Curr Opin Infect Dis 2016; 29(4):400–6.
17. Ochmann U, Wicker S. Needlestick injuries of healthcare workers. Anaesthesist 2019;68(8):569–80.

18. Occupational Safety and Health Administration. Bloodborne pathogens and needlestick prevention. Available at: https://www.osha.gov/SLTC/bloodbornepathogens/evaluation.html. Accessed October 6, 2019.
19. Tatelbaum MF. Needlestick safety and prevention act. Pain Physician 2001;4(2): 193–5.
20. The Canadian Committee on Antibiotic Resistance. Infection prevention and control best practices for small animal veterinary clinics 2008. Available at: https://www.wormsandgermsblog.com/files/2008/04/CCAR-Guidelines-Final2.pdf. Accessed October 6, 2019.
21. American Veterinary Medical Association. Waste disposal by veterinary practices: what goes where?. Available at: https://www.avma.org/PracticeManagement/Administration/Pages/Waste-Disposal-by-Veterinary-Practices-What-Goes-Where.aspx. Accessed October 6, 2019.

Update on Albumin Therapy in Critical Illness

Elisa M. Mazzaferro, MS, DVM, PhD[a,b,*], Thomas Edwards, DVM, MS, LTC, VC[c]

KEYWORDS

- Albumin • Colloid osmotic pressure • Endothelial glycocalyx
- Type III hypersensitivity reaction • Transfusion

KEY POINTS

- Albumin is among most important proteins in the body and plays a significant role in maintenance of colloid osmotic pressure, wound healing, decreasing oxidative damage, carrying drugs and endogenous substances, and coagulation.
- Hypoalbuminemia is common in a variety of acute and chronic illnesses. An albumin concentration of less than 2.0 g/dL is a negative prognostic indicator in veterinary patients.
- Replenishment of albumin can be in the form of fresh frozen, frozen, or cryopoor plasma or in the form of human or canine albumin concentrates.
- Infusion of human albumin concentrate to healthy and critically ill dogs can induce acute and delayed hypersensitivity reactions that range in signs from fever, urticaria, vomiting, peripheral edema, joint effusion, and renal failure. Death has been reported.

INTRODUCTION

Albumin is one of the most important proteins in the body. The functions of albumin are numerous and include maintenance of colloid osmotic pressure (COP) within the intravascular and extravascular body compartments and carrier of endogenous hormones and ions, as well as exogenous drugs, scavenger of oxygen-derived free radical species in sites of inflammation, participation in the acid–base balance within the body, contributor to waste product elimination, and mediator of coagulation.[1,2]

During states of health, albumin is synthesized exclusively in the liver in response to local COP and the presence of available amino acid nutrients.[3] During states of critical illness, however, hypoalbuminemia, which is defined as a serum albumin of less than 3.0 g/dL,[4] is common, and has a prevalence that ranges from 9.8%[5] to 25.2%.[6] The causes of hypoalbuminemia are numerous, and result from a lack of production with

[a] Cornell University Veterinary Specialists, 880 Canal Street, Stamford, CT 06902, USA; [b] Emergency and Critical Care, Cornell University Hospital for Animals; [c] Research Support Division, U.S. Army Institute of Surgical Research, JBSA Fort Sam Houston, 3698 Chambers Pass, San Antonio, TX 78234, USA
* Corresponding author.
E-mail address: emazzaferro@cuvs.org

Vet Clin Small Anim 50 (2020) 1289–1305
https://doi.org/10.1016/j.cvsm.2020.07.005
0195-5616/20/© 2020 Elsevier Inc. All rights reserved.

preferential synthesis of acute phase proteins,[1,7,8] as well as a lack of available nutrient stores for hepatic albumin synthesis. Increased loss into body cavities or from wound exudates, renal glomerular dysfunction, or gastrointestinal disease, as well as dilution caused by infusion of natural and synthetic colloids also contribute to hypoalbuminemia (**Box 1**). In both human and veterinary patients, hypoalbuminemia has been associated with impaired wound healing,[9] decreased binding of drugs,[10] increased risk of gastrointestinal surgical site dehiscence,[11] and increased patient morbidity and mortality.[12–18] In 1 study of human patients, the relative risk of mortality increased by 25% to 50% for each 0.25 g/dL decrease in serum albumin.[19] In another meta-analysis of hypoalbuminemia in acute illness in people, for each 10 g/L decrease in albumin, there was a 137% increase in odds of death, a 71% increase in length of hospital stay and an 89% increase in overall morbidity.[20]

Because of the negative consequences of hypoalbuminemia, restoration of total body albumin is encouraged. However, this can be challenging and controversial in both human and veterinary medicine. A Cochrane meta-analysis evaluated outcome in a heterogeneous population of critically ill human patients who received 4% or 5% human serum albumin (HSA) as a resuscitative fluid.[21] The resultant analyses determined that the use of HSA did not improve clinical outcome and may increase the relative risk of death in some patient populations. This study had a profound effect on the use of albumin in practice and it is estimated that subsequent to the publication of the Cochrane review, use of albumin decreased by more than 40% in the UK.[22] A later study, the Saline versus Albumin Fluid Evaluation (SAFE) trial, compared the use of 5% HSA with 0.9% saline for fluid resuscitation in human patients in the intensive care unit, and not only found lack of evidence to support detrimental effects of HSA, but found that its use may improve survival in human patients with sepsis.[23] Subsequent to the SAFE trial, a large meta-analysis of septic human patients found a decreased mortality for those patient who received albumin (odds ratio, 0.82; 95% confidence interval, 0.67–1.0).[24] This study and others have led the human health care community to recommend the use of HSA in conjunction with crystalloids for initial resuscitation in septic patients.[25] Veterinary advocates of albumin supplementation, therefore, have continued to support the supplementation and replenishment of albumin in critically ill small animal patients, provided that possible risks outweigh the perceived benefits.

Immunogenicity

Albumin shares 83% to 88% structural homology across animal species.[26–28] Canine albumin is approximately 79.3% structurally homologous to human albumin.[29] Species differences in the genetic amino acid sequence, molecular weight, net charge, and isoelectric set point of albumin are thought to contribute to antigenicity with the potential to develop adverse immediate and delayed hypersensitivity reactions in some dogs.[26,30] Even among different dog breeds, there seem to be small variations in the genetic sequencing of albumin,[31] which can result in variations in drug-binding capacity. It is unknown whether the small differences in amino acid sequencing in dog albumin can potentially contribute to its antigenicity at this time. Type I hypersensitivity reactions occur within minutes to hours of exposure to an antigen and requires prior exposure with subsequent sensitivity.[32] Type III or Arthus reactions are delayed and occur after soluble immune complexes adhere to the endothelium of vessels and other organs that then lead to the activation of the complement, with subsequent activation of the inflammatory cascade.[32] Type III hypersensitivity reactions are typically observed 1 to 3 weeks after antigenic exposure. The resultant widespread vasculitis with clinical signs

---

Box 1
Conditions associated with hypoalbuminemia

Albumin loss
  Renal loss
    Sepsis
    Diabetes mellitus
    Glomerulonephritis
    Amyloidosis
    Ehrlichia canis
  Gastrointestinal loss
    Inflammatory bowel disease
    Lymphangectasia
    Infectious
      Bacterial enteritis
      Parvoviral enteritis
      Histoplasmosis
      Parasitism
        Whipworm (*Trichuris vulpis*)
        Roundworms (*Toxocara canis, Toxocara cati*)
        Hookworms (*Ancylostoma caninum, Ancylostoma braziliense*)
        Giardia (*Giardia intestinalis, Giardia duodenalis, Giardia lamblia*)
        Coccidia (*Isospora* spp.)
      Panleukopenia virus
  Neoplasia
  Toxins
  Heat-induced illness/hyperthermia
  Pancreatitis
  Peritonitis
  Pleural space/pulmonary loss
    Pyothorax
    Noncardiogenic pulmonary edema
    Acute respiratory distress syndrome

Endocrinopathy
  Hypoadrenocorticism
  Hyperadrenocorticism

Decreased synthesis
  Malnutrition
  Hepatic disease
    Cholangiohepatitis
    Cirrhosis
    Lipidosis
    Phenobarbital toxicosis
    Portosystemic shunt
  Histoplasmosis
  Neoplasia

Increased hydrostatic pressure
  Heartworm caval syndrome (*D immitis*)
  Right sided cardiac disease
  Portal hypertension

Data from Mazzaferro EM, Rudloff E, Kirby R. The role of albumin replacement in the critically ill veterinary patient. J Vet Emerg Crit Care 2002; 12(2):113-124.

---

of fever, lethargy, joint effusion, polyarthralgia, lymphadenopathy, and urticaric skin lesions can be self-limiting or can lead to significant morbidity or mortality.

From the onset of considering using more concentrated forms of albumin for supplementation therapy in hypoalbuminemic patients, concern has been raised about the possible immunogenicity of xenotransfusions of non–species-specific albumin to veterinary patients.[33,34] Because canine-specific albumin was only sporadically available until recently, researchers initially investigated the use of bovine and human albumin concentrates to healthy and critically ill dogs. An early study that investigated the use of 500 mg/kg IV bovine albumin to healthy dogs,[19] 2 dogs demonstrated immediate adverse reactions that ranged from mild urticaria and pruritus to severe anaphylaxis during administration of a second dose 14 days after the initial administration. Five of the remaining 8 dogs that received only 1 initial infusion of bovine serum albumin developed clinical signs of mild to severe type III hypersensitivity reactions 15 to 18 days after bovine serum albumin administration.

In 2007, 2 separate groups of researchers performed prospective studies that investigated the use of 25% concentrated HSA in healthy dogs.[32,35] In the first study,[35] 6 healthy dogs received a single dose of 25% HSA (2 mL/kg IV over 1 hour) as a part of an investigation that compared the effects of various natural and synthetic colloids with crystalloids on coagulation, COP, and packed cell volume and total solids. One dog developed vomiting and facial edema within 15 minutes of the onset of HSA infusion. The remaining 5 dogs developed no immediate signs of adverse reaction; however, all 6 dogs developed delayed clinical signs that were consistent with a type III hypersensitivity reaction 5 to 37 days after HSA administration. Four dogs had mild clinical signs that did not require hospitalization, whereas, in 2 dogs, clinical signs progressed in severity and included protein-losing nephropathy, generalized severe vasculitis, and subsequent death. In both animals that died, the histopathology of the skin and kidneys demonstrated leukocytoclastic vasculitis and membranoproliferative glomerulonephritis, consistent with type III sensitivity reactions. An enzyme-linked immunosorbent assay test was developed to document anti-human albumin antibodies and found that all 6 dogs had developed antibodies directed against human albumin after initial exposure.

The second study[32] administered 50 g of 25% HSA to 9 healthy purpose-bred dogs at incremental doses of 0.5 mL/kg/h to a maximum of 4 mL/kg/h. One dog developed an acute anaphylactic reaction after receiving less than 1.5 mL/kg of 25% HSA and later developed facial edema and urticaria after HSA administration. A second dog developed urticaria and facial edema 7 days after HSA infusion. Two dogs received a second infusion of 25% HSA 14 days after the first and developed almost immediate signs of a hypersensitivity reaction. Although HSA infusion statistically increased serum albumin concentration and COP above baseline values, it also resulted in the production of IgG antibodies and positive skin testing supportive of IgE antibodies.[32]

A third study[29] measured anti-human albumin antibodies in 2 healthy dogs and 14 critically ill dogs that received 25% HSA as a part of therapy. The healthy dogs received 2 mL/kg 25% HSA over 2 hours, then a second infusion of 1 mL/kg over 1 hour 10 days later. One of the dogs developed facial edema and decreased appetite 8 days after the first infusion. Both dogs developed erythema, vomiting, and diarrhea during the second infusion. Serum IgG anti-human albumin antibodies were detected with 10 days of HSA administration and peaked at 3 weeks after administration.

The median dose of 25% HSA administered to critically ill dogs was 5.2 mL/kg (range, 1.8–47.1 mL/kg) over a median time of 0.8 mL/kg/h (range, 0.2–1.8 mL/kg/h). No acute or delayed hypersensitivity reactions were observed in the critically ill dogs. Critically ill dogs had no significant increase in anti-human antibodies at the time of hospital discharge but did develop increased anti-human albumin antibodies 4 and 6 weeks later. The duration of antibody response was prolonged through 6 months in both healthy and critically ill dogs tested. Five of 68 negative control dogs who did not receive HSA also tested positive for anti-human albumin antibodies.

The authors proposed a potential mechanism of cross-reactivity with bovine albumin when dogs are exposed to bovine albumin during the ingestion of food products or vaccination. Others have documented leukocytoclastic vasculitis and type III sensitivity reactions in critically ill dogs who received 25% HSA diluted to 5% and infused over 3 to 4 hours.[36] A case series of 2 critically ill dogs who received 25% HSA as part of therapy for septic peritonitis documented type III hypersensitivity reactions that progressed to acute glomerulonephritis, proteinuria, oligoanuria, and death.[37] This final article is the first to document death secondary to type III hypersensitivity reactions in critically ill dogs that had received 25% HSA.

Despite immune stimulation to HSA in critically ill dogs and cats, the majority of studies that have prospectively and retrospectively evaluated its use have demonstrated significant increases in serum albumin concentration, COP, and blood pressure in critically ill dogs without severe adverse sequelae.[34,38–42] Mathews and Barry[38] first reported the use of 25% serum albumin in 64 critically ill dogs and 2 cats in combination with fresh frozen and stored plasma, pentastarch and whole blood or packed red blood cells. Infusions were administered as a slow constant rate infusion (0.1–1.7 mL/kg/h) or more rapidly (2–4 mL/kg) for the treatment of hypoalbuminemia and hypotension, respectively. Facial edema was reported in 2 dogs during the 25% HSA infusion. Serum albumin, systolic blood pressure, and total solids significantly increased in treated patients, with a 71% survival to discharge.

Another retrospective case series[39] described the administration of 25% human albumin diluted to 10% in 73 critically ill dogs (1.4 g/kg median dose) that resulted in significantly higher serum albumin, total protein, and COP after infusion, with a 50.3% survival to hospital discharge. The serum albumin concentration was found to be higher in survivors versus nonsurvivors. Although some dogs experienced clinical signs of tachypnea, fever, peripheral edema, and tachycardia with ventricular dysrhythmias during or soon after administration of the HSA, the nature of their critical illness also could explain the same clinical signs. Three dogs did develop signs of a type III hypersensitivity reaction 5 to 14 days after the administration of the HSA.

A retrospective analysis of administration of HSA to dogs with septic peritonitis demonstrated statistically significant increases in serum albumin concentration, COP and total protein after albumin administration.[43] The postinfusion serum albumin concentrations were significantly higher in survivors versus nonsurvivors, with an overall survival rate of 46%. Despite these findings, the administration of HSA was not correlated with survival. No adverse reactions were reported, although the retrospective nature of the case series may have precluded follow-up.

The retrospective case series discussed administered concentrated human albumin as 25% or diluted to 10% solutions. Curiously, 2 studies[34,40] by the same veterinary researchers in Italy have documented no adverse reactions to HSA infusions diluted to 5% in a retrospective study of 418 dogs and 170 cats and in a prospective study of 40 critically ill cats. In both studies, 25% HSA was diluted to 5% then administered as a constant rate infusion of 2 mL/kg/h for 10 h/d until the patient's serum albumin reached 2.0 g/dL. In this study, 75.6% of dogs and 72.3% of cats survived to discharge. Similarly, the prospective study by the same group documented the apparent safety of 10 to 20 mL/kg 5% human albumin to 40 critically ill cats to significantly increase serum albumin, with no evidence of immediate or delayed hypersensitivity reactions through 28 days after the infusion.

The exact cause of immediate and delayed hypersensitivity reactions remains unknown. Despite lack of anti-human antibodies in healthy dogs that received 25% HSA, immediate reactions occurred after administration of a very small amount of infusion, suggesting previous sensitivity.[29] Further healthy animals naïve to HSA infusion also showed that some cross-reactivity, suggesting possible exposure to other species albumin (bovine, equine, other) in food products or vaccinations may sensitize the immune system to xenotransfusions with albumin. The majority of critically ill dogs in the United States and Canada received 25% HSA undiluted or diluted to 10% as a rapid infusion or as a slower constant rate infusion, but still had immediate and delayed hypersensitivity reactions.[29,32,35,36,38,39,44] Two large-scale studies from the researchers in Italy, who diluted 25% HSA to 5% and administered the product as a slow infusion over 10 hours each day, documented no adverse effects. Only 1 study in the United States that diluted 25% HSA to 5% documented type III hypersensitivity reactions. It is possible that the total dose of HSA administered, and rate of administration could potentially stimulate immune stimulation compared with smaller doses over a longer period of time. It is also possible that food and vaccine products in the United States and Canada differ from those in Italy, or that the albumin product pooled from human plasma differs, making animals in geographic locations more or less susceptible to immune stimulation. Because many critically ill patients have compromised immune systems and are hypoalbuminemic at the time of albumin replenishment therapies, the antigenic effects of infusion of non–species-specific albumin may be blunted or delayed, but still occur in a small population of patients. Clearly, more research must be performed to determine the cause of antigenicity and subsequent reactions using HSA before its use is advocated in our veterinary patients. When no other sources of albumin are available, clients must be informed of the potential adverse reactions including death before the infusion of HSA to critically ill dogs and cats.

CLINICAL SIGNS OF TYPE I AND TYPE III HYPERSENSITIVITY REACTIONS AND TREATMENT

Clinical manifestations of type I and type III hypersensitivity reactions have been documented in several articles following infusion of HSA to healthy and critically ill dogs. Although the manifestation of new-onset facial edema, anaphylaxis, and collapse during infusion seems to be directly associated with an immediate hypersensitivity reaction, other possible signs of infusion reactions are not as clear-cut, but have been described as tachypnea, vomiting, hypotension, fever, shaking, weakness, or tachycardia during or shortly after infusion. Cats may also manifest with bradycardia and hypothermia when experiencing an infusion reaction. Because many of the animals who receive albumin were not responding to more traditional therapies, one could argue that some of the reported signs of reaction could possibly be associated with the critical illness, and not a hypersensitivity reaction at all. More compelling evidence of type III hypersensitivity reactions 6 to 18 days after infusion include the clinical signs of lethargy, inappetence, facial and peripheral edema, urticaria, and skin lesions consistent with vasculitis, joint effusion, lameness, scleral hemorrhage, and the more serious developments of acute kidney injury and proteinuria that can progress to oligoanuria and death.

The early recognition of clinical signs of a hypersensitivity reaction is important for aggressive therapy. If clinical signs of an immediate anaphylactic reaction develop, dexamethasone-SP (0.15 mg/kg IV) or diphenhydramine (1–2 mg/kg IM, IV) should be administered. If collapse and hypotension develop, epinephrine (0.01 mg/kg IV) should also be administered. The treatment of more delayed hypersensitivity reactions includes administration of a glucocorticoid (predniso[lo]ne 1 mg/kg/d × 5 days, then 0.5 mg/kg/d × 7 days, then 0.5 mg/kg/d every other day for 1 week) along with diphenhydramine (1–2 mg/kg by mouth every 8 hours) should be administered, along with supportive care in the form of antiemetics, gastroprotectants, analgesia, and appetite stimulants as indicated.

ALBUMIN PRODUCTS

Until roughly the past decade, albumin replacement in small animals was largely in the form of large volumes of fresh frozen plasma or with concentrated human albumin products.[34] A 2001 study demonstrated that the replacement of albumin was the primary cause for administration of fresh frozen plasma in 63% of cases.[45] Another retrospective study that evaluated trends in use of fresh frozen plasma over 2 decades reported the primary reason for administration of fresh frozen plasma was to treat coagulopathies.[46] Curiously, that same study demonstrated that, when fresh frozen plasma was administered to treat hypoalbuminemia, the mean serum albumin concentration significantly decreased (17.4 g/L after the administration of fresh frozen plasma vs 21.5 g/L before infusion) after fresh frozen plasma administration.[46]

A recent study that solicited on-line feedback from more than 1000 veterinary practitioners in 42 countries found that the use of crystalloids and natural or synthetic colloids for intravascular volume replacement and maintenance of COP varies, possibly owing to clinician preference, geographic location, and the availability of the product.[47] More than 75% of practitioners use synthetic colloids such as hydroxyethyl starch for oncotic support despite recent concerns about the potential for contributing to acute kidney injury.[47–49] The same study found that 46% of respondents still used fresh frozen plasma for oncotic support, and 23% to 28% of respondents used some form of human or canine albumin concentrate, when available. Similarly, another Internet survey of transfusion practices in veterinary teaching hospitals and private referral hospitals showed that approximately 30% to 45% of these practices kept some form of lyophilized albumin product on hand. Unfortunately, the proportions of human versus canine albumin was not reported nor was the frequency that these products were used.[50]

ALLOGENIC ALBUMIN ADMINISTRATION

Canine fresh frozen and stored plasma contains 25 to 30 g of albumin per liter.[38] Plasma may be beneficial because it contains coagulation factors, alpha-2 macroglobulin, antithrombin, and fibrinogen in addition to albumin30, however, up to 25 mL/kg of plasma may be required to increase serum albumin by 0.5 g/dL.[51] Because of the dilutional effects of such as large volume of plasma required, hospital resource availability, and cost limitations for some clients, the administration of plasma is not an efficient means of albumin supplementation for many patients. Lyophilized canine specific concentrated albumin pooled from healthy donors available for use in the United States and Canada from multiple manufacturers. The product can be stored at room temperature and is stable for 36 months. The manufacturers recommend reconstitution to 5% to 25% solution using 0.9% NaCl or 5% dextrose in water, then administered within 6 hours or stored refrigerated for up to 24 hours. The manufacturers' indications for this product are for hypoproteinemia and shock or hypovolemia. Safety studies performed by Animal Blood Resources International administered the canine albumin product to healthy beagle dogs once weekly for 4 consecutive weeks without any immediate or delayed signs of hypersensitivity reaction. A prospective study that evaluated the use of canine-specific albumin in dogs with septic peritonitis documented a significant increase in serum albumin concentration, COP, and systolic blood pressure after administration.[52] A higher serum albumin concentration was positively associated with survival. The study documented no immediate or delayed adverse reactions in patients who received the canine albumin product. Similarly, the administration of canine-specific albumin to healthy dogs, with repeat infusions on days 2 and 14, had no immediate or delayed reactions, and significantly increased both COP and serum albumin concentration.[53] A list of veterinary studies using human serum and canine-specific albumin is provided in **Table 1**.

Given the cost and potential lack of availability of canine-specific albumin products in some countries, other resources have also been investigated for the replenishment of albumin in critically ill animals. A prospective study that evaluated albumin concentration, COP, and coagulation factors in fresh frozen plasma with cryoprecipitate and cryopoor plasma from healthy greyhound donor dogs found that cryopoor plasma had significantly higher albumin and COP compared with FFP,[54] suggesting that cryopoor plasma may be a viable alternative to FFP or species-specific albumin concentrates, depending on availability. The same researchers have successfully used cryopoor plasma to increase serum albumin concentrations in critically ill hypoalbuminemic dogs.[54,55] Despite its successful use, the volume of cryopoor plasma required (median 31 mL/kg) to increase serum albumin and replace whole body albumin deficit is still large compared with albumin concentrate.[54]

An alternative method has been reported to purify canine albumin from FFP or surplus stored plasma.[56] Briefly, this method, which was adapted from a similar method used to convert human plasma to albumin,[57] involves adding a stabilizing agent to the plasma, heating the plasma in a water bath to denature all but the stabilized albumin, and then acidifying the plasma to precipitate the denatured proteins. The purified albumin can then be expressed into a satellite bag and pH neutralized. Through this process, a roughly 5% canine albumin solution with a purity of greater than 91% can be obtained. At this point, in vivo research is still needed to determine the effects of this product on severely ill dogs.

Treatment Recommendations

Albumin can be replenished in hypoalbuminemic animals with infusion of fresh frozen or stored plasma, cryopoor plasma, concentrated HSA, or canine-specific albumin. Although a number of studies have documented that serum albumin, total solids, and COP can be successfully increased with use of HSA in critically ill dogs, there is a real risk of inciting both immediate and delayed hypersensitivity reactions in dogs. The serum albumin concentration in some studies was higher in survivors versus nonsurvivors; however, this finding was not necessarily associated with HSA infusion. Whenever possible, treatment of the primary critical illness and provision of early enteral nutrition is an important component of therapy. In many patients, however, clinicians reach for an albumin concentrate when the more traditional methods of replenishment of total protein, albumin, and oncotic support with natural and synthetic colloids is failing. It seems that critical illness results in a delayed immune response after HSA infusion compared with healthy dogs; however, all critically ill dogs who received HSA developed IgG and IgE antibodies after exposure, which can lead to immediate or delayed hypersensitivity reactions. The administration of glucocorticoids at the time of HSA infusion does not seem to blunt or prevent the occurrence of a hypersensitivity reaction.[44] The severity of documented acute and delayed hypersensitivity reactions to HSA range from self-limiting with administration of glucocorticoids and diphenhydramine, to progressive leading to death in some patients. For this reason, if alternate specific-specific albumin sources are available, their use is preferable and recommended.

As a general guideline, the authors consider colloid support when a patient's albumin approaches 2.0 g/dL or less, and albumin supplementation when serum albumin

Table 1
List of current retrospective and prospective studies using various concentrations of concentrated human and canine albumin, effects, and adverse reactions

Author	Type of Study	Animals	Albumin Product	Dose	Administration Rate	Concentration	Outcome	Adverse Reactions
Cohn et al,[32] 2007	Prospective	9 healthy dogs	ZLB Bioplasma	50 g	0.5–4 mL/kg/h	25%	Increased [albumin] at 7, 14, and 21 d	1 dog anaphylaxis immediately, facial edema and urticaria 6 d later 1 dog urticaria, edema 7 d after first infusion 8/9 dogs positive intradermal skin test
Craft & Powell,[52] 2012	Prospective	7 critically ill dogs, septic peritonitis	Canine albumin	800 mg/kg		5%	Increased [albumin], COP and BP, no effect on survival 79% survival	No adverse reactions
Francis et al,[35] 2007	Prospective	6 healthy dogs	Plasbumin	500 mg/kg	1 h	25%		1 dog facial edema, vomiting within 15 min 2 dogs died
Vigano et al,[40] 2019	Prospective	40 critically ill cats	Uman human albumin	10–20 mL/kg	2 mL/kg/h × 10 h/d	5%	Increased [albumin]	No reactions through 28 d after infusion
Powell et al,[36] 2013	Retrospective	2 critically ill dogs	Plasbumin	1300 mg/kg	4 h	25% diluted to 5%		Lymphocytoclastic biopsies

(continued on next page)

Table 1
(continued)

Author	Type of Study	Animals	Albumin Product	Dose	Administration Rate	Concentration	Outcome	Adverse Reactions
Mosley & Mathews,[19] 2005	Prospective	8 healthy dogs 2 dogs second infusion	Bovine albumin	500 mg/kg 500 mg/kg				5/8 mild to generalized signs type III hypersensitivity 15 d after infusion Immediate urticaria and pruritus in 1 dog, anaphylaxis in second dog
Martin et al,[29] 2008	Prospective	2 healthy dogs 14 critically ill dogs	Plasbumin	500 mg/kg 250 mg/kg 1300 mg/kg	2 h 1 h 0.8 mL/kg/h	25% 25% 25%		Decreased appetite, facial edema 8 d after albumin Increased anti-albumin IgG at 10 d after albumin, peak at 3–9 wk after infusion No acute or delayed reactions Increased anti-albumin IgG antibodies 4–6 wk after infusion

Study	Type	Population	Product	Dose	Rate	%	Outcome	Adverse reactions
Trow et al,[39] 2008	Retrospective	73 critically ill dogs	Baxter product	1400 mg/kg			Increased [albumin], TP	Increased [albumin] and TP
Vigano et al,[34] 2010	Retrospective	Critically ill dogs (418) and cats (170)	Albital	2 mL/kg/h × 10 h/d	5%	75.6% survival (dogs, 72.3% survival) (cats)	No hypersensitivity reactions observed or reported. 3 dogs lethargy, edema, urticaria, lameness, vomiting and inappetence 6–18 d after discharge
Mathews & Barry,[38] 2005	Retrospective	Critically ill dogs (n = 64) and cats (n = 2)	Plasbumin	2–4 mL/kg bolus or 0.1–1.7 mL/kg/h	25%	Increased [albumin], TS and BP 71% survival	2 dogs facial edema during infusion
Horowitz et al,[43] 2015	Retrospective	22 dogs septic peritonitis	Human	2550 mg/kg	25%	Increased [albumin], TP	No association between albumin administration and survival
Loyd et al,[44] 2016	Retrospective	21 dogs protein losing enteropathy	Human, Octapharma	500 mg/kg	20–30 min	1 dog with acute reaction euthanized 1 dog with delayed reaction euthanized	9.5% developed signs associated with acute reaction (vomiting or labored breathing). 9.5% developed signs of delayed reaction. Corticosteroids had no effect on occurrence of signs

(continued on next page)

Table 1
(continued)

Author	Type of Study	Animals	Albumin Product	Dose	Administration Rate	Concentration	Outcome	Adverse Reactions
Klainbart & Aroch,[41] 2005	Retrospective	8 dogs, 3 cats	Human		2 mL/kg, then 0.2–0.7 mL/kg/h	25%	Increase albumin in 3 dogs; 3 dogs survived, 5 dogs and 8 cats died	
Bell et al,[42] 2004	Retrospective	4 dogs, 1 cat	20% human, ALBA 20%		0.14–0.25 mL/kg/h, 5 mL/kg/h 1 dog hypovolemic shock	20%	Increased [albumin] from baseline, 3 dogs survived to discharge	
Enders et al,[53] 2018	Prospective	6 healthy dogs	Hemosolutions, canine albumin		1 g/kg over 2 h on days 0, 2, and 14	16%	Increased [albumin] and COP	

Abbreviation: BP, blood pressure.
Data from Refs. [19,29,32,34-36,38-44,52,53] .

is less than 1.5 g/dL. Albumin should be supplemented up to a goal of 2.0 g/dL, with additional colloidal support in the form of other natural or synthetic colloids. Any albumin administered will first replenish the interstitial albumin pool before serum albumin concentrations increase, making arbitrary administration of products challenging to meet goals and to alleviate clinical signs of peripheral edema, cavitary effusions and enteral feeding intolerance. As a general guideline, the following formula can be used to calculate an albumin deficit[4]:

Dose albumin (g) = 10 × (2.0 g/dL – patient albumin g/dL) × body weight in kg × 0.3.

As a general goal, a dose of 450 mg/kg canine albumin will increase the serum albumin by 0.5 g/dL.

If plasma products, rather than albumin concentrate are to be used, a clinician can use the following formula to help increase total solids, taking into consideration that albumin contributes roughly 50% of total solids:

mL of plasma to increase recipient TS (total solids) = desired recipient TS g/dL – recipient TS g/dL × weight (kg) × 50/donor TS g/dL.

Like other transfusions, the infusion of albumin products should be started slowly with careful monitoring for clinical signs of reaction. The canine albumin product should be reconstituted to a dilution of 5% according to manufacturer's recommendations, then initially administered at a rate of 1 to 2 mL/kg. If after 20 to 30 minutes no clinical signs of adverse reaction occur, the volume can be increased to administer a total dose over 3 to 4 hours. If volume expansion in addition to correction of hypoalbuminemia is needed, then the canine albumin product can be reconstituted with sterile water to a dilution of 10% to 16% according to manufacturer's recommendations. Then the reconstituted product can be administered through a dedicated central venous catheter initially at 0.5 to 1 mL/kg. If after 20 to 30 minutes no clinical signs of adverse reaction occur, the volume can be increased to administer the total dose over 3 to 4 hours.

SUMMARY

Albumin's functions are numerous and important for a wide variety of normal body functions. In critically ill small animal patients, hypoalbuminemia is associated with adverse consequences, including increased patient morbidity and mortality. Replenishment of albumin is recommended in hypoalbuminemic animals; however, cases must be selected carefully. The availability of albumin product, cost, volume required for infusion, and potential risk of immediate and delayed hypersensitivity reactions should be considered when choosing the method of albumin supplementation. The evidence to date indicates that species specific albumin should be considered the product of choice for correction of hypoalbuminemic patients. If plasma products or species specific albumin is not available, HSA can be considered if the risk to benefit ratio is low and provided that clients are informed of potential adverse sequelae that could occur after administration.

DISCLOSURE

The views expressed in this article are those of the authors and do not reflect the official policy or position of the US Army Medical Department, Departments of the Army, the Department of Defense, or the US Government.

REFERENCES

1. Mazzaferro EM, Rudloff E, Kirby R. The role of albumin replacement in the critically ill veterinary patient. J Vet Emerg Crit Care (San Antonio) 2002;12(2): 113–24.
2. Nicholson JP, Wolmarans MR, Park GR. The role of albumin in critical illness. Br J Anaesth 2000;85(4):599–610.
3. D'Angio RG. Is there a role for albumin in nutrition support. Ann Pharmacother 1994;28(4):478–82.
4. Conner BJ. Treating Hypoalbuminemia. Vet Clin North Am Small Anim 2017;47: 451–9.
5. Weinkle TK, Center SA, Randolph JF, et al. Evaluation of prognostic factors, survival rates and treatment protocols for immune-mediated hemolytic anemia in dogs:151 cases. J Am Vet Med Assoc 2005;226:1869–80.
6. Comazzi S, Pieralisi C, Bertazzolo W. Haematological and biochemical abnormalities in canine blood: frequency and associations in 1022 samples. J Small Anim Pract 2004;45:343–9.
7. O'Leary MJ, Koll M, Ferguson CN, et al. Liver albumin synthesis in sepsis in the rat: influence of parenteral nutrition, glutamine and growth hormone. Clin Sci (Lond) 2003;105(6):691–8.
8. Mathews KA. The therapeutic use of 25% human serum albumin in critically ill dogs and cats. Vet Clin North Am Small Anim 2008;38:595–605.
9. Chang CC, Lan YT, Joang JK, et al. Risk factors for delayed perineal wound healing and its impact on prolonged hospital stay after abdominoperineal resection. World J Surg Oncol 2019;17(1):226.
10. Ikenoue N, Saitu Y, Shimoda M, et al. Disease induced alterations in plasma drug-binding proteins and their influence on drug binding percentages in dogs. Vet Q 2000;22:43–9.
11. Ralphs SC, Jessen CR, Lipowitz AJ. Risk factors for leakage following intestinal anastomosis in dogs and cats: 115 cases (1991-2000). J Am Vet Med Assoc 2003;223(1):73–7.
12. Weil MH, Henning RJ, Puri VK. Colloid oncotic pressure: clinical significance. Crit Care Med 1979;7(3):113–6.
13. Foley EF, Borlase BC, Dzik WH, et al. Albumin supplementation in the critically ill. Arch Surg 1990;125(6):739–42.
14. Iseki K, Kawazoe N, Fukiyama K. Serum albumin is a strong predictor of death in chronic dialysis patients. Kidney Int 1993;44(1):115–9.
15. McEllistrum MC, Collins JC, Powers JS. Admission serum albumin level as a predictor of outcome among geriatric patients. South Med J 1993;86(12):1360–1.
16. Law MR, Morris JK, Wald NJ, et al. Serum albumin and mortality in the BUPA study. Int J Epidemiol 1994;23(1):38–41.
17. Guyton AC, Hall JE. The microcirculation and the lymphatic system, . Textbook of medical physiology. 9th edition. Philadelphia: WB Saunders Company; 1996. p. 170.
18. Doweiko JP, Nompleggi DJ. Use of albumin as a volume expander. JPEN J Parenter Enteral Nutr 1991;15(4):484–7.
19. Mosley CAE, Mathews KA. The use of concentrated bovine serum albumin in canines. Veterinary Anaesthesia and Analgesia 2005;32:1–19.
20. Vincent JL, Dubois MJ, Navickis RJ, et al. Hypoalbuminemia in acute illness: is there a rationale for intervention? A meta-analysis of cohort studies and controlled trials. Ann Surg 2003;237(3):319–34.

21. Cochrane Injuries Group Albumin Reviewers. Human albumin administration in critically ill patients: systematic review of randomized controlled trials. BMJ 1998;317:235–40.
22. Roberts I, Edwards P, McLelland B. More on albumin. Use of human albumin in UK fell substantially when systematic review was published. BMJ 1999; 318(7192):1214–5.
23. The SAFE Study Investigators. A comparison of albumin and saline for fluid resuscitation in the intensive care unit. N Engl J Med 2004;350:2247–56.
24. Delaney AP, Dan A, McCaffrey J, et al. The role of albumin as a resuscitation fluid for patients with sepsis: a systematic review and meta-analysis. Crit Care Med 2011;39(2):386–91.
25. Rhodes A, Evans LE, Alhazzani W, et al. Surviving sepsis campaign: international guidelines for management of sepsis and septic shock: 2016. Crit Care Med 2017;45(3):486–552.
26. Throop JL, Bingaman S, Huxley V. Differences between human and other mammalian albumins raises concerns over the use of human serum albumin in the dog. J Vet Intern Med 2004;18(3):439.
27. Throop JL, Kerl ME, Cohn LA. Albumin in health and disease: causes and treatment of hypoalbuminemia. Comp Contin Educ Pract Vet 2004;26(12):940–9.
28. Throop JL, Kerl ME, Cohn LA. Albumin in health and disease: protein metabolism and function. Comp Contin Educ Pract Vet 2004;26(12):932–9.
29. Martin LG, Luther TY, Alperin DC, et al. Serum antibodies against human albumin in critically ill and healthy dogs. J Am Vet Med Assoc 2008;232(7):1004–9.
30. Wong C, Koenig A. The colloid controversy – are colloids bad and what are the options? Vet Clin North Am Small Anim 2017;47:411–21.
31. Costa AP, Court MH, Burke NS, et al. Canine albumin polymorphisms and their impact on drug plasma protein binding. Drug Metab Dispos 2019;47:1024–31.
32. Cohn LA, Kerl ME, Lenox CE, et al. Response of healthy dogs to infusions of human serum albumin. Am J Vet Res 2007;68(6):657–63.
33. Adamantos S, Chan DL, Goggs R, et al. Risk of immunologic reactions to human serum albumin solutions. J Small Anim Pract 2009;50(4):206.
34. Vigano F, Perissinotto L, Bosco VRF. Administration of 5% human serum albumin in critically ill small animal patients with hypoalbuminemia: 418 dogs and 170 cats (1994-2008). J Vet Emerg Crit Care (San Antonio) 2010;20(2):237–43.
35. Francis AH, Martin LG, Haldorson GJ, et al. Adverse reactions suggestive of Type III hypersensitivity in six healthy dogs given human albumin. J Am Vet Med Assoc 2007;230(6):873–9.
36. Powell C, Thompson L, Murtaugh R. Type III hypersensitivity reaction with immune complex deposition in 2 critically ill dogs administered human serum albumin. J Vet Emerg Crit Care (San Antonio) 2013;23(6):598–604.
37. Mazzaferro EM, Balakrishnan A, Hackner SG, et al. Delayed Type-III hypersensitivity reaction with acute kidney injury in two dogs following administration of concentrated human albumin during treatment of hypoalbuminemia secondary to septic peritonitis. J Vet Emerg Crit Care (San Antonio) 2020 [Online ahead of print].
38. Mathews KA, Barry M. The use of 25% human serum albumin: outcome and efficacy in raising serum albumin and systemic blood pressure in critically ill dogs and cats. J Vet Emerg Crit Care (San Antonio) 2005;15(2):110–8.
39. Trow AV, Rozanski EA, delaforcade AM, et al. Evaluation of use of human albumin in critically ill dogs: 73 cases (2003-2006). J Am Vet Med Assoc 2008;233(4):607–12.

40. Vigano F, Blasi C, Carminato N, et al. Prospective review of clinical hypersensitivity reactions after administration of 5% human serum albumin in 40 critically ill cats. Top Companion Anim Med 2019;35:38–41.

41. Klainbart S, Aroch I. Use of albumin in critically ill dogs and cats. J Vet Emerg Crit Care (San Antonio) 2005;15(S1):S15.

42. Bell R, Tebb A, Knottenbelt C, et al. The use of human albumin transfusions in a veterinary critical care facility. J Vet Intern Med 2004;18(5):786.

43. Horowitz FB, Read RL, Powell LL. A retrospective analysis of 25% human serum albumin supplementation in hypoalbuminemic dogs with septic peritonitis. Can Vet J 2015;56:591–7.

44. Loyd KA, Cocayne CG, Cridland JM, et al. Retrospective evaluation of the administration of 25% human albumin to dogs with protein-losing enteropathy: 21 cases (2003-2013). J Vet Emerg Crit Care (San Antonio) 2016; 26(4):587–92.

45. Logan JC, Callan MB, Drew K, et al. Clinical indication for use of fresh frozen plasma in dogs: 74 dogs (October through December 1999). J Am Vet Med Assoc 2001;218(9):1449–55.

46. Snow SJ, Jutkowitz A, Brown AJ. Trends in plasma transfusion at a veterinary teaching hospital: 308 patients (1996-1998 and 2006 -2008). J Vet Emerg Crit Care (San Antonio) 2010;20(40):441–5.

47. Yozova ID, Howard J, Sigrist NE, et al. Current trends in volume replacement therapy and the use of synthetic colloids in small animals – an internet based survey (2016). Front Vet Sci 2016;4(140):1–12.

48. Hayes G, Benedicenti L, Mathews K. Retrospective cohort study on the incidence of acute kidney injury and death following hydroxyethyl starch (HES 10% 250/0.5/ 5:1) administration in dogs (2007-2010). J Vet Emerg Crit Care (San Antonio) 2016;26:35–40.

49. Sigrist NE, Kalin N, Dreyfus A. Changes in serum creatinine concentration and acute kidney injury (AKI) grade in dogs treated with hydroxyethyl starch 130/ 0.4 from 2013 to 2015. J Vet Intern Med 2017;31(2):434–41.

50. Jagodich TA, Holowaychuk MK. Transfusion practice in dogs and cats: an internet-based survey. J Vet Emerg Crit Care (San Antonio) 2016;26(3): 360–72.

51. Culler CA, Iazbik C, Guillaumin J. Comparison of albumin, colloid osmotic pressure, von Willebrand factor, and coagulation factors in canine cryopoor plasma, cryoprecipitate, and fresh frozen plasma. J Vet Emerg Crit Care (San Antonio) 2017;27(6):638–44.

52. Craft EM, Powell LL. The use of canine-specific albumin in dogs with septic peritonitis. J Vet Emerg Crit Care (San Antonio) 2012;22(6):631–9.

53. Enders B, Musulin S, Holowaychuk M, et al. Repeated infusion of lyophilized canine albumin safely and effectively increases serum albumin and colloid osmotic pressure in healthy dogs. J Vet Emerg Crit Care (San Antonio) 2018; 28(S1):S5.

54. Culler CA, Balakrishnan A, Yaxley PE, et al. Clinical use of cryopoor plasma continuous rate infusion in critically ill, hypoalbuminemic dogs. J Vet Emerg Crit Care (San Antonio) 2019;29:314–20.

55. Ropski MK, Guillaumin J, Monnig AA, et al. Use of cryopoor plasma for albumin replacement and continuous antimicrobial infusion for septic peritonitis. J Vet Emerg Crit Care (San Antonio) 2017;27(3):348–56.

56. Edwards TH, Koenig A, Thomas L, et al. Preparation of purified canine albumin by heat denaturation of stored plasma. J Vet Emerg Crit Care (San Antonio) 2017; 27(S1):S2.

57. Aghaie A, Khorsand Mohammed Pour H, Banazadeh S. Preparation of albumin from human plasma by heat denaturation method in plasma bag. Transfus Med 2012;22(6):44–445.

Update on Canine Parvoviral Enteritis

Elisa M. Mazzaferro, MS, DVM, PhD[a,b,*]

KEYWORDS

- Parvovirus • Enteritis • Fluid therapy • Outbreak • Outpatient therapy

KEY POINTS

- Canine parvoviral enteritis remains one of the most virulent and common enteric diseases of dogs worldwide.
- Canine parvovirus is endemic in many environments and can be carried by nonaffected hosts, contributing to spread of disease to domestic animals.
- Vaccination for canine parvovirus can effectively induce protective immunity in most dogs; however, vaccinations administered too early can interfere with maternal antibodies and result in a puppy being more susceptible to infection.
- Treatment currently involves administration of fluid to replenish hydration, early nutritional support, antiemetics, broad-spectrum antibiotics, and empiric deworming. Although inpatient therapy remains the gold standard, outpatient therapy protocols have been documented to have success rates of more than 80% survival.

PARVOVIRAL ENTERITIS

Introduction

Canine parvoviral enteritis is one of the most common causes of morbidity and mortality in young dogs worldwide.[1] Canine parvovirus belongs to the genus Protoparvovirus, family Parvoviridae, a single-stranded DNA virus that infects rapidly dividing cells of the gastrointestinal tract, bone marrow, lymphoid tissue, and cardiac myocytes.[2] The origin of canine parvovirus remains unknown. Because canine parvovirus (CPV) shares 98% structural homology with feline panleukopenia virus,[3] 1 theory is that CPV may have resulted from a genetic variant that later became capable of infecting dogs.[4] Because the family Parvoviridae is found in other wild mammals, including wild mink, genetic variation from other wildlife[5] may have also played a role in the evolution of CPV-1 and CPV-2.[6,7]

CPV-1, also known as minute virus of canines, was first discovered in the late 1960s as a cause of gastrointestinal and respiratory infection of dogs.[8] One decade later,

[a] Cornell University Veterinary Specialists, 880 Canal Street, Stamford, CT 06902, USA;
[b] Emergency and Critical Care, Cornell University Hospital for Animals, Ithaca, NY, USA
* Cornell University Veterinary Specialists, 880 Canal Street, Stamford, CT 06902.
E-mail address: emazzaferro@cuvs.org

Vet Clin Small Anim 50 (2020) 1307–1325
https://doi.org/10.1016/j.cvsm.2020.07.008
0195-5616/20/© 2020 Elsevier Inc. All rights reserved.

mutation of CPV-1 resulted in a distinctly different variant, CPV-2, and caused the first pandemic outbreak in both adult and young dogs previously naive to CPV.[8] Since the first isolation of CPV-1 and CPV-2, genetic drift during the 1980s has resulted in 2 variants (CPV-2a and CPV-2b), followed by a third variant (CPV-2c) more recently recognized since early 2000. Since the first emergence of CPV-2c in Italy, this isolate has spread worldwide.[9] Despite development and administration of vaccination against CPV-2 strains, the disease is still one of considerable veterinary and economic importance.

PATHOPHYSIOLOGY

CPV-2 strains are exquisitely robust in their strategies for infection in that they can infect mammalian hosts other than domestic dogs (raccoon, cat, coyote, wolves), are ubiquitous in the environment, and can remain viable for more than 1 year under favorable conditions.[1,10] Oronasal exposure and infection occurs in naive or poorly immunized dogs by ingestion of CPV-2 shed in the vomitus or feces of infected animals. The virus then replicates first in oropharyngeal and mesenteric lymph nodes and thymus, with infected animals becoming viremic within 1 to 5 days of exposure.[2] Next, CPV-2 targets rapidly dividing cells of the intestinal epithelial crypts, bone marrow, epithelium of the tongue, oral cavity, and cardiac myocytes, in addition to lung, spleen, liver, and kidneys.[11] Before widespread vaccination of dogs against CPV-2, myocarditis was a common cause of death in infected animals and can still rarely occur today.[11–13] Following exposure and an incubation period that can range from 4 to 14 days, virus shedding usually precedes the onset of clinical signs of vomiting and hemorrhagic diarrhea by several days.[14–16] The intestinal lining becomes denuded as enterocyte turnover is disrupted, resulting in blunting of the intestinal villi, which causes the clinical signs of vomiting and hemorrhagic diarrhea in addition to nutrient malabsorption and enteric bacterial translocation. Viral infection in the thymus results in destruction and collapse of thymic cortex. Along with destruction of leukocyte precursors in the bone marrow, this finding results in significant leukopenia in infected animals.[17,18] The lack of immunity, combined with bacteremia from translocation of gut bacteria, puts affected animals at high risk of developing septic shock, systemic inflammatory response syndrome, multiorgan failure, and death if left untreated.

Rare findings of erythema multiforme,[19] leukoencephalopathy,[20] and porencephaly with periventricular encephalitis[21] in puppies, as well as clinical disease and intracranial abscesses in cats,[22–24] infected with CPV-2 have been documented.

DIAGNOSTIC TESTING

Within 3 days of infection with CPV-2, animals can shed virus in their feces,[25] with peak shedding occurring 4 to 7 days after infection.[26] Accurate detection of viral shedding and infection is paramount to helping decrease spread of disease in veterinary hospitals, shelters, and breeding kennels by isolating infectious animals, because clinical signs are similar in dogs that test positive or negative by fecal enzyme-linked immunoabsorbent assay (ELISA) methodology.[18,27] Methodology to detect CPV-2 infection must therefore be widely accessible and accurate.

Antemortem, CPV-2 can be detected in feces, oropharyngeal swab, or whole blood.[15,28,29] Definitive diagnosis depends on the detection of virus particles in feces or from oropharyngeal swabs using a variety of detection methods that include ELISA, polymerase chain reaction (PCR), electron microscopy, hemagglutination, and virus isolation.[30,31] At this time, DNA-based PCR methods for virus detection are considered the most sensitive and specific but are not immediately available in the clinical setting.[31] Other methods, such as electron microscopy, hemagglutination, and virus isolation, are only available on a limited basis in specialized laboratories and are not as sensitive as more readily available cage-side ELISA or PCR methods.[31]

The most common method for initial screening and detection of canine parvovirus is the use of a cage-side, in-clinic immunochromatographic ELISA that has a high degree of sensitivity but intermediate to low specificity, compared with molecular methods such as PCR.[18] One study that compared PCR-positive CPV-2a, CPV-2b, and CPV-2c showed that a commonly used cage-side ELISA detected virus only 80.4%, 78.0%, and 77.0% for CPV 2a, CPV-2b, and CPV-2c, respectively.[32] Another study that compared the sensitivity and specificity of cage-side ELISA with PCR found a sensitivity of 81.8%.[30] The sensitivity of detection of both CPV-2b and CPV-2c was not statistically different, indicating that the cage-side ELISA, in addition to PCR, can detect the CPV-2c strain. The sensitivity and specificity of a second cage-side ELISA[2] compared with hemagglutination and PCR determine a sensitivity of 86.3% for ELISA and 65.3% for hemagglutination compared with PCR (100% sensitivity) for all CPV-2 strains.[31] A third cage-side ELISA test[3] was compared with PCR, and again showed lower sensitivity (76.5%) that seemed to decrease with storage time, but high specificity.[33] For all ELISA-positive animals with clinical signs of infection, the high specificity indicates that the animals should be considered true positive for means of isolation from other animals. Recent vaccination with modified live virus can result in false-positive results within 10 days; however, in puppies with clinical signs of vomiting and diarrhea who have been recently vaccinated, most cases are from true infection with field CPV strain or other gastrointestinal infection, rather than the vaccine itself.[34]

There are many reasons that fecal ELISA testing can be falsely negative. Investigation of fecal CPV viral load, serum antibody titers, and time of clinical signs to testing were compared, and dogs that had false-negative fecal ELISA characteristically were presented for evaluation earlier in the course of illness, had lower fecal virus loads, and had decreased frequency of defecation and higher serum antibody titers compared with dogs that tested CPV positive by fecal ELISA.[27] Fecal samples must contain a minimum of 10^6 copies of DNA per milligram of feces to test positive by ELISA methods.[31] CPV antibodies within the gastrointestinal tract can sequester virus particles and make them unavailable for detection by ELISA.[35–37] Fecal testing for parvovirus is warranted in any puppy with clinical signs of vomiting and diarrhea. If an animal tests negative by fecal ELISA and there is concern for infection of other animals in breeding kennels or shelters, additional testing by PCR should be considered.

CLINICAL SIGNS AND ADDITIONAL DIAGNOSTIC TESTING

In addition to fecal testing, physical examination findings, patient signalment, and clinician index of suspicion and other diagnostic testing can be supportive of but not pathognomonic for CPV infection. The most common clinical signs of parvoviral enteritis are lethargy, inappetence, vomiting, and diarrhea. The diarrhea can vary in appearance from soft to mucoid to liquid and hemorrhagic. Sloughing of the intestinal mucosal lining can give a red gelatinous appearance to the feces. With gastrointestinal fluid losses, interstitial dehydration that progresses to hypovolemic shock can occur quickly. Lack of enterocyte nutrient absorption, systemic bacteremia, and lack of sufficient hepatic and muscle glycogen stores also can result in significant hypoglycemia with neuroglycopenia and seizures. In addition, systemic inflammation and bacteremia can result in septic shock with hypotension and organ failure.

The severity of clinical signs can vary with age, protective antibody titer, and duration of illness. The diagnostic accuracy of using clinical signs and physical examination alone to make a presumptive diagnose of parvovirus is only 58%. The index of suspicion can increase based on an individual patient's age and vaccination status. In addition to the clinical signs listed earlier, physical examination can reveal mucosal pallor, delayed capillary refill time, fever or hypothermia, and abdominal discomfort. Small intestinal intussusception can occur and create a painful, firm, tubular soft tissue mass effect found on abdominal palpation.[38,39] The presence and severity of clinical signs can be predictive of the length of time required in hospital.[40]

COMPLETE BLOOD COUNT

Total white blood cell count and the presence of leukoneutropenia have previously been considered to be a hallmark in patients with CPV because the virus attacks actively replicating cells of the bone marrow, thymus, and other lymphoid tissues. Lymphopenia can occur in puppies infected with CPV as well as puppies affected with canine coronavirus,[41] so is used along with other testing to further support a diagnosis of CPV in affected patients. The presence of cytopenia during the course of illness can be useful for predicting outcome in CPV. One study documented no significant difference in neutropenia between survivors and nonsurvivors with CPV.[42] The same study found that maintenance of total leukocyte count greater than 4500/μL and a lymphocyte count greater than 1000/μL at the time of admission and through 48 hours of hospitalization were strongly predictive of survival.[42]

DIAGNOSTIC IMAGING

Diagnostic imaging is largely nonspecific for animals afflicted with CPV. Early in the course of illness, abdominal radiographs may appear normal, then develop radiographic signs of ileus with gas or fluid distension of the small intestine.[43] Findings of abdominal ultrasonography in 40 puppies with confirmed CPV infection were nonspecific, with signs of gas and fluid distension of all areas of the stomach and the small and large intestine, ileus with ineffective peristalsis, anechoic peritoneal effusion, in addition to a corrugated appearance to the duodenum with hyperechoic speckling.[44] However, ultrasonography is useful to rule out other causes of vomiting and diarrhea, such as gastrointestinal foreign body, obstruction, or intussusception, in animals with intractable discomfort or severe vomiting despite administration of antiemetic drugs. The degree of ultrasonographic abnormalities is positively correlated with the severity of illness in dogs with CPV.[44]

ENDOCRINE AND OTHER BIOMARKERS IN CANINE PARVOVIRUS INFECTION

Other researchers have investigated a variety of clinicopathologic biomarkers in dogs infected with CPV. As observed with other critical illnesses, animals infected with CPV have augmented stress response and cortisol concentrations and develop euthyroid sick syndrome, which can be predictive of mortality at 24 and 48 hours of hospitalization.[45,46] In naturally occurring infection, endogenous canine granulocyte colony-stimulating factor (G-CSF) levels have been found to be increased during the period of time that the animal is neutropenic.[47] This finding was extrapolated to consideration for use of G-CSF as a treatment of neutropenia in affected animals and is discussed later. Serum magnesium levels are often decreased, as is found in other critical illness in dogs; however, this finding is not correlated with disease outcome.[48] C-reactive protein,[49,50] total cholesterol, high-density lipoprotein, serum triglyceride,[51] lipid peroxidase, zinc,[52] pancreatic lipase, and plasma citrulline levels[53–55] have also been documented to change in response to CPV infection. The tests are not useful alone in predicting morbidity or mortality and are not easily available as cage-side tests; however, they may be predictive of the severity of infection.[45,49,50] In addition, the presence of inflammatory biomarkers as well as vascular endothelial damage, systemic inflammation, activation of coagulation, along with hypovolemia often predispose patients to a hypercoagulable state.[56] This possibility can be a factor in maintenance of intravenous (IV) catheters and the development of thrombophlebitis as well as contributing to end-organ damage in the most severe cases.

TREATMENT

Treatment of parvoviral enteritis largely is supportive until clinical signs of vomiting and diarrhea resolve. In general, improvement in clinical signs often correspond with rebound in leukocyte count; however, development of adverse sequelae such as aspiration pneumonia, ongoing hypoglycemia, hypoalbuminemia with edema, or intussusception can result in higher morbidity and increased length of hospitalization. One of the primary challenges and limiting factors for client owners in the treatment of parvovirus is the cost of hospitalization and treatment. Clusters of cases of parvovirus have been documented in socioeconomic underprivileged areas,[57–59] highlighting perhaps a lack of education and financial opportunity for vaccination, making these puppies at higher risk of contracting the disease. The decision whether to admit an affected animal to the hospital to receive gold-standard versus outpatient therapy or euthanasia is largely based on the client's ability and willingness to pay for the cost of care.

VASCULAR ACCESS AND FLUID THERAPY

The most aggressive therapy that involves administration of IV fluids to restore intravascular fluid volume status, replenish interstitial fluid losses, and maintain hydration is the gold standard of care for treatment of CPV. Ancillary therapies that minimize fluid loss in the form of antiemetics and gastroprotectant agents, provide analgesia and nutrition, and prevent secondary bacterial infection with antibiotics also are important factors for the best patient outcome. The mainstay of fluid therapy first involves establishing vascular access. In the most hypovolemic or interstitially dehydrated patients, this can sometimes be challenging, and may require placement of an intraosseous catheter or vascular cutdown. Because of the high risk of contamination of a catheter with vomitus and feces, placement of a jugular catheter is preferred. Jugular catheter placement not only provides a means of administration of IV fluids but can also allow for blood sample collection for glucose, acid-base, and electrolyte monitoring without the need for repeated percutaneous venipuncture. In the most hypovolemic patients, intraosseous access can be quicker with the same degree of success of jugular catheter placement,[60] and should be considered in the interest of time to start volume resuscitation strategies. When necessary, any fluid that can be administered intravenously can also be administered through an intraosseous catheter.[61,62]

Once vascular access is achieved, a balanced isotonic crystalloid fluid should be administered. The initial volume and rate of fluid administration largely depend on the degree of interstitial dehydration and whether hypovolemia is present. If a patient is showing clinical signs of hypovolemia (tachycardia or bradycardia, hypothermia, delayed capillary refill time, hypotension), IV fluid should be administered in incremental boluses (20 mL/kg) as quickly as possible while monitoring the perfusion parameters discussed earlier for normalization.

Once intravascular volume status has been restored, interstitial fluid losses can then be replenished. Despite some veterinarians' practice of multiplying a patient's maintenance fluid requirements by an arbitrary factor of 1.5 or 2 to replace interstitial fluid deficits, this practice often underestimates the needs of individual patients, particularly when ongoing losses are present. A more accurate and recommended approach is to calculate the patient's interstitial hydration deficit and replace that over the next 12 to 24 hours, taking care to also consider the maintenance fluid requirements and ongoing losses. A simple method of monitoring fluid loss is to weigh the patient frequently, because 1 g of body weight is equal to 1 mL of fluid lost. Once intravascular and interstitial volume have been restored, ongoing fluid gain or loss is equal to the patient's body weight, provided that third spacing of fluid is not occurring.

In addition to provision of fluid, crystalloid fluids can be used to help restore acid-base and electrolyte derangements observed in patients with CPV enteritis. Although most patients have normal acid-base status, the degree of hydrochloric acid loss in the vomitus can cause a hypochloremic metabolic alkalosis to develop.[34] Potassium[63] can be supplemented based on the individual patient's serum potassium concentration.[64] Hypoglycemia is common. Serum glucose concentration should be monitored frequently and supplemented as needed. If serum glucose level decreases to less than 60 mg/dL, administration of an IV (or intraosseous) dextrose (VetOne Dextrose 50%, Nova-Tech, Inc., Grand Island, NE) bolus (1–2 mL/kg 25% dextrose) should be administered, followed by addition of 2.5% to 5% dextrose in the crystalloid fluids.

ONCOTIC SUPPORT

Fluid loss in diarrheic feces, along with lack of enteral intake of nutrients and production of acute phase proteins in preference to albumin synthesis, all can result in significant hypoproteinemia in patients with CPV enteritis. The decision to provide oncotic support in the form of either natural or synthetic colloids usually depends on clinician preference, product availability, and patient size and need. Patient morbidity and mortality can increase when serum albumin concentration decreases to less than 2.0 g/dL.[65] Albumin also contributes to free radical scavenging and drug transport, making albumin replacement essential in puppies with CPV. Albumin can be restored by administration of either fresh or fresh-frozen plasma or concentrated albumin products. Roughly 20 mL/kg of plasma must be administered to increase serum albumin concentration by 0.5 g/dL. Anecdotal reports suggest that administration of fresh-frozen plasma (6.6–11 mL/kg IV or intraperitoneal, 3 doses administered 12 hours apart) may be prophylactic at preventing severe infection in exposed dogs.[66] Canine-specific albumin concentrate (Virbagen Omega, feline omega-interferon, Virbac Animal Health, Carros, France) is also available for administration and is a cost-effective method of restoring serum albumin without significant risk of immune stimulation observed with administration of concentrated human albumin products.[67–69] If further oncotic support is required, hydroxyethyl starch (20–30 mL/kg/d) can be administered, depending on clinician preference.

ANTIEMETICS

In addition to fluid therapy and enteral nutrition, the use of antiemetics is important in decreasing vomiting in patients with CPV. One prospective study that investigated antiemetic use in puppies with CPV enteritis documented an increased length of hospital stay in patients who did not receive antiemetics.[70] A randomized, prospective study that compared the use of metoclopramide (0.5 mg/kg IV every 8 hours), ondansetron (0.5 mg/kg IV every 8 hours), and maropitant (1 mg/kg subcutaneously every 24 hours) showed that all antiemetics were equally successful at reducing the number of vomiting events.[71] In contrast with the first study,[70] the second study[71] documented that the use of antiemetics decreased the number of vomiting events on day 1 and from day 3 onward. Another study[72] showed no difference in the duration of hospitalization, need for rescue antiemetics, duration of vomiting, or days to voluntary food consumption in puppies with CPV treated with ondansetron (0.5 mg/kg IV every 8 hours) or maropitant (1 mg/kg IV every 24 hours).

ANTIMICROBIAL USE

Patients with CPV enteritis are at high risk of bacterial translocation from intestinal villous collapse and lack of protective immune function. A variety of bacteria (*Escherichia coli, Clostridium difficile, Salmonella* spp) have been documented in septic patients with CPV enteritis.[73–77] Broad-spectrum antibiotics are recommended in all CPV-affected patients (**Table 1**). Ongoing fluid losses from vomiting and diarrhea, combined with the potential for hypotension and sepsis, make dogs with CPV enteritis at high risk of developing acute kidney injury (AKI). A study that investigated routine use of blood urea nitrogen (BUN), creatinine, urine specific gravity (SpGr), and urine protein/creatinine ratio (UPC) in dogs with CPV enteritis showed no change in BUN and creatinine; however, UPC and SpGr were higher compared with healthy controls. Other biomarkers of glomerular injury and renal tubular injury were significantly increased, showing occult AKI in dogs with CPV.[78] Because there are numerous other broad-spectrum antimicrobial combinations for use in patients with CPV enteritis, aminoglycoside antibiotics that have the inherent risk of nephrotoxicity are not recommended.

Puppies with CPV enteritis often have comorbidities, including gastrointestinal parasitism. With this in mind, antiparasite therapy should be initiated as soon as the puppy can tolerate oral therapies[79] (**Table 2**).

ENTERAL NUTRITION

Enteral nutrition is essential to help prevent enterocyte atrophy and to provide nutrients required for healing. Early provision of enteral nutrition in puppies with CPV enteritis was found to decrease patient morbidity and length of hospital stay.[80] A variety of formulae exist for calculation of resting energy expenditure (REE). A simple, linear formula for calculation of an individual patient's energy needs is REE = Kcal/d = $(30 \times BW_{kg}) + 70$, where BW_{kg} is body weight in kilograms. Because individual patients' REEs can vary from day to day during the course of hospitalization,[81] multiplication of arbitrary illness, injury, and infection factors is not accurate and is not generally recommended. Placement of a nasogastric tube in patients with CPV can be a means of provision of enteral nutrition as well as allowing for gastric suctioning

| Table 1 | | |
| Antibiotic choices for use in inpatient and outpatient treatment protocols for canine parvoviral enteritis | | |
Antibiotic	Dose (mg/kg)/Route/Frequency	In/Outpatient
Ampicillin	20–40/IV/Q 8 h	Inpatient
Ampicillin-sulbactam	30–50/IV/Q 6–8 h	Inpatient
Cefovecin	8/SQ/once	Outpatient
Cefoxitin	20–30/IV/Q 8 h	Inpatient
Enrofloxacin	10/IV/Q 24 h	Inpatient
Metronidazole	10/IV/Q 8 h	Inpatient

Abbreviations: Q, every; SQ, subcutaneous.

Table 2
Antiparasite strategies for dogs with canine parvovirus enteritis and coinfection with gastrointestinal parasites

Drug	Dosage	Efficacy Against
Pyrantel pamoate	5–10 mg/kg PO Q 24 h Repeat in 7–10 d	*Toxocara canis* *Ancylostoma* spp
Fenbendazole	50 mg/kg PO Q 24 h for 3–5 d	*Giardia duodenalis* *Ancylostoma* spp *Trichuris vulpis*[a] *T canis*
Sulfadimethoxine	50–60 mg/kg PO Q 24 h for 5–20 d	*Isospora* spp
Metronidazole	10–30 mg/kg PO Q 12 h for 5–7 d	*G duodenalis*

Abbreviation: PO, by mouth.
[a] For *T vulpis*, repeat dose of fenbendazole 3 weeks then 3 months after first therapy.

to prevent abdominal discomfort and vomiting or regurgitation. A recent article[82] documented little to no change in acid-base status in patients whose treatment protocols included gastric suctioning. Liquid enteral diets can be started at 25% of a patient's REE and administered either in intermittent boluses or as constant-rate infusions, depending on clinician preference and hospital resources. Other studies have documented that the use of an (Hydrolyte Advanced Nutritional Support, Hormel Health Labs, Austin, MN.) or commercially available enteral nutrition product (Viyo Recuperation, Viyo International, Antwerp, Belgium.) is palatable and can be voluntarily consumed by some puppies during their recovery period, and this may be beneficial in increasing caloric intake and influence the return of appetite.[83,84] Because aggressive early interventional nutrition is beneficial and the preferred method of providing calories and nutrients to patients infected with CPV, parenteral nutritional strategies are no longer needed.[1]

ANALGESIA

Many patients with CPV infection show abdominal discomfort caused by vomiting, ileus, and possible intussusception.[1] Opioid analgesics can promote ileus and vomiting. Partial agonists such as buprenorphine (0.01–0.02 mg/kg IV every 8 hours) or an agonist-antagonist such as butorphanol (0.1–0.2 mg/kg/h) may be preferred to pure mu agonists such as methadone (0.1–0.2 mg/kg IV every 6 hours), morphine (0.1–0.2 mg/kg IV, intramuscularly [IM], or subcutaneously every 8 hours), hydromorphone (0.1 mg/kg IV or IM every 8 hours), or fentanyl (1–5 μg/kg/h IV continuous-rate infusion [CRI]). Lidocaine (15–30 μg/kg/min IV CRI) can promote gastrointestinal motility and also provide some degree of analgesia. In addition to its actions as a centrally acting antiemetic, maropitant, a neurokinin-1 receptor antagonist, functions to provide visceral analgesia in puppies with CPV enteritis.[85] Alpha-2 agonists, which can promote extreme vasoconstriction and limit gastrointestinal perfusion, and nonsteroidal antiinflammatory drugs, which can impair gastrointestinal and renal perfusion, are both contraindicated.

MONITORING

Monitoring of patients with CPV involves careful and frequent assessment of their interstitial and intravascular volume status, blood pressure, blood glucose levels, acid-base and electrolyte status, level of comfort, and degree of nausea. By using Kirby's Rule of 20 monitoring,[86] clinicians can use a checklist to monitor the patient's status without overlooking important consideration of aspects of care (**Box 1**).

OUTPATIENT TREATMENT

The prognosis for animals infected with CPV is dismal without treatment. Because cost of hospitalization and therapy is a limiting factor that can influence patients' outcomes, recent prospective and retrospective studies have documented a 75% to 80% survival using outpatient strategies for CPV infection.[87,88] The similarities for both studies include the need for hydration in the form of subcutaneous fluids, use of an antiemetic, and essential need for enteral nutrition. The prospective study[88] recommends placement of an IV catheter, then to administer IV crystalloid fluid (15–45 mL/kg) until perfusion parameters (heart rate, capillary refill time, pulse quality, mentation, serum lactate concentration, and body temperature) normalize. When present, hypoglycemia was corrected using IV dextrose (25%, 1–2 mL/kg). Once intravascular volume status and perfusion had been restored, affected puppies received 1 dose of cefovecin (8 mg/kg subcutaneously), maropitant (1 mg/kg subcutaneously every 24 hours), buprenorphine (0.02 mg/kg subcutaneously), high-fructose corn

---

Box 1
Kirby's Rule of 20

1. Fluid balance
2. Oxygenation and ventilation
3. Blood pressure and perfusion
4. Heart rate, rhythm, and contractility
5. Glucose
6. Body temperature
7. Albumin/oncotic pressure
8. Electrolytes
9. Mentation
10. Hemoglobin/red blood cell mass
11. Gastrointestinal integrity and motility
12. Nutrition
13. Renal function
14. Coagulation
15. Immune status, antibiotic dose and selection
16. Drug doses and metabolism
17. Wound care and bandages
18. Pain control
19. Nursing care
20. Tender loving care

A checklist to use for treatment and monitoring of critical animals, including those with parvoviral enteritis.

syrup, a commercially available diet[89] (1 mL/kg by mouth every 6 hours), oral potassium supplementation, and subcutaneous fluids (30 mL/kg crystalloid every 6 hours). Dedicated owners whose financial limitations preclude inpatient therapy can be instructed how to administer subcutaneous fluids and other medications at home with a moderately good chance of success.

ANCILLARY THERAPIES

Discovery of viral replication strategies, immunosuppression, failure of protective immunity, presence of biomarkers and inflammatory cytokines, bacterial endotoxin, and disruption of the fecal microbiome have led to investigative strategies to improve outcomes in patients with CPV enteritis.

ANTIVIRAL STRATEGIES

Oseltamivir, an antiviral drug used primarily for the treatment of human influenza, is a neuraminidase inhibitor that has been studied in puppies with CPV enteritis.[90,91] Although 1 study documented increased body weight and maintenance of white blood cell counts in oseltamivir-treated animals,[90] neither study documented a decrease in morbidity, length of hospitalization, or mortality.[90,91] The role of interferons as a possible antiviral therapy has been investigated for dogs with CPV enteritis. Recombinant feline omega-interferon ($1–5 \times 10^6$ IU/kg/d IV for 3 days) has been shown to decrease the incidence of fever, vomiting, diarrhea, and mortality and to improve appetite.[92–95] The drug is not currently approved for use in the United States, but is available for use in Europe and Australia.

IMMUNE PLASMA

The decline in circulating antibodies derived from maternal passive immunity is a significant contributing factor in the risk of contracting CPV infection. Antibodies that bind with circulating parvovirus can theoretically neutralize the ability of parvovirus to bind with and attack cells, effectively decreasing infection and ability to replicate.[96] Strategies to increase circulating antiparvovirus antibodies have been investigated as a potential therapy.[96–99] Administration of canine CPV-hyperimmune plasma immediately after CPV inoculation to experimentally infected dogs effectively decreased the incidence of vomiting and diarrhea and improved survival.[97,98] In a randomized prospective study, a single dose of 12 mL of immune plasma obtained from dogs that survived natural infection with CPV was not successful at improving white blood cell count or weight, or decreasing viremia or length of hospital stay.[96] Feline antiparvovirus antibodies, too, failed to decrease gastrointestinal signs, fecal viral load and shedding, duration of hospitalization, morbidity, or mortality.[100] Lyophilized immunoglobulin G has been documented in 1 study to decrease clinical signs and length of hospital stay in naturally occurring CPV enteritis.[99] Despite inconclusive findings of parenteral administration of immune plasma, early enteral administration of CPV antibodies has been shown to be effective at reducing clinical signs in puppies with experimental CPV infection, suggesting that early administration of antibodies may be effective at reducing the risk of infection in exposed animals before the onset of clinical signs.[101]

GRANULOCYTE COLONY-STIMULATING FACTOR

Leukopenia is an important contributor to impaired immune function and morbidity associated with bacteremia in dogs with CPV infection. Increases in endogenous concentrations of canine G-CSF (cG-CSF) have been documented to improve neutrophil counts in puppies with experimental parvoviral infection.[47,102-106] Human G-CSF (hG-CSF)[102-104] and cG-CSF[105,106] have been investigated to promote bone marrow stimulation and release of neutrophils. Although 1 study[102] did show that the use of recombinant hG-CSF improved neutrophil counts in a small population of puppies infected with parvovirus, other studies showed no improvement in neutrophil count, length of hospitalization, or survival.[104,105] Two studies have shown that canine-specific G-CSF (5 μg/kg recombinant cG-CSF [recombinant canine Granulocyte-Colony Stimulating Factor] once daily) is effective at statistically increasing white blood cell and neutrophil count,[105] as well as monocyte and lymphocyte counts.[106] Despite these findings, the use of rcG-CSF may not necessarily improve survival.[105]

FECAL TRANSFAUNATION

The fecal microbiota has multipurpose benefits for the host, including enterocyte nutrition, protective barrier function, immune regulation, and gastrointestinal motility.[107] Disruption of host fecal bacteria and the microbiota occurs in acute gastroenteritis, including that observed with CPV enteritis.[108] Administration of probiotics to puppies with CPV has shown improved clinical scoring with respect to degree of dehydration, incidence of vomiting and diarrhea, fecal scoring, and appetite,[109] although a second study showed no benefit with respect to length of hospital stay or case fatality.[110] Other methods of restoring fecal microbiota include transfaunation, or administration of fecal transplants from a healthy host to animals with acute hemorrhagic diarrhea. A recent study that investigated rectal administration of 10 g of feces from a healthy canine donor, diluted in 10 mL of sterile 0.9% saline, to puppies with CPV enteritis showed earlier onset of resolution of diarrhea, decreased length of hospital stay, and improved survival in the fecal transplant group.[107]

PREVENTION

Subclinical infection in both wild and domestic dogs that shed virus in their feces can represent a significant potential source of infection to other dogs, particularly in crowded or unsanitary conditions such as shelters or some breeding kennels.[75] Dilute 0.75% sodium hypochlorite solution on environmental surfaces is effective at significantly reducing spread of CPV within crowded areas such as veterinary hospitals and shelters.[111] The only method of preventing infection is to isolate at-risk puppies from exposure to CPV. Client education to avoid exposure of at-risk puppies to other dogs until the puppy has received its full series of vaccinations is of paramount importance, because well-vaccinated adults with normal feces can still shed CPV virus and be a potential source of exposure. Within shelters and veterinary hospitals, personnel should adhere to careful handwashing and wearing of new gloves between each patient. Clothing, instrumentation, and environment such as thermometers, stethoscopes, fluid pumps, tables, cages, and bedding should be carefully cleaned and disinfected on a regular basis with a detergent and virucidal solutions that are effective at deactivating CPV. In any diarrheic patient, even with a negative fecal ELISA, barrier methods with disposable gloves, cap, gown, and booties should be worn when handling the patient to prevent cross-contamination and spread of infection.

VACCINATIONS

In addition to strict hygiene strategies, the most effective method of preventing CPV infection and disease is through careful and strategic inoculation with the development of protective antibodies. Dogs of any age and breed can be infected with parvovirus, but puppies between the ages of 6 and 16 weeks seem to be the most susceptible.[1] Young puppies that are born to and allowed to nurse colostrum from vaccinated bitches have maternally derived passive immunity.[112] As maternally derived antibody levels start to decrease at 8 to 12 weeks of age, neonates are at a higher risk of infection.[8,26] Earlier decreases in maternally derived antibodies can occur if maternal antibody dose is low. Vaccination strategies are therefore directed at stimulating innate immunity by administration of a series of vaccinations during the time period that maternal antibody is waning. In young animals, maternally derived antibodies can interfere with vaccine-induced protective antibodies,[6] particularly between 49 and 69 days of age. For this reason, the timing of vaccinations is important when considering a protocol to help prevent infection in puppies. Current vaccination guidelines recommend vaccination using a high-titer, low-passage, modified live vaccination starting at 6 weeks of age and repeated every 3 to 4 weeks through 16 weeks of age. For dogs with significantly increased risk of exposure (eg, those in shelters), vaccination as early as 4 weeks through 18 to 20 weeks of age may be recommended.[113] One study documented that even 1 vaccination can decrease the risk of developing CPV enteritis by 2.3 times.[40] Current vaccinations impart protective immunity against CPV-2, CPV-2b, and CPV-2c strains.[114–117] A booster vaccination is recommended at 1 year of age, then every 3 years.

Vaccination failure has been documented in both young and adult dogs. A recent study documented a high prevalence of CPV-seronegative dogs admitted to a veterinary critical care unit, despite receiving recent vaccination according to standard guidelines.[118] Others have reported lack of protective immunity in dogs that received the recommended series of vaccinations through adulthood but developed infection and were able to shed virus in their feces, posing a risk to other dogs.[119,120] Despite vaccination, animals with rare contact with other dogs also may have inadequate CPV antibodies, although this does not necessarily reflect an increased risk of infection.[121] CPV should be considered as a possible differential diagnosis in adult animals with clinical signs of gastroenteritis with no other cause. Dogs that test positive may lack the ability to develop protective immunity from routine vaccination or exposure and should be culled from breeding populations.

PROGNOSIS

The prognosis for survival often depends on the severity of clinical signs at the time that therapy is initiated. Clinical signs indicating hypovolemia and poor perfusion and fever, along with low protein C level, increased cortisol level, low thyroxine level, lymphocyte count less than $1000/\mu L$, and hypoalbuminemia have been associated with increased mortality.[40] Lymphopenia and hypoalbuminemia at the time of admission have been associated with increased length of hospitalization.[40] Overall, the prognosis for survival ranges from 60% to 90%, depending on the study, type of therapy, and individual patient response to treatment.[36,40,122,123] Comorbidities such as canine coronavirus and gastrointestinal parasitism also increased patient morbidity and mortality. Recent outpatient strategies[88] have improved outcomes when client financial limitations prevent hospitalization and aggressive care. Without therapy, prognosis is grim, with death occurring in more than 90% of patients.[36]

DISCLOSURE

The author has nothing to disclose.

REFERENCES

1. Mylonakis ME, Kalli I, Rallis TS. Canine parvoviral enteritis: an update on the clinical diagnosis, treatment and prevention. Vet Med 2016;11(7):91–100.
2. Goddard A, Leisewitz AL. Canine parvovirus. Vet Clin North Am Small Anim Pract 2010;40(6):1041–53.
3. Chang SF, Sgro JY, Parrish CR. Multiple amino acids in the structure of canine parvovirus coordinately determine the canine host range and specific antigenic and hemagglutination properties. J Virol 1992;66:6858–67.
4. Ohshima T, Mochizuki M. Evidence for recombination between feline panleukopenia virus and canine parvovirus Type 2. J Vet Med Sci 2009;71(4):403–8.
5. Wang J, Cheng S, Yi L, et al. Evidence for natural recombination between mink enteritis virus and canine parvovirus. Virol J 2012;30(9):252.
6. Pollack RV, Carmichael LE. Canine viral enteritis. In: Barlough JE, editor. Manual of small animal infectious diseases. London: Churchill Livingstone; 1988. p. 101–7.
7. Kramer JM, Meunier PC, Pollack RV. Canine parvovirus: update. Vet Med Small Anim Clin 1980;75(10):1541–55.
8. Lamm CG, Rezabek GB. Parvovirus infection in domestic companion animals. Vet Clin North Am Small Anim Pract 2008;38:837–50.
9. Decaro N, Desario C, Addie DD. The study of molecular epidemiology of canine parvovirus Europe. Emerg Infect Dis J 2007;13:1222–4.
10. Sykes JE. Canine parvovirus infections and other viral enteritides. In: Sykes JE, editor. Canine and feline infectious disease. 1st edition. St Louis (MO): Elsevier; 2014. p. 141–51.
11. Ford J, McEndaffer L, Renshaw R, et al. Parvovirus infection is associated with myocarditis and myocardial fibrosis in young dogs. Vet Pathol 2017;54(6):964–71.
12. Strom LM, Reis JC, Brown CC. Parvoviral myocarditis in a dog. J Am Vet Med Assoc 2015;246(8):853–5.
13. Sime TA, Powell LL, Schildt JC, et al. Parvoviral myocarditis in a 5-week-old dachshund. J Vet Emerg Crit Care (San Antonio) 2015;25(6):765–9.
14. Decaro N, Desario C, Campolo M, et al. Clinical and virological findings in pups naturally infected with canine parvovirus type 2 Gluc-426 mutant. J Vet Diagn Invest 2005;17(2):133–8.
15. Smith-Carr S, Macintire DK, Swango LJ. Canine parvovirus: Part I Pathogenesis and vaccination. Comp Cont Educ Pract 1997;19(2):125–33.
16. McCaw DM. Hoskins JD> Canine viral enteritis. In: Green CE, editor. Infectious diseases of the dog and cat. 4th edition. St Louis (MO): Saunders; 2006. p. 63–73.
17. Pollack RV. Experimental canine parvovirus infection in dogs. Cornell Vet 1982; 72:103–19.
18. Decaro N, Buonavoglia C. Canine parvovirus – a review of the epidemiological and diagnostic aspects, with emphasis on type 2c. Vet Microbiol 2012; 155:1–12.
19. Woldemskel M, Liggett A, Ilha M, et al. Canine parvovirus-2b associated erythema multiforme in a litter of English setter puppies. J Vet Diagn Invest 2011; 23(3):576–80.
20. Schaudien D, Polizopoulou Z, Koutinas A, et al. Leukoencephalopathy associated with parvovirus infection in Cretan hound puppies. J Clin Microbiol 2010; 48(9):3169–75.

21. Marenzoni ML, Calo P, Foiani G, et al. Porencephaly and periventricular encephalitis in a 4 month old puppy: detection of canine parvovirus type 2 and potential role in brain lesions. J Comp Pathol 2019;169:20–4.

22. Decaro N, Desario C, Amorisco F, et al. Canine parvovirus type 2c infection in a kitten with intracranial abscess and convulsions. J Feline Med Surg 2011;13(4): 231–6.

23. Gamoh K, Shimazaki Y, Macki H, et al. The pathogenicity of canine parvovirus type 2-b, FP84 strain isolated from a domestic cat. J Vet Med Sci 2003;65(9): 1027–9.

24. Miranda C, Parrish CR, Thompson G. Canine parvovirus 2c infection in a cat with severe clinical disease. J Vet Diagn Invest 2014;26(3):462–4.

25. Johnson RH, Smith JR. Epidemiology and pathogenesis of canine parvovirus. Aust Vet Pract 1983;13(1):31.

26. Pollack RV, Carmichael LE. Maternally derived immunity to canine parvovirus infection: transfer, decline, and interference with vaccination. J Am Vet Med Assoc 1982;204(8):37–42.

27. Proksch AL, Unterer S, Speck S, et al. Influence of clinical and laboratory variables on faecal antigen ELISA results in dogs with canine parvovirus infection. Vet J 2015;204(3):304–8.

28. Meunier PC, Cooper BJ, Appel MJ, et al. Pathogenesis of canine parvovirus: the importance of viremia. Vet Pathol 1985;22(1):60–71.

29. Decaro N, Campolo M, Desario C, et al. Maternally derived antibodies in pups and protection from canine parvovirus infection. Biologicals 2005;33:259–65.

30. Maarkovich JE, Stucker KM, Carr AH, et al. Effects of canine parvovirus strain variations on diagnostic test results and clinical management of enteritis in dogs. J Am Vet Med Assoc 2012;241(11):66–72.

31. Decaro N, Desario C, Billi M, et al. Evaluation of an in-clinic assay for the diagnosis of canine parvovirus. Vet J 2013;198:504–7.

32. Decaro N, Desario C, Beall MJ, et al. Detection of canine parvovirus type 2c by a commercially available in-house rapid test. Vet J 2010;184(3):373–5.

33. Kantere MC, Athanasiou LV, Spyrou V, et al. Diagnostic performance of a rapid in-clinic test for the detection of canine parvovirus under different storage conditions and vaccination status. J Virol Methods 2015;215-216:52–5.

34. Decaro N, Dessario C, Elia G, et al. Occurrence of severe gastroenteritis in pups after canine parvovirus vaccination administration: a clinical and laboratory diagnostic dilemma. Vaccine 2007;25(7):1161–6.

35. Pollack RV, Coyne MJ. Canine parvovirus. Vet Clin North Am Small Anim Pract 1993;23(3):555–68.

36. Prittie J. Canine parvoviral enteritis a review of diagnostic, management and prevention. J Vet Emerg Crit Care (San Antonio) 2004;13:167–76.

37. Macintire DK, Smith-Carr S. Canine parvovirus. II. Clinical signs, diagnosis and treatment. Comp Cont Educ Pract 1996;19(3):291–302.

38. Faz M, Martinez JS, Gomez LB, et al. Origin and genetic diversity of canine parvovirus 2c circulating in Mexico. Arch Virol 2019;164(2):371–9.

39. Rallis TS, Papazoglou LG, Adamama-Moraitou KK, et al. Acute enteritis or gastroenteritis in young dogs as a predisposing factor for intestinal intussusception: a retrospective study. J Vet Med A Physiol Pathol Clin Med 2000;47(8): 507–11.

40. Kalli I, Leontides LS, Mylonakis ME, et al. Factors affecting the occurrence, duration of hospitalization and final outcome in canine parvoviral enteritis. Res Vet Sci 2010;89:174–8.

41. Castro TX, Cubel Garcia Rde C, Goncalves LP, et al. Clinical, hematological and biochemical findings in puppies with coronavirus and parvovirus enteritis. Can Vet J 2013;54(9):885–8.
42. Goddard A, Leisewitz AL, Christopher MM, et al. Prognostic usefulness of blood leukocyte changes in canine parvoviral enteritis. J Vet Intern Med 2008;22: 309–16.
43. Farro CS. Radiographic appearance of canine parvoviral enteritis. J Am Vet Med Assoc 1982;180(1):43–7.
44. Stander N, Wagner WM, Goddard A, et al. Ultrasonographic appearance of canine parvoviral enteritis in puppies. Vet Radiol Ultrasound 2010;51(1):69–74.
45. Schoeman JP, Goddard A, Herrtage ME. Serum cortisol and thyroxine concentrations as predictors of death in critically ill puppies with parvoviral diarrhea. J Am Vet Med Assoc 2007;231:1534–9.
46. Schoeman JP, Herrtage ME. Serum thyrotropin, thyroxine and free thyroxine concentrations as predictors of mortality in critically ill puppies with parvovirus infection: a model for human paediatric illness? Microbes Infect 2008;10:203–7.
47. Cohn LA, Rewerts RM, McCaw D, et al. Plasma granulocyte-colony stimulating factor concentrations in neutropenic, parvoviral-enteritis infected puppies. J Vet Intern Med 1999;13:581–6.
48. Mann FA, Boon GD, Wagner-Mann CC, et al. Ionized and total magnesium concentrations in blood from dogs with naturally acquired parvovirus. J Am Vet Med Assoc 1998;212:1398–401.
49. Kocaturk M, Martinez S, Eralp O, et al. Prognostic value of serum acute-phase proteins in dogs with parvoviral enteritis. J Small Anim Pract 2010;51:478–83.
50. McClure V, van Schoor M, Goddard A, et al. Serial C-reactive protein measurements as a predictor of outcome in puppies infected with parvovirus. J Am Vet Med Assoc 2013;243(3):361–6.
51. Yilmaz Z, Senturk S. Characterisation of lipid profiles in dogs with parvoviral enteritis. J Small Anim Pract 2007;48:643–50.
52. Panda D, Patra R, Nandi S, et al. Oxidative stress indices in gastroenteritis in dogs with canine parvoviral infection. Res Vet Sci 2009;86:36–42.
53. Kalli IV, Adamama-Moraitou KK, Patsika MN. Prevalence of increased canine pancreas-specific lipase concentrations in young dogs with parvovirus enteritis. Vet Clin Pathol 2017;46(1):111–9.
54. Dossin O, Rupassara S, Weng HY, et al. Effect of parvoviral enteritis on plasma citrulline concentration in dogs. J Vet Intern Med 2011;25:215–21.
55. Otto CM, Drobatz KJ, Soter C. Endotoxemia and tumor necrosis factor activity in dogs with naturally occurring parvoviral enteritis. J Vet Intern Med 1997;11: 65–70.
56. Otto CM, Rieser TM, Brooks MB, et al. Evidence of hypercoagulability in dogs with parvoviral enteritis. J Am Vet Med Assoc 2000;217:1500–4.
57. Brady S, Norris JM, Kelman M, et al. Canine parvovirus in Australia: the role of socio-economic factors. Vet J 2012;193(2):522–8.
58. Zourkas E, Ward MP, Kelman M. Canine parvovirus in Australia: a comparative study of reported rural and urban cases. Vet Microbiol 2015;181(3–4):198–203.
59. Kelman M, Ward MP, Barrs VR, et al. The geographic distribution and financial impact of canine parvovirus in Australia. Transbound Emerg Dis 2019;66: 299–311.
60. Allukian AR, Abelson AL, Babyak J, et al. Comparison of time to obtain intraosseous versus jugular catheterization in canine cadavers. J Vet Emerg Crit Care (San Antonio) 2017;27(5):506–11.

61. Hughes D, Beal MW. Emergency vascular access. Vet Clin North Am Small Anim Pract 2000;30(3):491–507.
62. Macintire DK. Pediatric fluid therapy. Vet Clin North Am Small Anim Pract 2008; 38(3):621–7.
63. Ford RB, Larson LJ, McClure KD, et al. 2017 AAHA Canine Vaccination Guidelines. American Animal Hospital Association.
64. Heald RD, Jones BD, Schmidt DA. Blood gas and electrolyte concentrations in canine parvoviral enteritis. J Am Anim Hosp Assoc 1986;22:745–8.
65. Mazzaferro EM, Rudloff E, Kirby R. The role of albumin replacement in the critically ill veterinary patient. J Vet Emerg Crit Care (San Antonio) 2002;12(2): 113–24.
66. Dodd WJ. Immune plasma for treatment of parvoviral gastroenteritis. J Am Vet Med Assoc 2012;240(9):1056.
67. Cohn LA, Kerl ME, Lenox CE, et al. Response of healthy dogs to infusions of human serum albumin. Am J Vet Res 2007;68(6):657–63.
68. Martin LG, Luther TY, Alperin AC, et al. Serum antibodies against human albumin in critically ill dogs and cats. J Am Vet Med Assoc 2008;232(7):1004–9.
69. Mazzaferro EM, Balakrishnan A, Hackner SG, et al. Delayed Type-III hypersensitivity reaction with acute kidney injury in two dogs following administration of concentrated human albumin during treatment for hypoalbuminemia secondary to septic peritonitis. J Vet Emerg Crit Care (San Antonio) 2020. https://doi.org/10.1111/vec.12976.
70. Mantione NL, Otto CM. Characterization of the use of antiemetic agents in dogs with parvoviral enteritis treated at a veterinary teaching hospital: 77 cases (1997-2000). J Am Vet Med Assoc 2005;227(11):1787–93.
71. Yalcin E, Keser GO. Comparative efficacy of metoclopramide, ondansetron and maropitant in preventing parvoviral enteritis-induced emesis in dogs. J Vet Pharmacol Ther 2017;40(6):599–603.
72. Sullivan LA, Lenberg JP, Boscan P, et al. Assessing the efficacy of maropitant versus ondansetron in the treatment of dogs with parvoviral enteritis. J Am Anim Hosp Assoc 2018;54(6):338–43.
73. Sykes JE. Immunodeficiencies caused by infectious diseases. Vet Clin North Am Small Anim Pract 2010;40:409–23.
74. Silva ROS, Dorella FA, Figueriedo HCP, et al. Clostridium perfringens and C. difficile in parvovirus positive dogs. Anaerobe 2017;48:66–9.
75. Tupler T, Levy JK, Sabshin SJ, et al. Enteropathogens identified in dogs entering a Florida animal shelter with normal feces or diarrhea. J Am Vet Med Assoc 2012;241(3):338–43.
76. Duijvestijn M, Mughini-Gras L, Schuurman N, et al. Enteropathogen infections in canine puppies (co)occurrence, clinical relevance and risk factors. Vet Microbiol 2016;195:115–22.
77. Botha WJ, Schoeman JP, Marks SL, et al. Prevalence of salmonella in juvenile dogs affected with parvoviral enteritis. J S Afr Vet Assoc 2018;89:e1–6.
78. Van den Berg MF, Schoeman JP, Defauw P, et al. Assessment of acute kidney injury in canine parvovirus infection: comparison of kidney injury biomarkers with routine renal function parameters. Vet J 2018;242:8–14.
79. Brunner CJ, Swango LJ. Canine parvovirus infection: effects on the immune system and factors that predispose to severe disease. Comp Cont Educ Pract 1985;7(12):979–88.

80. Mohr AJ, Leisewitz AL, Jacobson LS, et al. Effect of early enteral nutrition on intestinal permeability, intestinal protein loss and outcome in dogs with severe parvoviral enteritis. J Vet Intern Med 2003;17:791–8.

81. O'Toole E, Miller CW, Wilson BA, et al. Comparison of the standard predictive equation for calculation of resting energy expenditure with indirect calorimetry in hospitalized and healthy dogs. J Am Vet Med Assoc 2004;225(1):58–64.

82. Chih A, Rudloff E, Waldner C, et al. Incidence of hypochloremic metabolic alkalosis in dogs and cats with and without nasogastric tubes over a period of up to 36 hours in the intensive care unit. J Vet Emerg Crit Care (San Antonio) 2018; 28(3):244–51.

83. Tenne R, Sullivan LA, Contreras ET, et al. Palatability and clinical effects of an oral recuperation fluid during recovery of dogs with suspected parvoviral enteritis. Top Companion Anim Med 2016;31(2):68–72.

84. Reineke EL, Walton K, Otto CM. Evaluation of an oral electrolyte solution for treatment of mild to moderate dehydration in dogs with hemorrhagic diarrhea. J Am Vet Med Assoc 2013;243(6):851–7.

85. Marquez M, Boscan P, Weir J, et al. Comparison of NK-1 receptor antagonist (maropitant) to morphine as a preanesthetic agent for canine ovariohysterectomy. PLoS One 2015;10(10):e0140734.

86. Purvis D, Kirby R. Systemic inflammatory response syndrome: septic shock. Vet Clin North Am Small Anim Pract 1994;24(6):1225–47.

87. Sarpong KJ, Lukowski JM, Knapp CG. Evaluation of mortality rate and predictors of outcome in dogs receiving outpatient treatment for parvoviral enteritis. J Am Vet Med Assoc 2017;251(9):1035–41.

88. Venn EC, Presinder K, Boscan PL, et al. Evaluation of an outpatient protocol in the treatment of canine parvoviral enteritis. J Vet Emerg Crit Care (San Antonio) 2017;27(1):52–65.

89. Hill's AD. Hill's Pet Nutrition. Topeka(KS).

90. Savigny MR, Macintire DK. Use of oseltamivir in the treatment of canine parvoviral enteritis. J Vet Emerg Crit Care (San Antonio) 2010;20(1):132–42.

91. Papaioannou E, Soubais N, Theodorou K, et al, The potential role of oseltamivir in the management of canine parvoviral enteritis in 50 natural cases. Abstract BSAVA Congress April 4–7, 20-13 Birmingham, UK.

92. Ishiwata K, Minagawa T, Kajimoto T. Clinical effects of feline interferon-omega on experimental parvovirus infection in beagle dogs. J Vet Med Sci 1998;72: 1145–51.

93. Minagawa T, Ishiwata K, Kajimoto T. Feline interferon-omega treatment on canine parvovirus infection. Vet Microbiol 1999;69:51–3.

94. Martin V, Najbar W, Gueguen S, et al. Treatment of canine parvoviral enteritis with interferon-omega in a placebo-controlled challenge trial. Vet Microbiol 2002;89:115–27.

95. De Mari K, Maynard L, Eun HM, et al. Treatment of canine parvoviral enteritis with interferon-omega in a placebo-controlled field trial. Vet Rec 2003;152: 105–8.

96. Bragg RF, Duffy AL, DeCecco FA, et al. Clinical evaluation of a single dose of immune plasma for treatment of canine parvovirus infection. J Am Vet Med Assoc 2012;240(6):700–4.

97. Meunier PC, Cooper BJ, Appel MJ, et al. Pathogenesis of canine parvoviral enteritis sequestration, virus distribution and passive immunization studies. Vet Pathol 1985;22:617–24.

98. Ishibashi K, Maede Y, Ohsugi T, et al. Serotherapy for dogs infected with canine parvovirus. Nippon Juigaku Zasshi 1983;45:59–66.

99. Macintire D, Smith-Carr S, Jones R, et al. Treatment of dogs naturally infected with canine parvovirus with lyophilized canine IgG. Proceedings 17th Annual Conference of the American College of Veterinary Internal Medicine, Chicago, USA, June 10–13, 1999, p 721.

100. Gerlach M, Proksch AL, Unterer S, et al. Efficacy of feline anti-parvovirus antibodies in the treatment of canine parvovirus infection. J Small Anim Pract 2017;58:408–15.

101. Van Nguyen S, Umeda K, Yokoyama H, et al. Passive protection of dogs against clinical disease due to canine parvovirus-2 specific antibody from chicken egg yolk. Can J Vet Res 2006;70:62–4.

102. Kraft W, Kuffer M. Treatment of severe neutropenia in dogs and cats with filgrastim. Tierarztl Prax 1995;23:609–13.

103. Rewerts JM, McCaw DL, Cohn LA, et al. Recombinant human granulocyte-colony stimulating factor for treatment of puppies with neutropenia secondary to canine parvovirus infection. J Am Vet Med Assoc 1998;213:991–2.

104. Mischke R, Barth T, Wohlsein P, et al. Effect of recombinant human granulocyte colony-stimulating factor (rhG-CSF) on leukocyte count and survival rate in dogs with parvoviral enteritis. Res Vet Sci 2001;70:221–5.

105. Duffy A, Dow S, Ogilvie G, et al. Hematologic improvement in dogs with parvovirus infection treated with recombinant canine granulocyte-colony stimulating factor. J Vet Pharmacol Ther 2010;33:352–6.

106. Armenise A, Trerotoli P, Cirone F, et al. Use of recombinant canine granulocyte-colony stimulating factor to increase leukocyte count in dogs naturally infected by canine parvovirus. Vet Microbiol 2019;231:177–82.

107. Pereira GQ, Gomes LA, Santos IS, et al. Fecal microbiota transplantation in puppies with canine parvovirus infection. J Vet Intern Med 2018;32:707–11.

108. Honneffer JB, Minamoto Y, Suchodolski JS. Microbiota alterations in acute and chronic gastrointestinal inflammation of cats and dogs. WJG 2014;20:16489–97.

109. Arslan HH, Saripinar AD, Terzi G, et al. Therapeutic effects of probiotic bacteria in parvoviral enteritis in dogs. Rev Med Vet 2012;163:55–9.

110. DeCamargo P, Ortolani M, Uenaka S, et al. Evaluation of the therapeutic supplementation with commercial powder probiotic to puppies with hemorrhagic gastroenteritis. Semin Cienc Agrar 2006;27:453–61.

111. Cavalli A, Marinaro M, Desario C, et al. In vitro virucidal activity of sodium hypochlorite against canine parvovirus type 2. Epidemiol Infect 2018;146(15):2010–3.

112. Mila H, Grellet A, Desario C, et al. Protection against canine parvovirus type 2 infection in puppies by colostrum-derived antibodies. J Nutr Sci 2014;3:e54.

113. De Cramer KG, Stylianides E, van Vuuren M. Efficacy of vaccination at 4 and 6 weeks in the control of canine parvovirus. Vet Microbiol 2011;149(1–2):126–32.

114. Larson LJ, Schulz RD. Do current canine parvovirus Type 2 and type 2b vaccinations provide protection against the new type 2c variant? Vet Ther 2008;9(2):94–101.

115. Wilson S, Stirling C, Borowski S, et al. Vaccination of dogs with duramune DAPPi-LC protects against pathogenic parvovirus type 2c challenge. Vet Rec 2013;172(25):662.

116. Wilson S, Illambas J, Siedek E, et al. Vaccination of dogs with canine parvovirus type 2b (CPV-2b) induces neutralizing antibody responses to CPV-2a and CPV-2c. Vaccine 2014;32(42):5420–4.
117. Siedek EM, Schmidt H, Sture GH, et al. Vaccination with canine parvovirus type 2 (CPV-2) protects against challenge with virulent CPV-2b and CPV-2c. Berl Munch Tierarztl Wochenschr 2011;124(1–2):58–64.
118. Mahon JL, Rozanski EA, Paul AL. Prevalence of serum antibody titers against canine distemper virus and canine parvovirus in dogs hospitalized in an intensive care unit. J Am Vet Med Assoc 2017;250(12):1413–8.
119. Miranda C, Thompson G. Canine parvovirus in vaccinated dogs: a field study. Vet Rec 2016;178(16):397–402.
120. Decaro N, Cirone F, Desario C, et al. Severe parvovirus in a 12 year old dog that had been repeatedly vaccinated. Vet Rec 2009;164:593–5.
121. Riedl M, Truyen U, Reese S, et al. Prevalence of antibodies to canine parvovirus and reaction to vaccination in client-owned healthy dogs. Vet Rec 2015; 177(23):597.
122. Miranda C, Carvalheira J, Parrish CR, et al. Factors affecting the occurrence of canine parvovirus in dogs. Vet Microbiol 2015;180:59–64.
123. Ling M, Norris JM, Kelman M, et al. Risk factors for death from canine parvoviral-related disease in Australia. Vet Microbiol 2012;158(3–4):280–90.

Therapeutic Strategies for Treatment of Immune-Mediated Hemolytic Anemia

Robert Goggs, BVSc, PhD, MRCVS

KEYWORDS

- Dogs • Glucocorticoids • Mycophenolate mofetil • Blood transfusion • Thrombosis
- Antithrombotics • Therapeutic plasma exchange • C1-INH

KEY POINTS

- Supportive therapies for canine immune-mediated hemolytic anemia (IMHA) including blood transfusion and antithrombotic drugs are vital to maximize patient survival.
- Glucocorticoids, potentially in combination with another immunosuppressive drug such as azathioprine, cyclosporine, or mycophenolate mofetil remain the primary means of treating canine IMHA.
- Therapeutic drug monitoring may enhance the utility and maximize the safety of cyclosporine and mycophenolate mofetil.
- Emerging therapies for canine IMHA include novel drug formulations and therapeutic plasma exchange.
- Future therapies may include anti-CD20 monoclonal antibodies and inhibitors of complement activation.

INTRODUCTION

Immune-mediated hemolytic anemia (IMHA) is among the most common hematologic disorders of dogs. Despite years of research, the disease continues to cause substantial morbidity and mortality.[1–3] Recently, an American College of Veterinary Internal Medicine (ACVIM) panel generated guidelines for the diagnosis of IMHA in dogs and cats[4] and for the management of IMHA in dogs.[5] These 2 statements were generated using the best available evidence, but large randomized clinical trials supporting most recommended therapies are lacking. The rarity of feline IMHA precludes evidence-based guidance on the management of IMHA in cats, and hence this review focuses solely on dogs. The treatment strategies discussed here are consistent with the ACVIM recommendations with an emphasis on management of the acute and severely affected patients who are more prevalent in Emergency and Critical Care (ECC)

Emergency and Critical Care, Department of Clinical Sciences, Cornell University College of Veterinary Medicine, 930 Campus Road, Ithaca, NY 14853, USA
E-mail address: r.goggs@cornell.edu

Vet Clin Small Anim 50 (2020) 1327–1349
https://doi.org/10.1016/j.cvsm.2020.07.010
0195-5616/20/© 2020 Elsevier Inc. All rights reserved.

settings. In addition, this review provides further discussion of emerging current treatments and speculative future therapies.

Primary or nonassociative IMHA is an autoimmune disorder characterized by loss of self-tolerance, immune dysregulation, and production of autoantibodies.[6] Thus, treatment presently depends on use of nonspecific immunosuppressive drugs including glucocorticoids and mycophenolate mofetil (MMF).[2,3,7–9] The recent ACVIM consensus statements discuss drug selection, but without high-quality evidence solid recommendations on specific drug choices cannot be made. Large, multicenter clinical trials are urgently required to address these knowledge gaps and to place the management of canine IMHA on a firmer footing.[10] Until these become available, reviews such as this most accurately reflect the biases and current practice of the author.

Venous thrombosis, particularly pulmonary thromboembolism, is an important cause of morbidity and mortality in IMHA.[11–13] Thromboprophylaxis is therefore crucial for management of canine IMHA. In addition to the recent ACVIM guidance on IMHA, the American College of Veterinary Emergency and Critical Care (ACVECC) also recently published consensus statements on the use of antithrombotics in small animals.[14] Both sets of guidelines strongly recommend the use of thromboprophylaxis for dogs with IMHA.[5,15] The guidelines are aligned in their recommendation of anticoagulants in preference to antiplatelet agents for IMHA, but there are some differences in the prioritization of particular drugs.[9,16]

Dogs with IMHA that are managed by ECC personnel are often severely affected, and their disease can be life-threatening. As such, it is appropriate that these patients receive maximal supportive care in order to buy time for immunosuppression to take effect. Blood transfusion is central to this support, but some patients may benefit from additional therapies including oxygen therapy and gastroprotectant drugs. Several innovative strategies such as therapeutic plasma exchange (TPE) and complement inhibition may provide novel ways to ameliorate the disease and to aid the immediate control of symptoms, but these are presently investigational treatments. In time, it is hoped that additional insights provided by ongoing investigations of the genetic basis,[17,18] and the pathogenesis of the disorder,[19] may offer new therapeutic options and modalities.

EXPEDITED DIAGNOSTIC EVALUATION

In ECC settings, where IMHA is life-threatening, diagnosis must be expedited in order to rapidly identify potential underlying disorders and prevent delays to the institution of treatment. The diagnostic approach to IMHA is extensively discussed in the recent ACVIM guidelines and will not be revisited in detail here. Complete blood counts with clinical pathologist review, serum chemistry panels, in-saline agglutination testing, or point-of-care Coombs testing are essential. Infectious disease testing adjusted to individual patient and geographic location is prudent. Coagulation testing including multiple markers of thrombosis or thrombotic risk is recommended in severely affected patients in order to better delineate risk, provide a baseline for reassessment, and to provide a rationale for adjusting or augmenting antithrombotic therapy.[20–23] Diagnostic imaging of thorax and abdomen should be performed rapidly in dogs with severe anemia and appropriate cytology or tissue samples collected in a timely manner if neoplasia is suspected. It is probable that in many cases these tests will be negative, but this remains a sensible and straightforward component of the diagnostic investigation.[24] It is unlikely that a single dose of glucocorticoids will preclude establishing a diagnosis of secondary or associative IMHA, but more caution should be exercised where test results are inconclusive or suggest neoplasia. If in doubt, provide maximal supportive care and attempt to achieve more certainty of the diagnosis before committing the patient and the client to the costs and consequences of immunosuppressive therapies.

BLOOD TRANSFUSION

In dogs with anemia, transfusion is the best method for increasing blood oxygen content. The decision to transfuse should be based on individual patient-specific factors including the speed of onset of disease, the current packed cell volume (PCV), and the nature and severity of clinical signs. It is prudent to transfuse dogs with a PCV less than 12% to 15%, even in the absence of clinical signs, because these dogs have limited physiologic reserve and may not tolerate increases in oxygen demand. Dogs with IMHA are typically euvolemic and hence packed red blood cells (pRBCs) are recommended for the provision of additional oxygen carrying capacity.[5] Fresh whole blood is a reasonable alternative if pRBC are unavailable, but patients should be monitored for intravascular volume overload. Packed red cells less than 7 to 10 days old are preferred because RBC age is associated with mortality risk in dogs with hemolysis.[25] Increasing age of transfused pRBC may also increase the risk of hemolytic transfusion reactions.[26] Administration of fresh frozen plasma to dogs with IMHA is not recommended because of a lack of proved benefit,[27] the risk of harm,[28] and the financial cost.

Transfusion naïve dogs do not express preformed alloantibodies against dog erythrocyte antigen (DEA) 1. Hence, dogs are often not typed or crossmatched before the first transfusion. However, because it is likely that dogs with severe IMHA may require multiple transfusions, it is preferable to transfuse DEA 1 type–specific blood. Thus, all IMHA dogs should be typed before transfusion. Some transfusion naïve dogs do express alloantibodies against some minor erythrocyte antigens such as DEA 7.[29,30] These antibodies are considered to be of limited clinical significance because they elicit minimal immune response,[31] but their presence could be responsible for shortened erythrocyte lifespans. In a recent study, 17% transfusion-naïve dogs were crossmatch incompatible with at least one potential donor unit. The study also demonstrated a significantly greater mean change in PCV after transfusion in dogs that had crossmatching performed.[32] Thus, there may be benefits from universally crossmatching dogs before transfusion. The financial and time costs of this approach should be weighed against the benefit of small mean difference in posttransfusion PCV, however. In the acute, severe IMHA patient timely intervention with blood products may be lifesaving and hence it may not be feasible or advisable to attempt crossmatching before first transfusion. All dogs will require crossmatching once 72 hours have elapsed since any prior transfusion. In dogs with IMHA, hemolysis, erythrocyte fragility, and agglutination can affect the results of both typing and crossmatching because hemolysis and agglutination are the endpoints for these tests. The point-of-care immunochromatographic blood typing kits may be less affected by agglutination than are card assays.[33] Point-of-care crossmatching kits are also available,[31] but a recent study found them to be inferior to the gel and tube methods.[34] In addition, some discordant results have been reported for the gel column versus the standard laboratory methods in dogs with IMHA.[35] Owing to these issues, use of a reference laboratory for crossmatching is encouraged whenever feasible.

SUPPORTIVE THERAPIES

Numerous symptomatic and supportive therapies have been administered to dogs with IMHA. However, the evidentiary base for these treatments is sparse. Gastrointestinal ulceration is a frequent concern for dogs receiving glucocorticoids, but there is actually minimal data suggesting corticosteroid therapy increases ulcerogenesis or gastrointestinal bleeding in dogs.[36,37] Likewise, in people, the risk is minimal.[38,39] As such, gastroprotectant therapy is only indicated in canine IMHA patients with demonstrable gastrointestinal ulceration or bleeding or in those with other risk factors such as concurrent liver disease, inflammatory bowel disease, or pancreatitis. If gastroprotectant therapy is indicated, current recommendations are to use proton pump inhibitors such as pantoprazole or omeprazole during the period of risk or until clinical signs resolve.[40,41] It should be noted that proton pump inhibitors may decrease the efficacy of oral MMF because gastric acidity is required for generation of the active metabolite.[42] If there is a medical need for use of proton pump inhibitors, injectable MMF can be administered during the period of concurrent use.

There is evidence of association between some infectious agents and IMHA.[4] Thus, efficacious antimicrobial drugs should be administered to dogs with evidence of infection by hemotropic or vector-borne pathogens (eg, babesiosis, ehrlichiosis). In some cases, these infections can be suspected or diagnosed based on point-of-care assays. In other situations, definitive diagnostic testing by a reference laboratory will be necessary. ECC clinicians should make a patient-specific risk assessment incorporating client and patient lifestyle factors, geographic location, and travel history. High-risk patients should be empirically treated pending diagnostic test results. Empirical antimicrobial drug therapy is not indicated where hemotropic pathogens are not endemic, absent any relevant travel history.

IMMUNOSUPPRESSION
Glucocorticoids

Intravenous or oral glucocorticoids are the first-line therapies for canine IMHA and are effective sole agents in many cases.[2,7,43–51] In patients who cannot tolerate oral drug therapy, intravenous dexamethasone sodium phosphate (0.2–0.4 mg/kg q24 h) is appropriate. There is likely no difference in efficacy between intravenous and oral routes, drugs, or formulations, and hence patient factors are more important. If the patient does not have gastrointestinal signs, then oral prednisolone is recommended for cost and ease of long-term management. A wide range of prednisolone dosages can be found in the literature, and there is considerable debate regarding the optimal dose to provide effective immunosuppression while minimizing the side effects that seem dose related. Typically, dosages of 2–3 mg/kg/d are acceptable and can be given as a single dose or divided. In people and in dogs, once daily dosing may reduce the polyuria associated with the mineralocorticoid effects, but a recent canine study found that twice daily dosing was associated with more rapid reductions in bilirubin concentrations.[52] The exact dosage may depend on the availability of sensible dosage forms (ie, tablet sizes). The most commonly reported side effects of glucocorticoids are polydipsia and polyuria, polyphagia, excessive panting, lethargy, and weakness. Because of the nonspecific, broad immunosuppressive effects of glucocorticoids, secondary infections are a prominent risk. Most clinicians recommend a maximum glucocorticoid dosage (2 mg/kg/d) or a body surface-area dosing scheme (40–60 mg/m²) for large-breed dogs weighing more than 25 kg to mitigate the risk of adverse effects. Similarly, reducing high oral prednisolone dosages to ~2 mg/kg/d 7 to 14 days after the patient responds to therapy may help to reduce side effects.

Second-Line Immunosuppressive Drugs

Additional immunosuppressive drugs are commonly used in ECC practice to manage canine IMHA (**Table 1**). The primary reasons for introducing a second-line drug early in

Table 1
A summary of therapeutic options for dogs with immune-mediated hemolytic anemia

Category	Therapy	Dose	Route	Potential Adverse Effects	Notes
Supportive	Packed red blood cell transfusion	Estimated volume (mL) = 1.5 × BW(kg) × desired PCV change (%)	IV	Transfusion reactions including fever, hemolysis, hypertension, hypotension, sepsis, circulatory overload, acute lung injury	Use units <7 d old whenever possible
Supportive	Omeprazole	0.5–1.0 mg/kg q12–24 h	PO	Occasional diarrhea. May cause increased liver enzymes	
Supportive	Pantoprazole	1.0 mg/kg q24 h	IV	Occasional diarrhea	
Antimicrobial	Doxycycline	5 mg/kg q12 h	PO or IV	Gastrointestinal upset Esophagitis (PO administration)	Only if documented or high risk of vector-borne disease
Immunosuppression	Dexamethasone sodium phosphate	0.2–0.4 mg/kg q24 h	IV	Polydipsia and polyuria, polyphagia, excessive panting, lethargy, weakness, secondary infection	
Immunosuppression	Prednisolone	2–3 mg/kg/d or 40–60 mg/m² for dogs >25 kg	PO	Polydipsia and polyuria, polyphagia, excessive panting, lethargy, weakness, secondary infection	Once daily dosing may decrease mineralocorticoid effects
Immunosuppression	Azathioprine	2 mg/kg q24 h or 50 mg/m² q24 h	PO	Gastrointestinal disturbances, myelosuppression, hepatotoxicity, pancreatitis, secondary infection	After 2–3 wk, dose every other day until discontinued
Immunosuppression	Cyclosporine	5 mg/kg q12 h	PO	Vomiting, diarrhea, anorexia, gingival hyperplasia, secondary infection. Freezing drug may reduce gastrointestinal side effects	Use of therapeutic drug monitoring is recommended
Immunosuppression	Mycophenolate mofetil (MMF)	8–12 mg/kg q12 h	PO or IV	Diarrhea, myelosuppression, secondary infection	Use of therapeutic drug monitoring is recommended

(continued on next page)

Table 1
(continued)

Category	Therapy	Dose	Route	Potential Adverse Effects	Notes
Immunosuppression	Human intravenous immunoglobulin (IVIG)	0.5–1.0 g/kg	IV	Hypotension, hypersensitivity, anaphylaxis, thrombosis, acute kidney injury	Single use only, recommended only as a salvage procedure
Thromboprophylaxis	Unfractionated heparin (UFH)	150–300 U/kg q6 h (dose adjustment required)	SC	Hemorrhage	Individual dose adjustment using anti-Xa or other assays is essential if UFH is used
Thromboprophylaxis	Dalteparin (LMWH)	150–175 U/kg q8 h	SC	Hemorrhage	Anti-Xa monitoring is available and may aid dose optimization
Thromboprophylaxis	Enoxaparin (LMWH)	0.8–1.0 mg/kg q6 h	SC	Hemorrhage	May not be effective in all breeds of dog, for example, Beagles
Thromboprophylaxis	Rivaroxaban	1–2 mg/kg q24 h	PO	Hemorrhage	Calibrated anti-Xa monitoring is available
Thromboprophylaxis	Clopidogrel	1.1–3.0 mg/kg q24 h	PO	Hemorrhage	

Abbreviation: LMWH, low-molecular-weight heparin.

the course of treatment are disease severity and lack of response to initial therapy. In some cases, a second immunosuppressive agent may be added early in order to facilitate reductions in the glucocorticoid dosage. All of these scenarios are commonly encountered by ECC practitioners, but there are no concrete guidelines on what constitutes the right situation for therapeutic escalation. The recent ACVIM guidelines suggested a second-line drug might be initiated if the dog's PCV decreases more than 5% in 24 hours despite glucocorticoids or if the dog depends on repeated transfusion to maintain safe PCV. Likewise, the presence of multiple indicators of severity[53] might justify augmenting glucocorticoids with another agent. In particular, increased serum bilirubin (or clinical icterus) and increased blood urea nitrogen concentrations have been consistently identified as independent mortality predictors.[54,55]

If the decision is made to administer a second immunosuppressive drug, there are multiple options. To date, no study has demonstrated superiority of any of these drugs and they are therefore discussed alphabetically later. The most data exist for azathioprine, cyclosporine, and MMF. The first-choice additional immunosuppressive drug in the author's practice is MMF, but this represents the author's own biases. Cyclosporine represents the most frequent second-line drug used by ACVIM and ACVECC diplomates based on self-reporting.[10] Although some specialists reported using 3 immunosuppressive drugs in dogs with IMHA, this should be avoided unless absolutely necessary. There is no evidence that use of multiple immunosuppressive drugs improves outcome, whereas there are data suggesting multiple immunosuppressive drug use increases the risk of severe adverse effects, including life-threatening secondary infection.[56,57]

Azathioprine

This drug is a cytotoxic synthetic imidazole derivative of 6-mercaptopurine[58] that acts to diminish lymphocyte number and T-cell–dependent antibody synthesis through disruption of the purine synthesis required for DNA and RNA replication. Data on the efficacy of azathioprine in IMHA is conflicting. There are 5 retrospective studies that suggest a potential outcome benefit of azathioprine (in combination with other drugs) in the management of canine IMHA.[7,9,46,59,60] However, the quality of evidence provided by these studies is limited by incomplete information, small sample size, and differences in illness severity between groups. In opposition is a large single-center study that suggests azathioprine may have no beneficial effect in IMHA.[2] That study used a before-after design to compare the efficacy of 2 treatment protocols. Specifically, the study found no difference between the outcomes of dogs treated with prednisolone only compared with a historical control population that received azathioprine and prednisolone. Changes in practice over time, the effects of unmeasured variables on outcome, and notable differences in the incidence of prognostic factors between the 2 groups potentially bias these results.[61] Ultimately, an adequately powered prospective randomized clinical trial will be needed to determine if azathioprine offers any benefit in IMHA. Oral azathioprine is typically dosed at 2 mg/kg or 50 mg/m^2 q24 h. After 2 to 3 weeks, the dosing interval may be increased to every other day until treatment is discontinued. The most frequent adverse effects associated with azathioprine are mild gastrointestinal disturbances, but azathioprine occasionally also causes severe myelosuppression, hepatotoxicity, and pancreatitis.

Cyclosporine

This calcineurin inhibitor prevents T-cell proliferation and maturation through suppression of cytokine transcription.[62] Although cyclosporine use in canine IMHA has been widely reported,[7,9,47,55,63–65] there is little objective evidence of efficacy. Two retrospective studies suggest that cyclosporine when added to prednisolone or when combined with other medications does not affect outcome in canine IMHA.[7,47] A double-blinded, randomized clinical trial comparing glucocorticoids alone with glucocorticoids and cyclosporine found no difference in survival between groups. That study was small and has only been reported in abstract form, however.[66] Oral cyclosporine is typically dosed at 5 mg/kg q12 h. Cyclosporine is a safe drug and adverse effects are uncommon. The most frequently reported effects include vomiting, diarrhea, and anorexia. Anecdotally, freezing capsules may reduce side effects, without altering drug pharmacokinetics.[67] Gingival hyperplasia is also occasionally reported. Therapeutic drug monitoring is likely of particular importance for achieving and maintaining cyclosporine efficacy, but it is presently not widely available.

Mycophenolate Mofetil

MMF is a prodrug for mycophenolic acid (MPA), a noncompetitive, selective, and reversible inhibitor of inosine 5′-monophosphate dehydrogenase (IMPDH).[68] Inhibition of IMPDH prevents proliferation of both B- and T-lymphocytes by preventing de novo guanine nucleotide synthesis.[69] Other potential immunosuppressive mechanisms include T-cell apoptosis and suppression of dendritic cell and monocyte activities.[70] MMF has been used to treat canine IMHA by multiple groups[8,55,64,65,71,72] and is an effective single-agent immunosuppressive for immune thrombocytopenia in dogs.[73] A small retrospective cohort study suggested equivalent efficacy of MMF with glucocorticoids compared with other second-agent combinations.[8] However, without randomization or inclusion of a control group it could also be concluded that all of the second-line drugs were equally ineffective! Clearly, prospective randomized trials are needed.

Oral MMF is typically dosed at 8 to 12 mg/kg q12 h. MMF is generally well tolerated in dogs, but myelosuppression is also occasionally seen. The principal limitation to the use of MMF in dogs is the incidence of gastrointestinal side effects (diarrhea in particular) that may be sufficiently severe as to require drug discontinuation. These signs likely result from the pharmacokinetic profile of MMF in dogs.[70] Controlled-release formulations of the drug might mitigate this limitation. An extended-release formulation of the active metabolite MPA is in development and was recently given MUMS (minor-use, minor species) designation by the FDA (Klotsman, M. Personal communication, 2020). Pilot studies investigating the efficacy of this novel formulation in canine IMHA patients are planned to commence in late 2020.

Intravenous Immunoglobulin

Early studies suggested that administration of IVIG might be a useful adjunctive treatment of canine IMHA. Specifically, these studies suggested IVIG administration might reduce transfusion requirements[74] or hasten PCV recovery.[75,76] However, these studies either lacked a control group or contained statistical errors. Several studies have since showed no effect of this treatment on survival when compared with other immunosuppressive regimens in dogs with IMHA.[51,72] A prospective blinded randomized controlled trial evaluating the addition of IVIG to corticosteroid treatment found no improvement in initial response to therapy or an effect on duration of hospitalization.[50] Current recommendations are therefore to use IVIG (0.5–1.0 g/kg) only as a salvage measure in dogs not responding to treatment. Additional limitations of IVIG include a lack of universal availability and high cost.

Splenectomy

Two retrospective case series have reported on the use of splenectomy for refractory or relapsing IMHA.[77,78] However, neither reported a control group that did not undergo splenectomy, precluding evaluation of the true influence of splenectomy on outcome in these dogs. Based on these 2 publications, splenectomy remains a salvage option for unresponsive cases. Care should be taken to screen patients for vector-borne disease before splenectomy,[4] and immunosuppressive and antithrombotic medications may need to be discontinued or reduced perioperatively.[79]

Therapeutic Drug Monitoring

Maximizing efficacy and minimizing adverse effects of immunosuppressive drugs requires optimization of drug dosage and thus therapeutic drug monitoring (TDM) may facilitate disease control. TDM should be considered for all dogs receiving cyclosporine and potentially also for dogs receiving MMF and is most important in dogs experiencing poor therapeutic responses, relapses, drug-specific adverse effects, or the development of secondary infections. It is well recognized that cyclosporine disposition in dogs is complex and variations in drug preparation combined with alterations of pharmacokinetics in disease states contribute to markedly variable blood concentrations within and between dogs.[80] TDM for cyclosporine may be achieved by monitoring blood cyclosporine concentrations, that is, cyclosporine pharmacokinetics, or perhaps preferably by functional assays analyzing T-cell activation and interleukin-2 and interferon-gamma expression, that is, pharmacodynamics.[81] For MMF, measurement of the catalytic activity of IMPDH is used for TDM in people. However, it is uncertain if IMPDH inhibition fully indicates the immunosuppressive effects of the active metabolite MPA. Studies in dogs suggest that IMPDH activity is suppressed by MPA,[82] but other indices of immune system activity such as lymphocyte proliferation assays may be superior.[83,84] The differences between pharmacodynamic assays may also underlie the apparent discrepancies in the reported onset and degree of immunosuppressive activity of MPA.[83,84]

Discontinuing Immunosuppression

It may take time for immunosuppression to be established, but once the disease is under control, thought should be given to withdrawal and eventual drug discontinuation. Abrupt, premature, or rapid dose deescalation can trigger relapse and must be avoided. It is prudent to wait for several weeks for the disease to stabilize before considering dose reduction. Stability might be defined as a stable PCV greater than 30% for 2 weeks with improvements in the disease including disappearance of agglutination and spherocytosis and reductions in serum bilirubin concentration. The first dose reductions are typically 20% to 25% depending on tablet sizes. If a second immunosuppressive drug was initiated to expedite glucocorticoid withdrawal, then a greater reduction in the dose of prednisone/prednisolone (eg, 25%–50%) may be possible. Provided the disease remains stable as dose reductions are conducted, then the glucocorticoid doses can be reduced by 20% to 25% every 2 to 3 weeks, depending on tablet sizes and the use of a second immunosuppressive drug. Most dogs will require 3 to 6 months of treatment. Second-line immunosuppressive drugs are typically stopped once the glucocorticoids are discontinued provided the disease remains in remission.

THROMBOPROPHYLAXIS

Considerable evidence supports an association between IMHA and thrombosis,[12,27,85–88] and thromboembolism causes substantial morbidity and mortality in dogs with the disease.[13,89,90] Dogs at particular risk include those with severe disease characterized by autoagglutination and intravascular hemolysis. These dogs often have a marked inflammatory response characterized by leukocytosis and hepatopathy.[12,13,53,91] Administration of high-dose glucocorticoids and IVIG likely increases the risk of thrombosis.[76,92–95] Universal thromboprophylaxis is recommended for dogs with IMHA, except those with severe thrombocytopenia defined as a platelet count less than 30,000/μL. The platelet count cutoff of 30,000/μL is somewhat arbitrary but was considered by the ACVIM panelists to represent the point of increased risk of spontaneous hemorrhage,[5] particularly in patients with concurrent inflammation. In IMHA, thrombocytopenia with platelet counts greater than 30,000/μL likely represents a consumptive process.[96,97] Dogs with IMHA seem to be at highest risk of death within the first 2 weeks of diagnosis,[61] when the disease is uncontrolled and patients are receiving blood products and immunosuppressive drugs that may increase the risk of thrombosis. Hence, antithrombotic drug therapy should be initiated at the time of diagnosis and continued until the patient is in remission and no longer receiving glucocorticoids. The genesis of thrombosis in dogs with IMHA is multifactorial.[11,98] The proinflammatory disease process drives intravascular expression of tissue factor,[99,100] endothelial activation,[98] and the release of procoagulant microparticles.[101] The homeostatic balance of pro- and anticoagulant factors is upset,[20,102,103] with secondary platelet activation.[104] Neutrophil extracellular trap formation may also contribute to the prothrombotic phenotype.[105–108]

Thrombosis in canine IMHA is predominantly venous, including pulmonary thromboembolism and splenic and portal vein thrombosis.[15,109,110] As such, thromboprophylaxis with anticoagulants is preferable to an antiplatelet regimen.[27,91,111] Given the risk of thrombosis, administration of an antiplatelet agent is preferable to no antithrombotic therapy, however. There is insufficient evidence to strongly recommend one specific anticoagulant for dogs with IMHA. The recent ACVIM guidelines recommended administration of unfractionated heparin (UFH) with individual dose adjustment using an anti-Xa assay. This was based on a small randomized controlled trial in which dogs that received individually dose-adjusted UFH therapy had lower mortality rates and longer median survival times. It should be noted that the trial has a fragility index of only 2[112] and hence would benefit from replication. In the trial, dogs required UFH doses between 150 and 566 U/kg q6 h to achieve target anti-Xa activities (0.35–0.7U/mL).[63] Initiating antithrombotic therapy at 150 to 300U/kg SC q6 h and individually incrementing the dose may provide a margin of safety for patients against hemorrhagic complications. Per the ACVIM guidelines, UFH should not be used at a constant dose based on the poor survival rate of the dogs in the constant dose arm of the trial. UFH is cheap and widely available, but the anti-Xa assay is available in only a handful of centers, which makes this recommendation hard to follow in practice. The most frequently available alternative monitoring tests include the activated partial thromboplastin time (aPTT) and the viscoelastic tests.[113–122] Nomograms for adjustment of UFH therapy using aPTT and thromboelastograph assays have been reported in abstract form.[123]

Alternatives to UFH proposed in the ACVIM guidelines include the use of low-molecular-weight heparins (LMWH) such as dalteparin and enoxaparin or the direct oral Xa inhibitors such as rivaroxaban. In contrast to the ACVIM guidelines on IMHA, the ACVECC CURATIVE guidelines suggest that the more dependable pharmacokinetics and better safety profiles of the LMWH drugs make them preferable to UFH.[14] Some data suggest that the LMWH compounds should also be dose-adjusted by anti-Xa assay.[124] The level of anti-Xa activity that confers thromboprophy-laxis remains uncertain, but, given the variation in pharmacokinetics and efficacy, monitoring of anti-Xa activity may be justifiable. It seems reasonable to target 0.5 to 1.0 U/mL activity for both enoxaparin and dalteparin.[118] Retrospective studies in canine IMHA suggest that both enoxaparin and rivaroxaban are safe and may be effi-cacious,[64,65] but randomized controlled trials comparing anticoagulant drugs in IMHA are urgently required. Variable anti-Xa activities have been reported for the LMWH preparations, and there is uncertainty regarding the efficacy of enoxaparin in some dog breeds.[65,120,125] Dalteparin does seem efficacious in dogs for venous and arterial thromboprophylaxis.[126,127]

If an antiplatelet agent is selected for thromboprophylaxis in IMHA, then clo-pidogrel (1.1–3.0 mg/kg PO q24 h) represents a better choice than aspirin,[14,128] and there is evidence for efficacy against arterial thrombosis in dogs.[129–133] Clo-pidogrel is likely a more efficacious antiplatelet agent than aspirin in dogs,[14] and a large proportion of dogs fail to respond to low-dose aspirin.[134,135] Further-more, aspirin doses greater than 2 mg/kg in dogs receiving concurrent prednis-olone may cause gastrointestinal bleeding.[136] It should be noted that evidence of clopidogrel efficacy for prevention of venous thrombosis in dogs is lacking, which suggests clopidogrel should be the last resort for thromboprophylaxis in IMHA.

EMERGING THERAPIES

The management of canine IMHA has remained largely unchanged over the last few decades. Recognition of the limitations of standard therapeutic approaches has driven investigation of other treatments including liposomal clodronate, melatonin, hy-perbaric oxygen therapy (HBOT), and most recently TPE. All of these therapies are investigational but they may establish themselves as viable options. If efficacy is demonstrated, further investigation will still be required to determine how they should be integrated with existing treatment modalities.

Liposomal clodronate is a bisphosphonate encapsulated into spherical lipid mem-brane vesicles that are phagocytosed by macrophages. Once the bisphosphonate moiety is released intracellularly it leads to apoptosis, thereby depleting blood and tis-sue macrophage populations.[137] In the context of canine IMHA, macrophages are responsible for extravascular erythrocyte breakdown. Hence macrophage depletion by liposomal clodronate may be equivalent to a temporary pharmaceutical splenec-tomy. In experimental mouse IMHA models liposomal clodronate significantly de-creases erythrocyte destruction,[138] and the compound seems to be well tolerated in dogs. The drug showed promise in early investigations but the efficacy of liposomal clodronate in canine IMHA is presently uncertain,[139] and although it can be purchased for research the drug is not available for medical use.

Melatonin is a hormone released from the pineal gland in response to day-night cy-cles. The hormone serves to control circadian rhythms and regulate sleep and wake-fulness. Melatonin may also have other effects including immunomodulation,[140] which has prompted investigations of its use in human immune-mediated thrombocyto-penia,[141] and IMHA,[142] with mixed results. Melatonin can be purchased as an over-the-counter supplement and anecdotally some veterinary criticalists are using it clin-ically. However, a recent study suggests that oral melatonin therapy does not signif-icantly affect interleukin 2 or interferon gamma expression in healthy dogs,[143] and presently there are no published reports of melatonin use in management of canine IMHA.

The severe anemia in dogs with IMHA can lead to tissue hypoxia due to severe reductions in blood oxygen content. Using a specialized chamber to increase the external environmental pressure, HBOT delivers oxygen at supraatmospheric pressure, thereby dramatically increasing the partial pressure of oxygen dissolved in plasma to enhance tissue oxygen delivery.[144] In addition, immunomodulatory effects are proposed for this modality.[145] Systematic reviews in people suggest HBOT has a role to play in the supportive treatment of severe anemia.[146] One case report of the use of HBOT in a person with autoimmune hemolytic anemia exists,[147] and anecdotally, HBOT has been suggested as a viable adjunctive therapy in canine IMHA patients. However, there are no published reports of the use of HBOT in canine IMHA.

TPE is the emerging therapy that holds the most promise. This extracorporeal therapy aims to remove high-molecular-weight compounds from the circulation by continuous flow centrifugation or membrane filtration. Centrifugation-based TPE requires very specialized equipment that is rare in veterinary medicine. Membrane filtration is much more widely available because it employs equipment typically used for renal replacement therapies. Membrane-based TPE involves filtration of blood through a large-pore hollow-fiber plasma separator to retain only the cellular elements of blood while removing the plasma. Replacement fluids including fresh-frozen plasma, albumin, cryopoor plasma, synthetic colloids, and crystalloids are used to reconstitute the filtered red cells before returning the blood to the patient.[148] This process rapidly reduces plasma antibody levels and hence may aid in the short-term stabilization of the acute, severe IMHA patient. In people, therapeutic plasmapheresis is typically used in patients with fulminant and refractory autoimmune hemolytic anemia in an attempt to attain temporary stabilization.[149] Various case reports have been published on TPE for immune-mediated diseases in small animals, including 3 on IMHA.[150–152] The efficacy of TPE in these dogs is hard to establish, however, because all were receiving other therapies simultaneously. Additional anecdotal reports suggest that TPE may reduce the degree of autoagglutination and the need for transfusion in dogs with severe IMHA.[5] Much more work needs to be done in this area, but it seems likely that this approach will become an important part of the management strategy for canine IMHA in the coming years.

NOVEL THERAPIES AND FUTURE DIRECTIONS

Various novel immunotherapies are in development for the management of immune-mediated and neoplastic diseases in dogs.[153,154] Some of these therapies may provide new treatment options for canine IMHA in the future. The furthest advanced of these are medications targeting B-cell populations. The treatment of people with glucocorticoid-resistant autoimmune hemolytic anemia involves administration of rituximab, a chimeric anti-CD20 monoclonal antibody.[155,156] Monoclonal antibodies offer the potential to target one specific aspect of the immune system while preserving other elements of host immunity. Rituximab binds the cell surface CD20 expressed on B-lymphocytes leading to complement and antibody-mediated cytotoxicity and the specific depletion of B-cells throughout the body.[157] Unfortunately, rituximab is highly specific for human CD20. Because of variations in the extracellular domain between dogs and people, the drug does not bind canine CD20, precluding its use in dogs.[158] A caninized Mab against CD20 was developed by Aratana Pharmaceuticals and 2 preliminary studies presented in 2014 seemed to suggest efficacy in dogs with B-cell lymphoma.[154] The drug (Blontress) was licensed by the FDA in 2015, but it is currently unavailable because the company has stated it is not as specific to the CD20 target as expected.[159] Aratana was recently acquired by Elanco,[160] which along with Kindred Biosciences are reportedly working on alternative canine anti-CD20 monoclonal antibodies for canine lymphoma.[161]

In its most severe intravascular form, erythrocytes are lysed in the bloodstream, which is profoundly inflammatory. Intravascular hemolysis is mediated by activation of the complement system culminating in the formation of the membrane attack complex (C5b-9). In the human disease paroxysmal nocturnal hemoglobinuria (PNH) uncontrolled complement activation results in episodic intravascular hemolysis.[162,163] Management of PNH now successfully uses pharmaceutical complement inhibitors.[164] Although the pathophysiology of PNH and intravascular canine IMHA are distinct, they both result in complement-mediated hemolysis, suggesting that complement inhibition might effectively treat canine IMHA. In vitro investigations suggest that C1 esterase inhibitor (C1-INH) prevents canine complement-mediated hemolysis.[165] The safety and pharmacokinetics of a commercial formulation of C1-INH have been evaluated in dogs.[166] Data from transplantation studies in dogs suggest that C1-INH protects against complement-mediated ischemia-reperfusion injury[167] and reduces endotoxin-induced pulmonary dysfunction and coagulation activation.[168] C1-INH has also been used successfully in people to manage autoimmune hemolytic anemia.[169,170] These data suggest that C1-INH might be an effective treatment of canine IMHA, and an interventional trial to test this hypothesis is now underway.[171]

Looking to the future, additional prospective, randomized, multicenter clinical trials will be necessary to determine key questions in the management of canine IMHA. In particular, large trials will be needed to determine the comparative efficacy of second-line immunosuppressive drugs, to evaluate antithrombotic drug regimens, to determine the utility of therapeutic drug monitoring, and to evaluate the potential of novel therapies to augment existing treatments. In the interim, the recently published ACVIM guidelines will provide clinicians with guidance now while the much needed additional research is conducted. It is hoped that the future for canine IMHA patients is indeed bright.[172]

DISCLOSURE

The author declares he has no commercial or financial relationships that could be construed as a potential conflict of interest.

REFERENCES

1. Lewis RM, Schwartz RS, Gilmore CE. Autoimmune diseases in domestic animals. Ann N Y Acad Sci 1965;124(1):178–200.
2. Piek CJ, van Spil WE, Junius G, et al. Lack of evidence of a beneficial effect of azathioprine in dogs treated with prednisolone for idiopathic immune-mediated hemolytic anemia: a retrospective cohort study. BMC Vet Res 2011;7(1):15.
3. Swann JW, Skelly BJ. Systematic review of evidence relating to the treatment of immune-mediated hemolytic anemia in dogs. J Vet Intern Med 2013;27(1):1–9.
4. Garden OA, Kidd L, Mexas AM, et al. ACVIM consensus statement on the diagnosis of immune-mediated hemolytic anemia in dogs and cats. J Vet Intern Med 2019;33(2):313–34.
5. Swann JW, Garden OA, Fellman CL, et al. ACVIM consensus statement on the treatment of immune-mediated hemolytic anemia in dogs. J Vet Intern Med 2019;33(3):1141–72.

6. Corato A, Shen CR, Mazza G, et al. Proliferative responses of peripheral blood mononuclear cells from normal dogs and dogs with autoimmune haemolytic anaemia to red blood cell antigens. Vet Immunol Immunopathol 1997;59(3–4): 191–204.

7. Swann JW, Skelly BJ. Evaluation of immunosuppressive regimens for immune-mediated haemolytic anaemia: a retrospective study of 42 dogs. J Small Anim Pract 2011;52(7):353–8.

8. Wang A, Smith JR, Creevy KE. Treatment of canine idiopathic immune-mediated haemolytic anaemia with mycophenolate mofetil and glucocorticoids: 30 cases (2007 to 2011). J Small Anim Pract 2013;54(8):399–404.

9. Weinkle TK, Center SA, Randolph JF, et al. Evaluation of prognostic factors, survival rates, and treatment protocols for immune-mediated hemolytic anemia in dogs: 151 cases (1993-2002). J Am Vet Med Assoc 2005;226(11):1869–80.

10. Goggs R, Rishniw M. Developing randomized clinical trials to evaluate treatment effects in canine IMHA. J Vet Emerg Crit Care 2016;26(6):763–5.

11. Scott-Moncrieff JC, Treadwell NG, McCullough SM, et al. Hemostatic abnormalities in dogs with primary immune-mediated hemolytic anemia. J Am Anim Hosp Assoc 2001;37(3):220–7.

12. Carr AP, Panciera DL, Kidd L. Prognostic factors for mortality and thromboembolism in canine immune-mediated hemolytic anemia: a retrospective study of 72 dogs. J Vet Intern Med 2002;16(5):504–9.

13. Klein MK, Dow SW, Rosychuk RA. Pulmonary thromboembolism associated with immune-mediated hemolytic anemia in dogs: ten cases (1982-1987). J Am Vet Med Assoc 1989;195(2):246–50.

14. Goggs R, Blais MC, Brainard BM, et al. American College of Veterinary Emergency and Critical Care (ACVECC) Consensus on the Rational Use of Antithrombotics in Veterinary Critical Care (CURATIVE) guidelines: Small animal. J Vet Emerg Crit Care 2019;29(1):12–36.

15. deLaforcade A, Bacek L, Blais MC, et al. Consensus on the rational use of antithrombotics in veterinary critical care (CURATIVE): domain 1-defining populations at risk. J Vet Emerg Crit Care 2019;29(1):37–48.

16. Mellett AM, Nakamura RK, Bianco D. A prospective study of clopidogrel therapy in dogs with primary immune-mediated hemolytic anemia. J Vet Intern Med 2011;25(1):71–5.

17. Friedenberg SG, Buhrman G, Chdid L, et al. Evaluation of a DLA-79 allele associated with multiple immune-mediated diseases in dogs. Immunogenetics 2016; 68(3):205–17.

18. Kennedy LJ, Barnes A, Ollier WE, et al. Association of a common dog leucocyte antigen class II haplotype with canine primary immune-mediated haemolytic anaemia. Tissue Antigens 2006;68(6):502–8.

19. Swann JW, Woods K, Wu Y, et al. Characterisation of the Immunophenotype of Dogs with Primary Immune-Mediated Haemolytic Anaemia. PLoS One 2016; 11(12):e0168296.

20. Bauer N, Moritz A. Characterisation of changes in the haemostasis system in dogs with thrombosis. J Small Anim Pract 2013;54(3):129–36.

21. Bauer N, Eralp O, Moritz A. Reference intervals and method optimization for variables reflecting hypocoagulatory and hypercoagulatory states in dogs using the STA Compact (R) automated analyzer. J Vet Diagn Invest 2009;21(6): 803–14.

22. Wiinberg B, Jessen LR, Tarnow I, et al. Diagnosis and treatment of platelet hyperactivity in relation to thrombosis in dogs and cats. J Vet Emerg Crit Care 2012;22(1):42–58.

23. Jeffery U, Staber J, LeVine D. Using the laboratory to predict thrombosis in dogs: An achievable goal? Vet J 2016;215:10–20.

24. Andres M, Hostnik E, Green E, et al. Diagnostic utility of thoracic radiographs and abdominal ultrasound in canine immune-mediated hemolytic anemia. Can Vet J 2019;60(10):1065–71.

25. Hann L, Brown DC, King LG, et al. Effect of duration of packed red blood cell storage on morbidity and mortality in dogs after transfusion: 3,095 cases (2001-2010). J Vet Intern Med 2014;28(6):1830–7.

26. Maglaras CH, Koenig A, Bedard DL, et al. Retrospective evaluation of the effect of red blood cell product age on occurrence of acute transfusion-related complications in dogs: 210 cases (2010-2012). J Vet Emerg Crit Care 2017;27(1):108–20.

27. Thompson MF, Scott-Moncrieff JC, Brooks MB. Effect of a single plasma transfusion on thromboembolism in 13 dogs with primary immune-mediated hemolytic anemia. J Am Anim Hosp Assoc 2004;40(6):446–54.

28. Griebsch C, Arndt G, Kohn B. Evaluation of different prognostic markers in dogs with primary immune-mediated hemolytic anemia. Berl Munch Tierarztl Wochenschr 2010;123(3–4):160–8.

29. Spada E, Proverbio D, Vinals Florez LM, et al. Prevalence of naturally occurring antibodies against dog erythrocyte antigen 7 in a population of dog erythrocyte antigen 7-negative dogs from Spain and Italy. Am J Vet Res 2016;77(8):877–81.

30. Spada E, Proverbio D, Baggiani L, et al. Activity, specificity, and titer of naturally occurring canine anti-DEA 7 antibodies. J Vet Diagn Invest 2016;28(6):705–8.

31. Zaremba R, Brooks A, Thomovsky E. Transfusion medicine: an update on antigens, antibodies and serologic testing in dogs and cats. Top Companion Anim Med 2019;34:36–46.

32. Odunayo A, Garraway K, Rohrbach BW, et al. Incidence of incompatible crossmatch results in dogs admitted to a veterinary teaching hospital with no history of prior red blood cell transfusion. J Am Vet Med Assoc 2017;250(3):303–8.

33. Seth M, Jackson KV, Winzelberg S, et al. Comparison of gel column, card, and cartridge techniques for dog erythrocyte antigen 1.1 blood typing. Am J Vet Res 2012;73(2):213–9.

34. Spada E, Perego R, Vinals Florez LM, et al. Comparison of cross-matching method for detection of DEA 7 blood incompatibility. J Vet Diagn Invest 2018;30(6):911–6.

35. Guzman LR, Streeter E, Malandra A. Comparison of a commercial blood crossmatching kit to the standard laboratory method for establishing blood transfusion compatibility in dogs. J Vet Emerg Crit Care 2016;26(2):262–8.

36. Neiger R, Gaschen F, Jaggy A. Gastric mucosal lesions in dogs with acute intervertebral disc disease: characterization and effects of omeprazole or misoprostol. J Vet Intern Med 2000;14(1):33–6.

37. Dowdle SM, Joubert KE, Lambrechts NE, et al. The prevalence of subclinical gastroduodenal ulceration in Dachshunds with intervertebral disc prolapse. J S Afr Vet Assoc 2003;74(3):77–81.

38. Conn HO, Poynard T. Corticosteroids and peptic ulcer: meta-analysis of adverse events during steroid therapy. J Intern Med 1994;236(6):619–32.

39. Caplan A, Fett N, Rosenbach M, et al. Prevention and management of glucocorticoid-induced side effects: A comprehensive review: Gastrointestinal and endocrinologic side effects. J Am Acad Dermatol 2017;76(1):11–6.

40. Tolbert K, Bissett S, King A, et al. Efficacy of oral famotidine and 2 omeprazole formulations for the control of intragastric pH in dogs. J Vet Intern Med 2011; 25(1):47–54.

41. Tolbert MK, Odunayo A, Howell RS, et al. Efficacy of intravenous administration of combined acid suppressants in healthy dogs. J Vet Intern Med 2015;29(2): 556–60.

42. Miura M, Satoh S, Inoue K, et al. Influence of lansoprazole and rabeprazole on mycophenolic acid pharmacokinetics one year after renal transplantation. Ther Drug Monit 2008;30(1):46–51.

43. Bennett D, Finnett SL, Nash AS, et al. Primary autoimmune haemolytic anaemia in the dog. Vet Rec 1981;109(8):150–3.

44. Day MJ. Serial monitoring of clinical, haematological and immunological parameters in canine autoimmune haemolytic anaemia. J Small Anim Pract 1996; 37(11):523–34.

45. Schwendenwein I. The autoimmune hemolytic-anemia (AIHA) in dogs - A survey of the clinical picture, diagnosis and therapy of 8 cases. Wien Tierarztl Monatsschr 1988;75(4):121–7.

46. Reimer ME, Troy GC, Warnick LD. Immune-mediated hemolytic anemia: 70 cases (1988-1996). J Am Anim Hosp Assoc 1999;35(5):384–91.

47. Grundy SA, Barton C. Influence of drug treatment on survival of dogs with immune-mediated hemolytic anemia: 88 cases (1989-1999). J Am Vet Med Assoc 2001;218(4):543–6.

48. Gerber B, Steger A, Hassig M, et al. Use of human intravenous immunoglobulin in dogs with primary immunmediated hemolytic anemia. Schweiz Arch Tierheilkd 2002;144(4):180–5.

49. Mason N, Duval D, Shofer FS, et al. Cyclophosphamide exerts no beneficial effect over prednisone alone in the initial treatment of acute immune-mediated hemolytic anemia in dogs: a randomized controlled clinical trial. J Vet Intern Med 2003;17(2):206–12.

50. Whelan MF, O'Toole TE, Chan DL, et al. Use of human immunoglobulin in addition to glucocorticoids for the initial treatment of dogs with immune-mediated hemolytic anemia. J Vet Emerg Crit Care 2009;19(2):158–64.

51. Park S, Kim H, Kang B, et al. Prognostic factors and efficacy of human intravenous immunoglobulin G in dogs with idiopathic immune-mediated hemolytic anemia: a retrospective study. Korean J Vet Res 2016;56(3):139–45.

52. Swann JW, Szladovits B, Threlfall AJ, et al. Randomised controlled trial of fractionated and unfractionated prednisolone regimens for dogs with immune-mediated haemolytic anaemia. Vet Rec 2019;184(25):771.

53. Piek CJ. Canine idiopathic immune-mediated haemolytic anaemia: a review with recommendations for future research. Vet Q 2011;31(3):129–41.

54. Swann JW, Skelly BJ. Systematic review of prognostic factors for mortality in dogs with immune-mediated hemolytic anemia. J Vet Intern Med 2015; 29(1):7–13.

55. Goggs R, Dennis SG, Di Bella A, et al. Predicting outcome in dogs with primary immune-mediated hemolytic anemia: results of a multicenter case registry. J Vet Intern Med 2015;29(6):1603–10.

56. Gregory CR, Kyles AE, Bernsteen L, et al. Results of clinical renal transplantation in 15 dogs using triple drug immunosuppressive therapy. Vet Surg 2006; 35(2):105–12.
57. Hopper K, Mehl ML, Kass PH, et al. Outcome after renal transplantation in 26 dogs. Vet Surg 2012;41(3):316–27.
58. Whitley NT, Day MJ. Immunomodulatory drugs and their application to the management of canine immune-mediated disease. J Small Anim Pract 2011;52(2): 70–85.
59. Burgess K, Moore A, Rand W, et al. Treatment of immune-mediated hemolytic anemia in dogs with cyclophosphamide. J Vet Intern Med 2000;14(4):456–62.
60. Goggs R, Boag AK, Chan DL. Concurrent immune-mediated haemolytic anaemia and severe thrombocytopenia in 21 dogs. Vet Rec 2008;163(11): 323–7.
61. Piek CJ, Junius G, Dekker A, et al. Idiopathic immune-mediated hemolytic anemia: treatment outcome and prognostic factors in 149 dogs. J Vet Intern Med 2008;22(2):366–73.
62. Halloran PF. Molecular mechanisms of new immunosuppressants. Clin Transplant 1996;10(1 Pt 2):118–23.
63. Helmond SE, Polzin DJ, Armstrong PJ, et al. Treatment of immune-mediated hemolytic anemia with individually adjusted heparin dosing in dogs. J Vet Intern Med 2010;24(3):597–605.
64. Morassi A, Bianco D, Park E, et al. Evaluation of the safety and tolerability of rivaroxaban in dogs with presumed primary immune-mediated hemolytic anemia. J Vet Emerg Crit Care 2016;26(4):488–94.
65. Panek CM, Nakamura RK, Bianco D. Use of enoxaparin in dogs with primary immune-mediated hemolytic anemia: 21 cases. J Vet Emerg Crit Care 2015; 25(2):273–7.
66. Husbands B, Polzin D, Armstrong PJ, et al. Prednisone and cyclosporine vs. prednisone alone for treatment of canine immune mediated hemolytic anemia (IMHA). J Vet Intern Med 2004;18(3):389.
67. Bachtel JC, Pendergraft JS, Rosychuk RA, et al. Comparison of the stability and pharmacokinetics in dogs of modified ciclosporin capsules stored at -20 degrees C and room temperature. Vet Dermatol 2015;26(4):228.e50.
68. Allison AC, Eugui EM. Mycophenolate mofetil and its mechanisms of action. Immunopharmacology 2000;47(2–3):85–118.
69. Hedstrom L. IMP dehydrogenase: structure, mechanism, and inhibition. Chem Rev 2009;109(7):2903–28.
70. Klotsman M, Sathyan G, Anderson WH, et al. Mycophenolic acid in patients with immune-mediated inflammatory diseases: From humans to dogs. J Vet Pharmacol Ther 2019;42(2):127–38.
71. West LD, Hart JR. Treatment of idiopathic immune-mediated hemolytic anemia with mycophenolate mofetil in five dogs. J Vet Emerg Crit Care 2014;24(2): 226–31.
72. Oggier D, Tomsa K, Mevissen M, et al. Efficacy of the combination of glucocorticoids, mycophenolate-mofetil and human immunoglobulin for the therapy of immune mediated haemolytic anaemia in dogs. Schweiz Arch Tierheilkd 2018; 160(3):171–8.
73. Yau VK, Bianco D. Treatment of five haemodynamically stable dogs with immune-mediated thrombocytopenia using mycophenolate mofetil as single agent. J Small Anim Pract 2014;55(6):330–3.

74. Link M, Dorsch R. Therapy of immune-mediated haemolytic anaemia in the dog using human immunoglobulin. Tierarztl Prax Ausg K Kleintiere Heimtiere 2001; 29(4):229–33.

75. Kellerman DL, Bruyette DS. Intravenous human immunoglobulin for the treatment of immune-mediated hemolytic anemia in 13 dogs. J Vet Intern Med 1997;11(6):327–32.

76. Scott-Moncrieff JC, Reagan WJ, Snyder PW, et al. Intravenous administration of human immune globulin in dogs with immune-mediated hemolytic anemia. J Am Vet Med Assoc 1997;210(11):1623–7.

77. Feldman BF, Handagama P, Lubberink AA. Splenectomy as adjunctive therapy for immune-mediated thrombocytopenia and hemolytic anemia in the dog. J Am Vet Med Assoc 1985;187(6):617–9.

78. Horgan JE, Roberts BK, Schermerhorn T. Splenectomy as an adjunctive treatment for dogs with immune-mediated hemolytic anemia: ten cases (2003-2006). J Vet Emerg Crit Care 2009;19(3):254–61.

79. Brainard BM, Buriko Y, Good J, et al. Consensus on the rational use of antithrombotics in veterinary critical care (CURATIVE): domain 5-discontinuation of anticoagulant therapy in small animals. J Vet Emerg Crit Care 2019;29(1):88–97.

80. Archer TM, Boothe DM, Langston VC, et al. Oral cyclosporine treatment in dogs: a review of the literature. J Vet Intern Med 2014;28(1):1–20.

81. Fellman CL, Archer TM, Stokes JV, et al. Effects of oral cyclosporine on canine T-cell expression of IL-2 and IFN-gamma across a 12-h dosing interval. J Vet Pharmacol Ther 2016;39(3):237–44.

82. Langman LJ, Shapiro AM, Lakey JR, et al. Pharmacodynamic assessment of mycophenolic acid-induced immunosuppression by measurement of inosine monophosphate dehydrogenase activity in a canine model. Transplantation 1996;61(1):87–92.

83. Guzera M, Szulc-Dabrowska L, Cywinska A, et al. In vitro influence of mycophenolic acid on selected parameters of stimulated peripheral canine lymphocytes. PLoS One 2016;11(5):e0154429.

84. Grobman M, Boothe DM, Rindt H, et al. Pharmacokinetics and dynamics of mycophenolate mofetil after single-dose oral administration in juvenile dachshunds. J Vet Pharmacol Ther 2017;40(6):e1–10.

85. de Laforcade A. Diseases associated with thrombosis. Top Companion Anim Med 2012;27(2):59–64.

86. Laurenson MP, Hopper K, Herrera MA, et al. Concurrent diseases and conditions in dogs with splenic vein thrombosis. J Vet Intern Med 2010;24(6): 1298–304.

87. Respess M, O'Toole TE, Taeymans O, et al. Portal vein thrombosis in 33 dogs: 1998-2011. J Vet Intern Med 2012;26(2):230–7.

88. Vanwinkle TJ, Bruce E. Thrombosis of the portal-vein in 11 dogs. Vet Pathol 1993;30(1):28–35.

89. Bunch SE, Metcalf MR, Crane SW, et al. Idiopathic pleural effusion and pulmonary thromboembolism in a dog with autoimmune hemolytic anemia. J Am Vet Med Assoc 1989;195(12):1748–53.

90. Johnson LR, Lappin MR, Baker DC. Pulmonary thromboembolism in 29 dogs: 1985-1995. J Vet Intern Med 1999;13(4):338–45.

91. McManus PM, Craig LE. Correlation between leukocytosis and necropsy findings in dogs with immune-mediated hemolytic anemia: 34 cases (1994-1999). J Am Vet Med Assoc 2001;218(8):1308–13.

92. Flint S, Abrams-Ogg A, Kruth S, et al. Thromboelastography in dogs with immune-mediated hemolytic anemia treated with prednisone, azathioprine and low-dose aspirin. J Vet Intern Med 2010;24(3):681.

93. Flint SK, Abrams-Ogg ACG, Kruth SA, et al. Independent and combined effects of prednisone and acetylsalicylic acid on thromboelastography variables in healthy dogs. Am J Vet Res 2011;72(10):1325–32.

94. Spurlock NK, Prittie JE. A review of current indications, adverse effects, and administration recommendations for intravenous immunoglobulin. J Vet Emerg Crit Care 2011;21(5):471–83.

95. Tsuchiya R, Akutsu Y, Ikegami A, et al. Prothrombotic and inflammatory effects of intravenous administration of human immunoglobulin G in dogs. J Vet Intern Med 2009;23(6):1164–9.

96. Bateman SW, Mathews KA, Abrams-Ogg AC, et al. Diagnosis of disseminated intravascular coagulation in dogs admitted to an intensive care unit. J Am Vet Med Assoc 1999;215(6):798–804.

97. Wiinberg B, Jensen AL, Johansson PI, et al. Thromboelastographic evaluation of hemostatic function in dogs with disseminated intravascular coagulation. J Vet Intern Med 2008;22(2):357–65.

98. Kidd L, Mackman N. Prothrombotic mechanisms and anticoagulant therapy in dogs with immune-mediated hemolytic anemia. J Vet Emerg Crit Care 2013; 23(1):3–13.

99. Kjelgaard-Hansen M, Goggs R, Wiinberg B, et al. Use of serum concentrations of interleukin-18 and monocyte chemoattractant protein-1 as prognostic indicators in primary immune-mediated hemolytic anemia in dogs. J Vet Intern Med 2011;25(1):76–82.

100. Piek CJ, Brinkhof B, Teske E, et al. High intravascular tissue factor expression in dogs with idiopathic immune-mediated haemolytic anaemia. Vet Immunol Immunopathol 2011;144(3–4):346–54.

101. Kidd L, Geddings J, Hisada Y, et al. Procoagulant microparticles in dogs with immune-mediated hemolytic anemia. J Vet Intern Med 2015;29(3):908–16.

102. Fenty RK, Delaforcade AM, Shaw SE, et al. Identification of hypercoagulability in dogs with primary immune-mediated hemolytic anemia by means of thromboelastography. J Am Vet Med Assoc 2011;238(4):463–7.

103. Goggs R, Wiinberg B, Kjelgaard-Hansen M, et al. Serial assessment of the coagulation status of dogs with immune-mediated haemolytic anaemia using thromboelastography. Vet J 2012;191(3):347–53.

104. Weiss DJ, Brazzell JL. Detection of activated platelets in dogs with primary immune-mediated hemolytic anemia. J Vet Intern Med 2006;20(3):682–6.

105. Jeffery U, LeVine DN. Canine neutrophil extracellular traps enhance clot formation and delay lysis. Vet Pathol 2018;55(1):116–23.

106. Lawson C, Smith SA, O'Brien M, et al. Neutrophil extracellular traps in plasma from dogs with immune-mediated hemolytic anemia. J Vet Intern Med 2018; 32(1):128–34.

107. Jeffery U, Ruterbories L, Hanel R, et al. Cell-Free DNA and DNase activity in dogs with immune-mediated hemolytic anemia. J Vet Intern Med 2017;31(5): 1441–50.

108. Jeffery U, Kimura K, Gray R, et al. Dogs cast NETs too: Canine neutrophil extracellular traps in health and immune-mediated hemolytic anemia. Vet Immunol Immunopathol 2015;168(3–4):262–8.

109. Goggs R, Bacek L, Bianco D, et al. Consensus on the Rational Use of Antithrombotics in Veterinary Critical Care (CURATIVE): Domain 2-Defining rational therapeutic usage. J Vet Emerg Crit Care 2019;29(1):49–59.

110. Aird WC. Vascular bed-specific thrombosis. J Thromb Haemost 2007;5283–91. https://doi.org/10.1111/j.1538-7836.2007.02515.x.

111. Mackman N. New insights into the mechanisms of venous thrombosis. J Clin Invest 2012;122(7):2331–6.

112. Ridgeon EE, Young PJ, Bellomo R, et al. The fragility index in multicenter randomized controlled critical care trials. Crit Care Med 2016;44(7):1278–84.

113. Green RA. Activated coagulation time in monitoring heparinized dogs. Am J Vet Res 1980;41(11):1793–7.

114. Hellebrekers LJ, Slappendel RJ, van den Brom WE. Effect of sodium heparin and antithrombin III concentration on activated partial thromboplastin time in the dog. Am J Vet Res 1985;46(7):1460–2.

115. Mischke R. Heparin in vitro sensitivity of the activated partial thromboplastin time in canine plasma depends on reagent. J Vet Diagn Invest 2003;15(6): 588–91.

116. Babski DM, Brainard BM, Ralph AG, et al. Sonoclot(R) evaluation of single- and multiple-dose subcutaneous unfractionated heparin therapy in healthy adult dogs. J Vet Intern Med 2012;26(3):631–8.

117. Jessen LR, Wiinberg B, Jensen AL, et al. In vitro heparinization of canine whole blood with low molecular weight heparin (dalteparin) significantly and dose-dependently prolongs heparinase-modified tissue factor-activated thromboelastography parameters and prothrombinase-induced clotting time. Vet Clin Pathol 2008;37(4):363–72.

118. Lynch AM, deLaforcade AM, Sharp CR. Clinical experience of anti-Xa monitoring in critically ill dogs receiving dalteparin. J Vet Emerg Crit Care 2014; 24(4):421–8.

119. McLaughlin CM, Marks SL, Dorman DC, et al. Thromboelastographic monitoring of the effect of unfractionated heparin in healthy dogs. J Vet Emerg Crit Care 2017;27(1):71–81.

120. Pouzot-Nevoret C, Barthelemy A, Cluzel M, et al. Enoxaparin has no significant anticoagulation activity in healthy Beagles at a dose of 0.8 mg/kg four times daily. Vet J 2016;210:98–100.

121. Allegret V, Dunn M, Bedard C. Monitoring unfractionated heparin therapy in dogs by measuring thrombin generation. Vet Clin Pathol 2011;40(1):24–31.

122. Gara-Boivin C, Del Castillo JRE, Dunn ME, et al. Effect of dalteparin administration on thrombin generation kinetics in healthy dogs. Vet Clin Pathol 2017;46(2): 269–77.

123. Hanel RM, Birkenheuer AJ, Hansen B, et al. Thromboelastography or activated partial thromboplastin time for heparin anticoagulation to prevent thrombosis: the TOPHATT trial. J Vet Emerg Crit Care 2017;27(S1):S4.

124. Sharp CR, deLaforcade AM, Koenigshof AM, et al. Consensus on the Rational Use of Antithrombotics in Veterinary Critical Care (CURATIVE): Domain 4-Refining and monitoring antithrombotic therapies. J Vet Emerg Crit Care 2019; 29(1):75–87.

125. Lunsford KV, Mackin AJ, Langston VC, et al. Pharmacokinetics of subcutaneous low molecular weight heparin (enoxaparin) in dogs. J Am Anim Hosp Assoc 2009;45(6):261–7.

126. Mestre M, Clairefond P, Mardiguian J, et al. Comparative effects of heparin and PK 10169, a low molecular weight fraction, in a canine model of arterial thrombosis. Thromb Res 1985;38(4):389–99.

127. Morris TA, Marsh JJ, Konopka R, et al. Anti-thrombotic efficacies of enoxaparin, dalteparin, and unfractionated heparin in venous thrombo-embolism. Thromb Res 2000;100(3):185–94.

128. Blais MC, Bianco D, Goggs R, et al. Consensus on the Rational Use of Antithrombotics in Veterinary Critical Care (CURATIVE): Domain 3-Defining antithrombotic protocols. J Vet Emerg Crit Care 2019;29(1):60–74.

129. Brainard BM, Kleine SA, Papich MG, et al. Pharmacodynamic and pharmacokinetic evaluation of clopidogrel and the carboxylic acid metabolite SR 26334 in healthy dogs. Am J Vet Res 2010;71(7):822–30.

130. Borgarelli M, Lanz O, Pavlisko N, et al. Mitral valve repair in dogs using an ePTFE chordal implantation device: a pilot study. J Vet Cardiol 2017;19(3): 256–67.

131. Hasa AA, Schmaier AH, Warnock M, et al. Thrombostatin inhibits cyclic flow variations in stenosed canine coronary arteries. Thromb Haemost 2001;86(5): 1296–304.

132. van Giezen JJ, Berntsson P, Zachrisson H, et al. Comparison of ticagrelor and thienopyridine P2Y(12) binding characteristics and antithrombotic and bleeding effects in rat and dog models of thrombosis/hemostasis. Thromb Res 2009; 124(5):565–71.

133. Bjorkman JA, Zachrisson H, Forsberg GB, et al. High-dose aspirin in dogs increases vascular resistance with limited additional anti-platelet effect when combined with potent P2Y12 inhibition. Thromb Res 2013;131(4):313–9.

134. Dudley A, Thomason J, Fritz S, et al. Cyclooxygenase expression and platelet function in healthy dogs receiving low-dose aspirin. J Vet Intern Med 2013; 27(1):141–9.

135. Sharpe KS, Center SA, Randolph JF, et al. Influence of treatment with ultralow-dose aspirin on platelet aggregation as measured by whole blood impedance aggregometry and platelet P-selectin expression in clinically normal dogs. Am J Vet Res 2010;71(11):1294–304.

136. Whittemore J, Mooney A, Mawby D, et al. Platelet function and endoscopic changes after clopidogrel, aspirin, prednisone, or combination therapy in dogs. J Vet Intern Med 2017;31:1282.

137. van Rooijen N, van Nieuwmegen R. Elimination of phagocytic cells in the spleen after intravenous injection of liposome-encapsulated dichloromethylene diphosphonate. An enzyme-histochemical study. Cell Tissue Res 1984;238(2): 355–8.

138. Jordan MB, van Rooijen N, Izui S, et al. Liposomal clodronate as a novel agent for treating autoimmune hemolytic anemia in a mouse model. Blood 2003; 101(2):594–601.

139. Mathes M, Jordan M, Dow S. Evaluation of liposomal clodronate in experimental spontaneous autoimmune hemolytic anemia in dogs. Exp Hematol 2006;34(10): 1393–402.

140. Carrillo-Vico A, Reiter RJ, Lardone PJ, et al. The modulatory role of melatonin on immune responsiveness. Curr Opin Investig Drugs 2006;7(5):423–31.

141. Todisco M, Rossi N. Melatonin for refractory idiopathic thrombocytopenic purpura: a report of 3 cases. Am J Ther 2002;9(6):524–6.

142. Posadzki PP, Bajpai R, Kyaw BM, et al. Melatonin and health: an umbrella review of health outcomes and biological mechanisms of action. BMC Med 2018; 16(1):18.

143. Peace AC, Kumar S, Wills R, et al. Pharmacodynamic evaluation of the effects of oral melatonin on expression of the T-cell cytokines interleukin-2 and interferon gamma in the dog. J Vet Pharmacol Ther 2019;42(3):278–84.

144. Edwards ML. Hyperbaric oxygen therapy. Part 1: history and principles. J Vet Emerg Crit Care 2010;20(3):284–8.

145. Edwards ML. Hyperbaric oxygen therapy. Part 2: application in disease. J Vet Emerg Crit Care 2010;20(3):289–97.

146. Van Meter KW. A systematic review of the application of hyperbaric oxygen in the treatment of severe anemia: an evidence-based approach. Undersea Hyperb Med 2005;32(1):61–83.

147. Myking O, Schreiner A. Hyperbaric oxygen in hemolytic crisis. JAMA 1974; 227(10):1161–2.

148. Francey T, Schweighauser A. Membrane-based therapeutic plasma exchange in dogs: Prescription, anticoagulation, and metabolic response. J Vet Intern Med 2019;33(4):1635–45.

149. Padmanabhan A, Connelly-Smith L, Aqui N, et al. Guidelines on the Use of Therapeutic Apheresis in Clinical Practice - Evidence-Based Approach from the Writing Committee of the American Society for Apheresis: the eighth special issue. J Clin Apher 2019;34(3):171–354.

150. Crump KL, Seshadri R. Use of therapeutic plasmapheresis in a case of canine immune-mediated hemolytic anemia. J Vet Emerg Crit Care 2009;19(4):375–80.

151. Scagnelli AM, Walton SA, Liu CC, et al. Effects of therapeutic plasma exchange on serum immunoglobulin concentrations in a dog with refractory immune-mediated hemolytic anemia. J Am Vet Med Assoc 2018;252(9):1108–12.

152. Heffner GG, Cavanagh A, Nolan B. Successful management of acute bilirubin encephalopathy in a dog with immune-mediated hemolytic anemia using therapeutic plasma exchange. J Vet Emerg Crit Care 2019;29(5):549–57.

153. Swann JW, Garden OA. Novel immunotherapies for immune-mediated haemolytic anaemia in dogs and people. Vet J 2016;207:13–9.

154. Regan D, Guth A, Coy J, et al. Cancer immunotherapy in veterinary medicine: Current options and new developments. Vet J 2016;207:20–8.

155. Zaja F, Iacona I, Masolini P, et al. B-cell depletion with rituximab as treatment for immune hemolytic anemia and chronic thrombocytopenia. Haematologica 2002; 87(2):189–95.

156. Reynaud Q, Durieu I, Dutertre M, et al. Efficacy and safety of rituximab in autoimmune hemolytic anemia: A meta-analysis of 21 studies. Autoimmun Rev 2015; 14(4):304–13.

157. Reff ME, Carner K, Chambers KS, et al. Depletion of B cells in vivo by a chimeric mouse human monoclonal antibody to CD20. Blood 1994;83(2):435–45.

158. Jubala CM, Wojcieszyn JW, Valli VE, et al. CD20 expression in normal canine B cells and in canine non-Hodgkin lymphoma. Vet Pathol 2005;42(4):468–76.

159. Aratana. Aratana therapeutics provides product updates. 2015. Available at: https://aratana.investorroom.com/2015-09-24-Aratana-Therapeutics-Provides-Product-Updates. Accessed January 11, 2020.

160. Aratana. Aratana Therapeutics to be Acquired by Elanco Animal Health. 2019. Available at: https://aratana.investorroom.com/2019-04-26-Aratana-Therapeutics-to-be-Acquired-by-Elanco-Animal-Health. Accessed January 11, 2020.

161. Rue SM, Eckelman BP, Efe JA, et al. Identification of a candidate therapeutic antibody for treatment of canine B-cell lymphoma. Vet Immunol Immunopathol 2015;164(3–4):148–59.
162. Brodsky RA. Complement in hemolytic anemia. Hematology Am Soc Hematol Educ Program 2015;126(22):2459–65.
163. Brodsky RA. Paroxysmal nocturnal hemoglobinuria. Blood 2014;124(18): 2804–11.
164. Hillmen P, Muus P, Duhrsen U, et al. Effect of the complement inhibitor eculizumab on thromboembolism in patients with paroxysmal nocturnal hemoglobinuria. Blood 2007;110(12):4123–8.
165. Hernandez DM, Goggs R, Behling-Kelly E. In vitro Inhibition of Canine Complement-Mediated Hemolysis. J Vet Intern Med 2018;32(1):142–6.
166. Wong C, Muguiro DH, Lavergne S, et al. Pharmacokinetics of human recombinant C1-esterase inhibitor and development of anti-drug antibodies in healthy dogs. Vet Immunol Immunopathol 2018;203:20366–72.
167. Salvatierra A, Velasco F, Rodriguez M, et al. C1-esterase inhibitor prevents early pulmonary dysfunction after lung transplantation in the dog. Am J Respir Crit Care Med 1997;155(3):1147–54.
168. Guerrero R, Velasco F, Rodriguez M, et al. Endotoxin-induced pulmonary dysfunction is prevented by C1-esterase inhibitor. J Clin Invest 1993;91(6): 2754–60.
169. Wouters D, Stephan F, Strengers P, et al. C1-esterase inhibitor concentrate rescues erythrocytes from complement-mediated destruction in autoimmune hemolytic anemia. Blood 2013;121(7):1242–4.
170. Berentsen S, Sundic T. Red blood cell destruction in autoimmune hemolytic anemia: role of complement and potential new targets for therapy. Biomed Res Int 2015;2015:363278.
171. Goggs R, Behling-Kelly E. C1 inhibitor in canine intravascular hemolysis (C1INCH): study protocol for a randomized controlled trial. BMC Vet Res 2019;15(1):475.
172. Mizuno T. A brighter future for dogs with immune-mediated haemolytic anaemia. Vet J 2016;209:1–2.

The Use of Antithrombotics in Critical Illness

Alexandra Pfaff, MedVet, Armelle M. de Laforcade, DVM,
Elizabeth A. Rozanski, DVM*

KEYWORDS

- Anticoagulant • Antiplatelet agent • Cats • Dogs • Therapeutic monitoring
- Low molecular weight heparin • Anti -Xa inhibitor

KEY POINTS

- Despite growing awareness of the importance of hypercoagulability and thrombosis, there is limited evidence for anticoagulation protocols for dogs and cats with critical illness.
- Immune-mediated hemolytic anemia, protein-losing nephropathy, severe/necrotizing pancreatitis, and feline cardiomyopathy are associated with a high risk of thromboembolic complications, and routine anticoagulation is recommended.
- Corticosteroid administration, hyperadrenocorticism, neoplasia, and sepsis are associated with a low to moderate risk for thromboembolic complications. Routine anticoagulation should be considered in cases in which hypercoagulability is demonstrated, or where other risk factors for thrombosis exist.
- The administration of anticoagulant medications seems most prudent in patients with venous thromboembolism, whereas antiplatelet agents are indicated in arterial thrombosis. Combination therapy is reasonable in patients with a high risk of thrombosis.
- Therapeutic drug monitoring is a valuable tool for safe and effective anticoagulant drug therapy, but is not always easily available.

INTRODUCTION

Coagulation abnormalities are commonly encountered in critical illness. Traditionally, these disorders have mostly been viewed as bleeding disorders associated with advanced stages of disseminated intravascular coagulation (DIC).[1,2] It is recognized that early (occult) DIC is associated with hypercoagulability, and additionally certain disease states (eg, immune-mediated hemolytic anemia) may be more commonly associated with a tendency toward the formation of clots.[3–5] In recent years, growing awareness of hypercoagulability and thrombosis as contributors to multiple diseases in veterinary medicine has led to a plethora of publications culminating in the creation of the CURATIVE guidelines that provide evidence-based guidelines for anticoagulation/antithrombotic uses in dogs and cats.[6]

Tufts University, Cummings School of Veterinary Medicine, 200 Westboro Road, North Grafton, MA 01536, USA
* Corresponding author.
E-mail address: Elizabeth.Rozanski@tufts.edu

Vet Clin Small Anim 50 (2020) 1351–1370
https://doi.org/10.1016/j.cvsm.2020.07.011
0195-5616/20/© 2020 Elsevier Inc. All rights reserved.

This article aimed to explore the human recommendation, the CURATIVE guidelines, as well as further information about the pathophysiology of hypercoagulability in critical illness and, finally, a brief overview of the available therapeutic agents.

Pathophysiology of Hypercoagulability in Critical Illness

Historically, hemorrhage associated with DIC has been considered the biggest threat affecting the coagulation system during critical illness, because the development of microthrombosis and macrothrombosis will worsen blood flow to vital organs, perpetuate acidosis, and promote organ failure.[7-9] In the past 2 decades, an increasing number of research and publications on coagulation with new information has allowed for the introduction of a new model of hemostasis. In 2001, Hoffman and Monroe[10] introduced the cell-based model of hemostasis, which emphasizes the importance of tissue factor (TF)-bearing cells and platelets in normal hemostasis.[11] It is a dynamic model that describes the activation of hemostasis in 3 phases: initiation, amplification, and propagation. Research has confirmed the key role of TF in the initiation of hemostasis and has also shown that TF-bearing cells and activated platelets act as the main cellular surfaces for assembly of the procoagulant complexes.[11,12]

Systemic inflammation has been found to be a potent trigger of coagulation. Recent and ongoing research shows a close link between inflammation, the innate immune system, and the hemostatic system.[5,10] This is mainly created through cytokine-mediated TF expression on the surface of activated inflammatory cells and the damaged vascular endothelium. In addition, in inflammatory or pathologic states, monocytes, endothelium, and platelets express TF, which perpetuates the process of thrombin production, which is a very potent platelet activator.[11,13-15]

This new knowledge allows for a new understanding of the key role platelets have in the etiology of hypercoagulable states and thromboembolic disease. Following endothelial injury, platelets bind to the exposed subendothelial collagen. Platelet binding initiates platelet activation and further binding. Activation results in the release of ADP and serotonin that further assist in platelet activation and recruitment. The arachidonic acid cascade results in synthesis of inflammatory mediators (such as thromboxane A2). The platelet fibrinogen receptor glycoprotein (GP)IIb-IIIa becomes activated and crosslinks fibrinogen into a stable clot.[16]

Damaged red cells, activated platelets, and small cell-derived membrane vesicles called microparticles may contribute to coagulation by providing membrane surfaces that serve as docking sites for prothrombinase (factor Va–factor Xa) and tenase (factor VIIIa–factor IXa) complexes of the coagulation cascade. Some microparticles also contain TF, which further activates coagulation.[17]

In addition to excessive activation of the procoagulant pathways during systemic inflammation, endogenous anticoagulant systems such as protein C, antithrombin, and TF pathway inhibitor are simultaneously activated to control coagulation but are ultimately overwhelmed when severe systemic inflammation predominates, leading to fibrin deposition in the microvasculature and reduced oxygen delivery to capillary beds. This clinically silent phenomenon may be only be identifiable by a mildly reduced platelet count on the complete blood count.[17]

Thrombosis can occur in either arteries or veins. Some diseases also result in a generalized microvascular thrombosis.[17-19] As inflammation continues and consumptive mechanisms play a larger role, the initial hypercoagulability commonly transitions into a global hypocoagulable state. This dilemma makes the decision for anticoagulation therapy even more challenging, as early introduction of anticoagulants may prevent transition to overt DIC, but introducing anticoagulants/antiplatelet therapy too late may magnify hemorrhage.

THE HUMAN EXPERIENCE

The American College of Chest Physicians (ACCP) provides a frequently updated set of guidelines for the prevention and management of thrombotic disorders in people.[20,21] Certain guidelines cannot be extrapolated to dogs and cats because of differences in disease processes and lack of availability of certain interventions. For the purpose of this article, we focused on the recommendations that might be applicable for our patient population.

The CHEST grading system considers the balance of risks and benefits as well as the level of evidence supporting their recommendations. Recommendations are strong when benefits clearly outweigh risks and are labeled as "we recommend." When benefits and risks are closely balanced and additional research might change the direction or recommendation, it is considered weak evidence, and is labeled as "we suggest."[22]

VENOUS THROMBOEMBOLISM

In people, venous thromboembolism (VTE) is typically divided into deep-vein thrombosis (DVT) and pulmonary thromboembolism (PTE). The major key difference between small animals and people is that most human thrombotic disease is associated with the development of DVT. DVT is uncommon in dogs and cats. In veterinary patients that develop PTE, it is usually unclear if the thrombus developed "in situ" or indicates embolism that has traveled from distant vasculature. Splenic and portal vein thrombosis on the other hand are well-described in dogs and cats, and likely share some of the same pathophysiology as DVT.[21]

In patients with a high clinical suspicion of acute VTE, the ACCP **suggests** initiation of treatment with parenteral anticoagulants while awaiting the results of diagnostic tests while treatment should not be initiated for patients with low index of suspicion until confirmatory testing is completed.

In patients with VTE, the ACCP in the latest update of their guidelines **recommends** anticoagulant therapy for 3 months and **suggests** the use of Factor Xa inhibitor or thrombin inhibitors over vitamin K antagonist (eg, warfarin) therapy. In people with VTE associated with cancer, the ACCP **suggests** low molecular weight heparin (LMWH) over other anticoagulants. Those patients should be treated indefinitely.[20,21]

People with an unprovoked VTE (eg, not associated with surgery or prolonged bed rest) should be reevaluated after 3 months to assess the risk-benefit ratio of extended therapy. In patients with a first VTE and who have a low or moderate bleeding risk, the ACCP **suggests** indefinite anticoagulant therapy. For patients with a first VTE and a high bleeding risk, discontinuation of anticoagulant therapy after 3 months is **recommended.** In patients with recurrent VTE, indefinite therapy is **suggested** even in the face of a moderate to high bleeding risk. The same applies to patients with active cancer.

In patients with VTE who are stopping anticoagulant therapy the ACCP **suggests** long-term aspirin therapy unless there is a contraindication. Aspirin is not considered an alternative to anticoagulant therapy but is considered preferable to no therapy to prevent recurrence.[20,21]

PULMONARY THROMBOEMBOLISM

Advances in computed tomography (CT) pulmonary angiography (CTPA) have increased the number of patients diagnosed with subsegmental PTE. Those PTEs are confined to the subsegmental pulmonary arteries. For patients with subsegmental

PTE and a low risk for recurrence, the ACCP **suggests** clinical surveillance over anti-coagulation. Whereas patients with a high risk for recurrence should receive anticoagulation. In patients with acute PTE associated with systemic hypotension or acute deterioration who do not have a high bleeding risk, the ACCP **suggests** systemically administered thrombolytic therapy. In patients with acute PTE without hypotension, thrombolytic therapy is **not recommended**. Routine echocardiography and biomarker measurement may not be necessary in all patients, but close monitoring of patients with signs of right heart dysfunction and repeated echocardiography and biomarkers measurement is appropriate to identify early those patients who should receive thrombolytics.[20,21]

In patients who have recurrent VTE while on therapy with anti X-a inhibitor or warfarin the ACCP **suggests** switching to LMWH at least temporarily. In patients who have recurrent VTE on long-term LMWH, the ACCP **suggests** increasing the dose of LMWH by about one-quarter to one-third.[20,21]

There is also concrete evidence about patient populations at increased risk of bleeding while on anticoagulant therapy. Known risk factors for bleeding in people include age older than 65, previous bleeding, cancer (including metastatic cancer), kidney failure, liver failure, thrombocytopenia, previous stroke, diabetes mellitus, anemia, concurrent antiplatelet therapy, poor anticoagulant control, recent surgery, and nonsteroidal anti-inflammatory drugs.[23,24]

Disease Processes Associated with a Hypercoagulable State

The CURATIVE guidelines have evaluated the association between disease and thrombosis in a number of conditions identified as potential risk factors in the current veterinary literature. The goal was the identification of medical conditions that warrant standard antithrombotic therapy due to the increased risk of thrombosis. A standardized Population, Intervention, Comparison, Outcome (PICO) question format was used to investigate these questions. Risk for thrombosis was further classified as "high," "moderate," or "low."[25] For this article, we focus on critical illness–associated recommendations.

Immune-mediated hemolytic anemia (IMHA), protein-losing nephropathy (PLN), severe/necrotizing pancreatitis, and feline cardiomyopathy are associated with a high risk of thromboembolic complications and routine anticoagulation is recommended based on the guidelines. Corticosteroid administration, hyperadrenocorticism, neoplasia, and sepsis are associated with a low to moderate risk for thromboembolic complications. Routine anticoagulation should be considered in cases in which hypercoagulability is demonstrated, or where other risk factors for thrombosis exist. Sepsis is an especially challenging situation as it is associated with the development of thrombosis but also commonly leads to a systemic hypocoagulable state during its later stages.[25,26]

It is debatable if dogs should undergo anticoagulation therapy after splenectomy.[27]

Cerebrovascular disease is more likely considered a consequence of hypercoagulability rather than the cause. Antithrombotic therapy should be considered when an ischemic stroke is identified, and a concurrent medical condition associated with a risk for thrombosis is present. Brain surgery and inflammatory brain disease may be associated with an increased risk of thrombosis, but this has been poorly explored in dogs.

Canine cardiac disease (degenerative mitral valve disease/dilated cardiomyopathy) do not seem to be associated with a high risk of thrombosis. The guidelines suggest antithrombotic therapy in individual dogs where other risk factors for thrombosis exist, but this would be expected to be uncommon.[25]

Diagnosis of Hypercoagulability and Thrombosis

Recognizing the presence of thromboembolism (TE) is often challenging, as the clinical signs are highly variable and they may be overlooked or attributed to the underlying disease. TE should be suspected whenever there is an unexplained clinical deterioration in a patient with a disease associated with hypercoagulability. Specific diagnosis typically relies on visualization of a thrombus or infarcted area on imaging studies, surgery, or postmortem; such investigations may have a low sensitivity or be technically challenging to perform.

BASELINE LABORATORY TESTING

Complete blood counts and chemistry panels are not discriminating for TE, but may identify predisposing conditions such as hyperadrenocorticism, PLN, diabetes mellitus, or hypothyroidism. Complete blood counts may identify abnormal circulating blood cells or myeloproliferative disorders such as polycythemia or essential thrombocytosis that can predispose to thrombosis. Thrombocytopenia or schistocytosis, as markers of DIC, may increase the index of suspicion for TE.[28] Arterial blood-gas can help to deepen suspicion for PTE in dogs that are hypoxemic, hypocapnic, and have an increased A-a gradient.[29]

COAGULATION TESTING

TE can be suspected based on certain laboratory tests that are considered markers of hemostasis activation. A recent retrospective study found that a shortened prothrombin time (PT) or activated partial thromboplastin time (aPTT) in dogs may be indicative of a hypercoagulable state as evidenced by an increased incidence of thrombosis, frequency of suspected PTE, and increased circulating D-dimers.[30] Fibrin degradation products (FDPs) detect the breakdown of both fibrin and fibrinogen and are therefore not very sensitive indicators for inappropriate coagulation.

D-dimers require activation of both thrombin and plasmin for their formation and are therefore considered more specific for fibrinolysis following thrombosis than FDPs. Rapid, accurate, bedside D-dimer assays are integral to decision making in humans with possible TE.[31] Unfortunately, there is no convenient and accurate D-dimer assay available for small animals and test results usually take several days to return. This makes the test inconvenient in a clinical setting. Also, D-dimers should be evaluated within 1 to 2 hours of the suspected embolic event because in experimental canine PTE, D-dimers were increased by 30 minutes, peaked at 1 to 2 hours before returning to normal after 24 hours.[32] In one study, D-dimers have been shown to be insensitive for PTE.[33]

Measuring patient levels of AT activity may allow thrombosis risk stratification. In people, patients with reductions of AT activity between 50% and 75% are considered at moderately risk, whereas activities below 30% to 50% markedly increase thrombosis risk.[34]

Viscoelastic testing, mostly thromboelastography (TEG; commonly used in North America), and rotational thromboelastometry (ROTEM), which is more common in Europe, can measure global hemostatic function in human and veterinary patients.

Viscoelastic testing has gained progressive popularity over the past decade due to its function as a point of care test and the global assessment of a patient's coagulation status. The test measures coagulation in whole blood and thus incorporates both cellular and plasma components. The assay provides information about the speed of clot formation as well as clot maintenance in vitro. The measured parameters provide information on initiation and kinetics (R, K, and alpha), strength (MA and G), and breakdown (LY30 and LY60) of the clot.[11] For more information on viscoelastic monitoring, readers are referred to the Karl E. Jandrey and Andrew G. Burton's article, "Use of Thromboelastography in Clinical Practice,"elsewhere in this issue.

Confirming that a patient is hypercoagulable through viscoelastic testing can be useful to support a suspicion of TE, but a hypercoagulable state does not confirm that TE has occurred. A recent study by Marschner and colleagues[11] showed a correlation between hypercoagulability and inflammatory parameters as well as hematocrit in dogs. But clear clinical correlates between TEG and confirmed TE have not been established to date. In fact, a recent retrospective study found no association between any TEG parameter and the presence of thrombosis on postmortem examination. In the same study, D-dimers were significantly higher in dogs with thrombosis[35] in contrast to the Epstein study.[34]

Modification of the TEG and ROTEM assays by the addition of tissue plasminogen activator (tPA) has been explored in both human and veterinary medicine as a means to better assess the fibrinolytic system. Several veterinary studies have suggested that the tPA-modified TEG may provide valuable information not only in dogs at risk of bleeding but could also be used for the assessment of their thrombosis risk. A recent study found that patients with thrombotic diseases were more "resistant" to the lytic effects of t-PA-modified TEGs than healthy controls. This suggests that occult hypofibrinolysis or delayed hypofibrinolysis may contribute to an increased thrombotic risk in some patients.[36]

DIAGNOSTIC IMAGING

In patients with new-onset respiratory distress and risk factors for PTE, thoracic radiography occasionally might show alveolar or alveolar-interstitial pulmonary infiltrates that increase suspicion for PTE, but are nonspecific. Hypovascular lung areas, known as the Westermark sign, are hyperlucent regions representing zones of reduced blood flow distal to sites of vascular occlusion. These changes are rare but considered pathognomonic for PTE.[37] Most patients will require additional imaging for a definitive diagnosis in form of a CT with angiography, which is considered the gold standard for diagnosis of PTE in people.[38,39]

In humans, rapid, multislice spiral computed tomography pulmonary angiography (CTPA) is central to making a diagnosis of PTE.[38] CTPA studies are obtained by simultaneous thoracic CT scanning and bolus injection of contrast media.[40] Diagnostic criteria for PTE using CT-angiography are failure to enhance the entire pulmonary arterial lumen due to occlusive or partial filling defects.[41] A normal study essentially rules out PTE, unless the index of suspicion is very high.[42] Multidetector-row or multislice CT scanners are increasingly available in veterinary medicine and allow imaging without the need for general anesthesia. A recent study found that CTPA can be successfully performed in dogs under mild sedation, even in patients with respiratory distress and can both confirm and rule out pulmonary thromboembolism.[43] Abdominal ultrasound or abdominal CT can help to identify intraabdominal thrombosis such as portal vein thrombosis, splenic thrombi, or infarction of other organs.

CARDIOVASCULAR FUNCTION ASSESSMENTS

Echocardiography is useful for identification and quantification of the cardiovascular compromise that occurs secondary to acute PTE. Changes associated with massive PTE include right atrial and right ventricular enlargement, paradoxic septal motion, pulmonary hypertension, and thrombi in the heart or pulmonary artery. In patients where PTE is suspected and hemodynamic instability exists, a normal echocardiogram can exclude massive or submassive PTE as the cause of the shock.[44–46]

Therapeutic Options and Monitoring of Therapy

Therapies for TE can be divided into prevention (antithrombotics) or treatment. Prevention is often advised in cases in which TE has already been documented (to minimize further TE or clot extension) or in cases with a high risk of TE (based on the underlying disease or tests of hypercoagulability).

Direct treatment of TE can be attempted through the use of thrombolytic drugs such as streptokinase, urokinase, or tissue plasminogen activator (tPA), or through more direct interventions such as thrombectomy. All thrombolytic therapies are associated with a high complication rate and their beneficial effects are questionable. As such, TE is often managed with supportive care and antithrombotics rather than lysis of existing clots. Preventive drugs include antiplatelet drugs, and anticoagulants (heparins, warfarin, and direct inhibitors of factor Xa).

Warfarin

Warfarin inhibits the synthesis of vitamin K–dependent clotting factors, which include factors II, VII, IX, and X, and the anticoagulant proteins C and S. Warfarin inhibits the vitamin K epoxide reductase enzyme complex, thereby reducing the regeneration of vitamin K_1 epoxide in the liver. Therapeutic doses of warfarin decrease the active form of each vitamin K–dependent clotting factor by approximately 30% to 50%.[47] Because of its narrow therapeutic index and the development of newer and safer anticoagulants, it has been largely replaced. The CURATIVE initiative suggests against the use of warfarin in dogs (and cats).[48]

Unfractionated Heparin

Heparin is a heterogeneous mixture of glycosaminoglycans with a molecular weight ranging from 3,00 to 30,000 Da. It complexes with and amplifies the inhibitory activity of antithrombin against FIIa (thrombin) and FXa, although factors IXa, XIa, XIIa and XIII are also inhibited. Variation in the size of heparin molecules and unpredictable bioavailability in critical illness cause variation in heparin dose responses necessitating therapeutic monitoring. The plasma half-life of heparin is 1 to 2 hours but increase in liver and renal failure. Due to lack of intestinal absorption and rapid inactivation by intestinal heparinase, oral administration is not effective.[49] The most common side effect of heparin use is hemorrhage. In people, an immune thrombocytopenia has been noted with heparin use, although this has not been described in dogs.[50]

Low Molecular Weight Heparins

LMWHs derive from depolymerization of unfractionate heparin (UFH) with a mean molecular weight of 4000 to 5000 Da. LMWHs are less protein-bound than UFH, have more predictable pharmacokinetic profiles and better bioavailability after subcutaneous injection. The reduced size of the LMWH polysaccharides limits their ability to simultaneously bind AT and thrombin. Because of that difference in size, LMWHs have a reduced anti-IIa activity relative to anti-Xa (approximately one-third that of UFH).[51]

Factor Xa inhibitors

Rivaroxaban is an orally administered direct inhibitor of activated factor X (FXa) that is useful for chronic anticoagulant therapy.[52] Based on available data, rivaroxaban appears safe and well tolerated in dogs and cats with predictable pharmacokinetics and anticoagulant effects.[53,54]

The peak anticoagulant effect is reached at 1.5 to 2.0 hours, and available studies showed no further increase in peak anticoagulation effect with twice daily administration versus once daily in studies.[53]

Antiplatelet Drugs

Antiplatelet agents are widely used in thromboprophylaxis for both arterial and venous thrombi, likely because of their low cost, ease of administration, and minimal monitoring requirements. In small animals, antiplatelet agents are typically used for long-term oral maintenance therapy or as thromboprophylaxis for at-risk patients.[16,55]

Aspirin

The nonselective cyclooxygenase (COX) inhibitor aspirin irreversibly inhibits platelet thromboxane A2 (TXA2) synthesis by inhibiting COX-1 for the lifetime of the platelet. Thromboxane mediates platelet activation through the G-protein signaling pathway.[16] Aspirin is the most widely used antiplatelet drug in both veterinary and human medicine. Studies have demonstrated that up to 70% of normal dogs have a defect in the G-protein signaling, raising concerns about limited and inconsistent therapeutic efficacy. Aspirin resistance is also well documented in people.[56–58]

In dogs, the dose required to inhibit platelet function varies and ranges from 0.5 to 20 mg/kg. This may be related to heritable variability in canine thromboxane responsiveness.[48,59] Feline aspirin pharmacokinetics, in contrast, are different because of a relative deficiency of glucuronate in cats. Aspirin has a prolonged elimination half-life of approximately 38 hours in cats compared with 15 to 20 minutes in people and approximately 7 hours in dogs.[60]

Thienopyridines

Thienopyridines are direct platelet agonist receptor inhibitors and are antagonists of the ADP receptor (P2Y12). Ticlopidine, clopidogrel, and prasugrel are all prodrugs and must be activated in the liver via cytochrome P450-dependent oxidation. The active metabolite irreversibly binds to the ADP receptor and causes impaired release of serotonin, thromboxane, and ADP as well as inhibition of ADP-mediated activation of the GPIIb/IIIa receptor.[61]

Due to the conversion needed, the onset of action of these drugs is dose dependent, takes a few hours, and is sensitive to variations in the P450 efficiency, which can translate into drug resistance.[16,62,63]

In dogs, clopidogrel may provide more consistent antiplatelet effects than aspirin.[55] A multicenter double-blinded prospective study (FATCAT study) comparing aspirin with clopidogrel in cats with arterial thromboemboli (ATE) recently demonstrated that clopidogrel significantly increased the time to ATE recurrence and significantly prolonged median survival time for cats with a history of thrombosis compared with aspirin.[64] A recent study in cats with a genetic mutation that predisposed them to develop hypertrophic cardiomyopathy found that clopidogrel is effective at attenuating platelet activation and aggregation in some cats. Other cats in the study with the mutation had increased platelet activation and were considered nonresponders based on flow cytometry.[65]

The oral bioavailability of clopidogrel in dogs is reportedly only 10%. As such, the oral dosages that are reported effective may produce substantially lower plasma concentrations than intravenous dosages.[53] Several newer P2Y12-inhibitors have been investigated but no veterinary clinical studies are available to date. Ticlopidine has been associated with myelosuppression in people and is now rarely used. Prasugrel has been used for pilot investigations in dogs, and very effectively inhibits ADP-induced platelet aggregation, but raises concern about a potentially increased risk of hemorrhage compared to clopidogrel. Cangrelor and ticagrelor have been demonstrated to be effective in dogs and especially ticagrelor seemed to have a promising safety profile.[66–68]

Integrin Gp IIb/IIIa Inhibitors

The platelet receptor complex Gp IIb/IIIa is integral in platelet aggregation and binding of Gp IIb/IIIa with fibrinogen is the final major step in platelet aggregation. The commercially available Gp IIb/IIIa antagonists are abciximab, tirofiban, and eptifibatide and they are all for intravenous use only.

In clinical trials, Abciximab has been used in canine and feline models of arterial injury and has not been associated with adverse effects. Eptifibatide has been shown to induce a toxic reaction in cats and is therefore contraindicated in this species. In people, Gp IIb/IIIa antagonists fare an important part of the management of patients undergoing percutaneous coronary intervention but bleeding complications and thrombocytopenia are relatively common side effects.[16,69,70]

Rationale for Use of Antithrombotics in Critical Illness

It remains challenging to determine which patients should receive antithrombotic medications and which antithrombotic medications are deemed necessary and appropriate. The second domain of the CURATIVE guidelines sought to establish what drug or drug combination should be administered in venous and arterial thromboembolic disease settings.[48]

In diseases associated with VTE, such as PLN and IMHA, thrombi form under low-shear conditions. Such thrombi are typically fibrin rich and their formation is less dependent on platelet number or function.[71]

In contrast, in diseases associated with arterial thrombosis (such as feline cardiomyopathies), thrombi form under high-shear conditions. ATE are typically platelet rich and hence drugs that limit the ability of platelets to activate, aggregate, or adhere may be most effective. Because of this pathophysiologic rationale, anticoagulant drugs are most commonly recommended in venous thrombosis and antiplatelet agents in arterial thrombosis.[72,73]

Newer evidence and knowledge about the cell-based model of hemostasis has shown that platelets are integral to hemostasis.[10,74] and therefore the use of antiplatelet drugs in venous thrombosis seems reasonable.[75,76] Experimental data support this practice,[77] and antiplatelet drugs have been shown to reduce the risk of venous thrombosis in people.[78,79] Furthermore, many hypercoagulable states in small animals can result in venous or arterial thrombosis and because definitive location and diagnosis of thrombi is challenging to determine, the judicious use of anticoagulants and antiplatelet drugs concurrently might be clinically indicated.[48]

The CURATIVE working group suggests that anticoagulants may be more effective than antiplatelet agents for VTE prevention in dogs in general and in dirofilariasis specifically. No evidence-based recommendations could be made regarding antiplatelet agents for VTE in cats, but anticoagulants rather than antiplatelet agents were suggested for the prevention of VTE in cats.[48]

Along the same lines, the working group suggests that antiplatelet agents may be more effective than anticoagulants for the prevention of ATE in dogs but that anticoagulants may also be effective. For the prevention and treatment of ATE in cats, the group recommends the use of antiplatelet agents. No evidence-based recommendations were made regarding the use of anticoagulants for ATE in cats.[48]

There was insufficient evidence to formulate strong recommendations regarding clopidogrel versus aspirin in dogs. According to CURATIVE, clopidogrel may be more effective than aspirin but there is good evidence for the efficacy of both drugs for the prevention of arterial thrombosis in dogs (**Table 1**).

For ATE in cats, the group strongly recommends clopidogrel over aspirin use.

No recommendations could be made regarding aspirin versus clopidogrel in cats at risk for VTE.[48]

The guidelines comment on the fact that both abciximab and ticagrelor appear safe and may be efficacious antiplatelet agents in dogs but at this point, insufficient evidence is available to formulate treatment recommendations.

Regarding anticoagulants, there was insufficient evidence available to make strong recommendations regarding the use of UFH versus LMWH in dogs or cats. The guidelines suggest that LMWH may be used in preference to UFH because of the positive safety profile and more reliable bioavailability. Direct Xa inhibitors may be used in preference to UFH based on evidence of equivalent efficacy, combined with reliable pharmacokinetics and the ease of oral dosing in dogs and cats, even though there is also insufficient information to formulate clear recommendations.

When looking at the use of warfarin versus other anticoagulants, the investigators state that there is insufficient evidence to make strong recommendations but advise that UFH, LMWH, or direct Xa inhibitors be used in preference to warfarin.

The guidelines also looked at combination anticoagulant and antiplatelet therapy for VTE in dogs and cats. The investigators suggest aspirin or clopidogrel in addition to LMWH or individually adjusted UFH therapy for dogs at high risk of VTE, where the risk of clot formation is felt to outweigh the increased risk of bleeding with combination therapy.[48]

SAFETY CONCERNS AND DRUG MONITORING OF ANTITHROMBOTIC THERAPY IN VETERINARY CRITICAL CARE

Therapeutic drug monitoring can be a valuable tool for guiding safe and effective anticoagulant drug therapy regimens in individual patients.[80]

Therapeutic drug monitoring is most appropriately implemented for drugs with significant individual variation in pharmacokinetics and pharmacodynamics or a narrow safety margin. This is particularly important for older generation drugs such as warfarin and UFH. The introduction of newer thromboprophylactic drugs with more reliable pharmacokinetics and pharmacodynamics has led to a reduced need for therapeutic drug monitoring in people.[80,81]

Due to species specific differences in disease processes and drug pharmacokinetics and pharmacodynamics, veterinary guidelines are needed to direct clinical use of antithrombotics. The CURATIVE guidelines therefore include a domain that is focused on drug monitoring recommendations.[81]

Platelet Inhibitors

No routine drug monitoring is recommended for platelet inhibitors at this time.

According to the CURATIVE guidelines, adjusting therapy to achieve platelet inhibition via platelet aggregometry in dogs receiving aspirin can be considered.

Guidelines for clopidogrel monitoring were not formulated, given the lack of literature addressing this question.[81]

Table 1
Summary of drugs, drug class, the conditions they treat, and the doses needed to treat them

Drug	MOA	Dosing Dog		Dosing Cat		Drug Monitoring	Possible Adverse Effects/Side Notes
		Plumb's	CURATIVE	Plumb's	CURATIVE		
Warfarin	Vitamin K epoxide reductase inhibitor	0.05–0.2 mg/kg PO q24 until INR 2–3, 0.22 mg/kg/d	0.05–0.5 mg/kg q24 h loading doses 0.05 mg/kg to 0.3 mg/kg	Not recommended	Not specified	Goal: prolong PT by 1.5- to 2-fold (109) or to attain an INR of 2.0–3.0. (113) Goggs, domain 2	Narrow therapeutic index, high bleeding risk, not recommended, uneven distribution within tablets, thrombo-cytopenia in humans
Unfractionated heparin (UFH)	Thrombin (factor IIa) and factor Xa inhibitor	IV dosing: 100 U/kg bolus, 20–50U/kg/h IV CRI 150–300U/kg SC Q6-8	IV dosing: 100 U/kg bolus, then 480–900 U/kg/24h (20–37.5 U/kg/h) CRI SC dosing: 150–300 U/kg q6h	200–250U/kg IV bolus, 12–25U/kg/h IV CRI 50–100 U/kg (low dose) or 200–300 U/kg SC Q6-8	250 U/kg SC q6h	Target unfractionated heparin specific anti-Xa activity range (0.35–0.7 U/mL) PTT 1.5–2-fold increased from baseline	Bleeding, thrombo-cytopenia, unpredictable bioavailability, oral admini-stration is not effective, reversible with protamine
Dalteparin	Factor Xa and IIa inhibitor	150 U/kg SC Q8, Q12 dosing might be effective	100–175 U/kg q8h SC	100–175 U/kg SC Q8-12	75 U/kg SC q6h	Human target therapeutic anti-Xa activity range (eg, 0.5–1.0)	Minor bleeding
Enoxaparin	Factor Xa and IIa inhibitor	0.8–1 mg/kg SC q6–8	0.8 mg/kg SC q6h	1–1.25 mg/kg SC Q6-12	0.75–1 mg/kg SC q6	Drug-specific anti-Xa activity	Minor bleeding

(continued on next page)

Table 1
(continued)

Drug	MOA	Dosing Dog		Dosing Cat		Drug Monitoring	Possible Adverse Effects/Side Notes
		Plumb's	CURATIVE	Plumb's	CURATIVE		
Fondaparinux	Factor Xa and IIa inhibitor	Not available	Not available	Not available	0.06 or 0.20 mg/kg SC q12 h	Drug-specific anti-Xa activity	Minor bleeding
Rivaroxaban	Factor Xa inhibitor	0.5–0.67 mg/kg PO Q24, 0.5–1 mg/kg PO q24, q12 may be more appropriate	1–2 mg/kg/d PO	1.25 mg total PO Q24	0.5–1 mg/kg/d PO	Drug-specific anti-Xa activity, peak anticoagulant effect at 1.5–2 h	Minor bleeding
Aspirin	COX-1 inhibitor	0.5–1 mg/kg PO q24, up to 10 mg/kg	No specific dosing recommendations, 0.5–15 mg/kg/d PO likely effective	5 mg/cat Q72 (low dose), 10 mg/kg (40.5 mg total) q24–72 (high dose)	No specific dosing recommendations, 5 mg/kg twice weekly to 25 mg/kg/d PO described in cats	No routine monitoring recommended	Minor bleeding, many dogs seem aspirin resistant
Clopidogrel	ADP receptor (P2Y12) antagonist	1–4 mg/kg PO q24, can consider 10 mg/kg loading dose, reduce to 0.5 mg/kg if used with aspirin	Loading dose: 4–10 mg/kg PO, Maintenance: 1.1–3 mg/kg PO q24 h	10–18.75 mg total PO Q24	Loading dose: 37.5 mg PO total, Maintenance: 18.75 mg PO q24 h	No routine monitoring recommended	Minor bleeding, prodrug, cytochrome P450-dependent activation, risk of drug resistance

Abbreviations: CRI, constant rate infusion; INR, international normalized ratio; IV, intravenous; MOA, mechanism of action; PO, by mouth; PT, prothrombin time; PTT, partial thromboplastin time; q, every; SC, subcutaneous.

Warfarin

According to the guidelines, warfarin should not be used in dogs or in cats. If warfarin is used, warfarin therapy should ideally be monitored with PT or international normalized ratio (INR) to achieve a target of 2 to 3 INR, or 1.5 to 2.0 times the baseline PT. Close therapeutic monitoring is indicated to maximize efficacy and reduce the risk of complications.[81]

Unfractionated Heparin

The CURATIVE group recommends anti-Xa activity monitoring for UFH in dogs because of the lack of evidence supporting the use of other monitoring tests (eg, ACT, aPTT, TEG, and Sonoclot). Dose adjustments should be performed to achieve the anti-Xa target range of 0.35 to 0.7 IU/mL.[81]

The test that is routinely used in clinical practice to measure UFH effect is aPTT, with an accepted therapeutic target range of 1.5 to 2.5 times the normal baseline aPTT value.[82] Therapeutic monitoring has also been reported using the ACT, thrombin generation, or viscoelastic testing.[83]

Low Molecular Weight Heparin

LMWH therapy can be monitored in dogs by use of a chromogenic anti-Xa assay (specific for the particular LMWH used), which is commercially available (but not widespread).[84] According to the CURATIVE working group, there is insufficient evidence to make strong recommendations for therapeutic monitoring of LMWH in dogs or cats given the relative safety profile at recommended dosing ranges. If drug monitoring is implemented, the guidelines suggest the measurement of anti-Xa levels 2 to 4 hours post dosing with a target range of 0.5 to 1.0 U/mL.[83]

LMWH at standard doses has minimal effect on aPTT.[85]

In people, TEG has been investigated as a potential method of monitoring LMWH therapy and may offer some advantages over anti-Xa assessment.[84]

Anti-Xa Inhibitors

Guidelines for rivaroxaban monitoring were not formulated given the lack of literature.

In people, both PT and aPTT are prolonged at therapeutic plasma concentrations but the PT is a more accurate measure.[53] In a recent study, a rivaroxaban-specific anti-Xa activity was much more sensitive to detect the anticoagulant activity of rivaroxaban in dogs than PT, aPTT, or TEG.[86]

DISCONTINUATION OF ANTICOAGULANT THERAPY

For every patient that is started on anticoagulant therapy, the question arises when and if to stop treatment. Discontinuation of therapy may be temporary to facilitate invasive medical or surgical procedures or may be permanent in case of resolution of the thrombus and the underlying disease process.

The CURATIVE working group evaluated these questions in one of their domains and formulated evidence-based recommendations.[87]

The guidelines state that in patients at high risk for thrombosis, anticoagulation should not be discontinued for invasive procedures. In patients at low to moderate risk for thrombosis, discontinuation of anticoagulation can be considered before procedures.[87]

In all cases, the risk for bleeding must be balanced with the risk for thrombosis. This means that for procedures in which hemorrhage may be catastrophic (eg, neurosurgery) or unable to be easily controlled (eg, percutaneous renal biopsy), discontinuation or alteration of therapy is necessary to limit the risk of hemorrhage. In contrast, for less-invasive procedures (eg, dental extraction, skin mass removal), or procedures in which hemorrhage may be addressed through tamponade (eg, surgery on a peripheral limb), it might be reasonable to continue anticoagulant therapy through the procedure.[87]

Clinicians should consider the risk of rebound hypercoagulability when planning complete or temporary cessation of therapy.[87]

ANTIPLATELET THERAPY

With regard to discontinuation of irreversible platelet antagonists (eg, aspirin and clopidogrel) in dogs and cats, the CURATIVE guidelines recommend that for patients undergoing elective surgery and at high risk of thrombosis, a single antiplatelet agent should be continued. If patients are receiving dual antiplatelet therapy, one of the agents can be discontinued. Close attention needs to be paid to surgical hemostasis in those patients. For low to moderate risk patients, the guidelines recommend that antiplatelet agents be discontinued 5 to 7 days before the planned procedure to allow time for replacement of inhibited platelets. This interval may be shorter in cats.[88]

ANTICOAGULANT THERAPY

In dogs and cats at high risk for thrombotic events and receiving UFH or LMWH and undergoing routine surgery, the guidelines recommend that heparin therapy should not be discontinued. Surgery should be planned to occur at the nadir of the anticoagulant effect (approximately 6–8 hours after prior dose). These patients are obviously at increased risk of bleeding and close attention needs to be paid to surgical hemostasis.

For patients with low to moderate risk of thrombosis, CURATIVE recommends that consideration may be given to taper UFH or stop LMWH therapy prior to a procedure.[87]

RESTARTING ANTITHROMBOTIC THERAPY FOLLOWING SURGERY

The guidelines recommend that in patients at high risk, antithrombotic therapy should be restarted as soon as possible after surgery as long as there is no evidence of ongoing bleeding. For patients at low/moderate risk the guidelines suggest that antithrombotic therapy should be restarted once there is no evidence of ongoing bleeding. Antithrombotic therapy should be initiated immediately in patients that develop thrombosis in the postoperative period.[87]

PERMANENT DISCONTINUATION OF ANTITHROMBOTIC THERAPY

Regarding discontinuation of antithrombotic therapy in patients with either an arterial or venous blood clot, the guidelines came to the following conclusion: If the blood clot is no longer identifiable and the underlying causative conditions have resolved, antithrombotic therapy should be discontinued following thrombus resolution. In patients with unknown underlying conditions or where these conditions cannot be cured or resolved, antithrombotic therapy should be continued indefinitely.

CURATIVE guidelines recommend that UFH in patients on intravenous constant rate infusion should be tapered rather than abruptly discontinued to prevent rebound hypercoagulability. For patients who receive UFH via subcutaneous injection, weaning should be considered.[87]

Clinicians do not need to wean LMWH therapy before discontinuation but should consider weaning direct oral Xa inhibitors.

In patients with venous thrombosis and low or moderate risk of recurrence, the risk of hemorrhage should be weighed against the risk of recurrence of the thromboembolism. In general, there is more evidence supporting the indefinite use of antithrombotics for the treatment of venous thrombi.[87]

SUMMARY

Antithrombotics role in critically ill veterinary patients is continuing to expand. Although certain key conditions (IMHA and marked left atrial enlargement in cats) are clear indications for therapy, in other cases it is far less clear what is the risk to benefit ratio. In addition, ideal approaches to dosing and monitoring remain to be determined, specifically the impact of critical illness (eg, inflammation and hypoalbuminemia) on drug metabolism and function as well as species and potential genetic differences in response to therapy. The role of antifibrinolytics remains to be determined, but could increase the risk of thromboembolic diseases, so should not be administered empirically to animals with hemorrhage.

Each critically ill patient should be carefully evaluated for risk factors for thromboembolic disease and daily decisions about the indications for starting or stopping medications should be made. Early return to activity may limit the effect of venous stasis.

Diagnostic testing should be focused on early detection of occult DIC before the development of overt hemorrhage. The astute clinician should continue to carefully monitor the patient, and also support research efforts to better stratify disease and therapeutic approaches.

DISCLOSURE

The authors have nothing to disclose.

REFERENCES

1. Brooks M. Coagulopathies and thrombosis. In: Ettinger SJ, Feldman EC, editors. Textbook of veterinary internal medicine. 5th edition. Philadelphia: WB Saunders; 2000. p. 1829–41.
2. Feldman BF, Kirby R, Caldin M. Recognition and treatment of disseminated intravascular coagulation. In: Bonagura JD, editor. Kirk's current veterinary therapy XIII: small animal practice. Philadelphia: WB Saunders; 2000. p. 190–4.
3. Piek CJ, Brinkhof B, Teske E, et al. High intravascular tissue factor expression in dogs with idiopathic immune-mediated haemolytic anaemia. Vet Immunol Immunopathol 2011;144(3–4):346–54.
4. Weiss DJ, Brazzell JL. Detection of activated platelets in dogs with primary immune-mediated hemolytic anemia. J Vet Intern Med 2006;20(3):682–6.
5. Fenty RK, de Laforcade AM, Shaw SE, et al. Identification of hypercoagulability in dogs with primary immune-mediated hemolytic anemia by means of thromboelastography. J Am Vet Med Assoc 2011;238(4):463–7.
6. Goggs R, Blais MC, Brainard BM, et al. American College of Veterinary Emergency and Critical Care (ACVECC) Consensus on the Rational Use of Antithrombotics in Veterinary Critical Care (CURATIVE) guidelines. J Vet Emerg Crit Care 2019;29(1):12–36.
7. Wiinberg B, Jensen AL, Johansson PI, et al. Thromboelastographic evaluation of hemostatic function in dogs with disseminated intravascular coagulation. J Vet Intern Med 2008;22(2):357–65.

8. Goggs R, Mastrocco A, Brooks MB. Retrospective evaluation of 4 methods for outcome prediction in overt disseminated intravascular coagulation in dogs (2009-2014): 804 cases. J Vet Emerg Crit Care 2018;28(6):541–50.

9. Hopper K, Bateman S. An updated view of hemostasis: mechanisms of hemostatic dysfunction associated with sepsis. J Vet Emerg Crit Care 2005;15(2):83–91.

10. Hoffman M, Monroe DM. A cell-based model of hemostasis. Thromb Haemost 2001;85(6):958–65.

11. Marschner CB, Wiinberg B, Tarnow I, et al. The influence of inflammation and hematocrit on clot strength in canine thromboelastographic hypercoagulability. J Vet Emerg Crit Care 2018;28(1):20–30.

12. McKenzie SB, Clare CN, Smith LA, et al. Laboratory test utilization in the diagnosis of hypercoagulability. Clin Lab Sci 2000;13(4):215–21.

13. Sinnott VB, Otto CM. Use of thromboelastography in dogs with immune-mediated hemolytic anemia: 39 cases (2000–2008). J Vet Emerg Crit Care 2009;19(5): 484–8.

14. Vilar Saavedra P, Lara Garcia A, Zaldivar Lopez S, et al. Hemostatic abnormalities in dogs with carcinoma: a thromboelastographic characterization of hypercoagulability. Vet J 2011;190(2):e78–83.

15. Goggs R, Wiinberg B, Kjelgaard-Hansen M, et al. Serial assessment of the coagulation status of dogs with immune-mediated haemolytic anaemia using thromboelastography. Vet J 2012;191(3):347–53.

16. Wiinberg B, Jessen LR, Tarnow I, et al. Diagnosis and treatment of platelet hyperactivity in relation to thrombosis in dogs and cats. J Vet Emerg Crit Care 2012; 22(1):42–58.

17. Kidd L, Mackman N. Prothrombotic mechanisms and anticoagulant therapy in dogs with immune-mediated hemolytic anemia. J Vet Emerg Crit Care 2013; 23(1):3–13.

18. Turpie AG, Esmon C. Venous and arterial thrombosis–pathogenesis and the rationale for anticoagulation. Thromb Haemost 2011;105(4):586–96.

19. Tufano A, Guida A, Di Minno MN, et al. Prevention of venous thromboembolism in medical patients with thrombocytopenia or with platelet dysfunction: a review of the literature. Semin Thromb Hemost 2011;37(3):267–74.

20. Kearon C, Akl EA, Ornelas J, et al. Antithrombotic therapy for VTE disease: CHEST guideline and expert panel report. Chest 2016;149(2):p315–52.

21. Kearon C, Akl EA, Comerota AJ, et al. Antithrombotic therapy for VTE disease: antithrombotic therapy and prevention of thrombosis, 9th ed: American College of Chest Physicians evidence-based clinical practice guidelines. Chest 2012; 141(2 Suppl):e419S–94S.

22. Lewis SZ, Diekemper R, Ornelas J, et al. Methodologies for the development of CHEST guidelines and expert panel reports. Chest 2014;146(1):182–92.

23. Brass LM, Lichtman JH, Wang Y, et al. Intracranial hemorrhage associated with thrombolytic therapy for elderly patients with acute myocardial infarction - Results from the Cooperative Cardiovascular Project. Stroke 2000;31(8):1802–11.

24. Mehta RH, Stebbins A, Lopes RD, et al. Race, bleeding, and outcomes in STEMI patients treated with fibrinolytic therapy. Am J Med 2011;124(1):48–57.

25. de Laforcade A, Bacek L, Blais MC, et al. Consensus on the Rational Use of Antithrombotics in Veterinary Critical Care (CURATIVE): Domain 1-Defining populations at risk. J Vet Emerg Crit Care 2019;29:37–48.

26. Marschner CB, Kristensen AT, Rozanski EA, et al. Diagnosis of canine pulmonary thromboembolism by computed tomography and mathematical modelling using haemostatic and inflammatory variables. Vet J 2017;229:6–12.

27. Phipps WE, de Laforcade AM, Barton BA, et al. Postoperative thrombocytosis and thromboelastographic evidence of hypercoagulability in dogs undergoing splenectomy for splenic masses. J Am Vet Med Assoc 2020;256(1):85–92.

28. Neel JA, Snyder L, Grindem CB. Thrombocytosis: a retrospective study of 165 dogs. Vet Clin Pathol 2012;41(2):216–22.

29. Johnson LR, Lappin MR, Baker DC. Pulmonary thromboembolism in 29 dogs: 1985-1995. J Vet Intern Med 1999;13(4):338–45.

30. Song J, Drobatz KJ, Silverstein DC. Retrospective evaluation of shortened pro-thrombin time or activated partial thromboplastin time for the diagnosis of hyper-coagulability in dogs: 25 cases (2006-2011). J Vet Emerg Crit Care 2016;26(3): 398–405.

31. Wells PS, Anderson DR, Rodger M, et al. Derivation of a simple clinical model to categorize patient's probability of pulmonary embolism: increasing the models utility with the SimpliRED D-dimer. Thromb Haemost 2000;83(3):416–20.

32. Ben SQ, Ni SS, Shen HH, et al. The dynamic changes of LDH isoenzyme 3 and D-dimer following pulmonary thromboembolism in canine. Thromb Res 2007; 120(4):575–83.

33. Epstein SE, Hopper K, Mellema MS, et al. Diagnostic utility of D-dimer concentra-tions in dogs with pulmonary embolism. J Vet Intern Med 2013;27(6):1646–9.

34. Feldman BF. Thrombosis - diagnosis and treatment. In: Kirk RW, editor. CVT IX: small animal practice. 1986. p. 505–9.

35. Thawley VJ, Sanchez MD, Drobatz KJ, et al. Retrospective comparison of throm-boelastography results to postmortem evidence of thrombosis in critically ill dogs: 39 cases (2005-2010). J Vet Emerg Crit Care 2016;26(3):428–36.

36. Spodsberg EH, Wiinberg B, Jessen LR, et al. Endogenous fibrinolytic potential in tissue-plasminogen activator-modified thromboelastography analysis is signifi-cantly decreased in dogs suffering from diseases predisposing to thrombosis. Vet Clin Pathol 2013;42(3):281–90.

37. Fluckiger MA, Gomez JA. Radiographic findings in dogs with spontaneous pul-monary thrombosis or embolism. Vet Radiol 1984;25(3):124–31.

38. Fesmire FM, Brown MD, Espinosa JA, et al. Critical issues in the evaluation and management of adult patients presenting to the emergency department with sus-pected pulmonary embolism. Ann Emerg Med 2011;57(6):628–52.

39. Goggs R, Benigni L, Fuentes VL, et al. Pulmonary thromboembolism. J Vet Emerg Crit Care 2009;19(1):30–52.

40. Habing A, Coelho JC, Nelson N, et al. Pulmonary angiography using 16 slice mul-tidetector computed tomography in normal dogs. Vet Radiol Ultrasound 2011; 52(2):173–8.

41. Wittram C, Maher MM, Yoo AJ, et al. CT angiography of pulmonary embolism: diagnostic criteria and causes of misdiagnosis. Radiographics 2004;24(5): 1219–38.

42. Torbicki A, Perrier A, Konstantinides S, et al. Guidelines on the diagnosis and management of acute pulmonary embolism: The Task Force for the Diagnosis and Management of Acute Pulmonary Embolism of the European Society of Car-diology (ESC). Eur Heart J 2008;29(18):2276–315.

43. Goggs R, Chan DL, Benigni L, et al. Comparison of computed tomography pul-monary angiography and point-of-care tests for pulmonary thromboembolism diagnosis in dogs. J Small Anim Pract 2014;55(4):190–7.

44. Bunch S, Metcalf M, Crane S, et al. Idiopathic pleural effusion and pulmonary thromboembolism in a dog with autoimmune hemolytic anemia. J Am Vet Med As-soc 1989;195(12):1748–53.

45. Palmer KG, King LG, Van Winkle TJ. Clinical manifestations and associated disease syndromes in dogs with cranial vena cava thrombosis: 17 cases (1989-1996). J Am Vet Med Assoc 1998;213(2):220–4.

46. Venco L, Calzolari D, Morini S. Pulmonary thromboembolism in a dog with renal amyloidosis. Vet Radiol Ultrasound 1998;39(6):564–5.

47. Horton JD, Bushwick BM. Warfarin therapy: evolving strategies in anticoagulation. Am Fam Physician 1999;59(3):635–46.

48. Goggs R, Bacek L, Bianco D, et al. Consensus on the Rational Use of Antithrombotics in Veterinary Critical Care (CURATIVE): Domain 2-Defining rational therapeutic usage. J Vet Emerg Crit Care 2019;29(1):49–59.

49. Mischke RH, Schuttert C, Grebe S. Anticoagulant effects of repeated subcutaneous injections of high doses of unfractionated heparin in healthy dogs. Am J Vet Res 2001;62:1887–91.

50. Ahmed I, Majeed A, Powell R. Heparin induced thrombocytopenia: diagnosis and management update. Postgrad Med J 2007;83(983):575–82.

51. Grebe S, Jacobs C, Kietzmann M, et al. Pharmacokinetics of low-molecular-weight heparins Fragmin D in dogs. Berl Munch Tierarztl Wochenschr 2000; 113(3):103–7.

52. Kubitza D, Becka M, Voith B, et al. Safety, pharmacodynamics, and pharmacokinetics of single doses of BAY 59-7939, an oral, direct factor Xa inhibitor. Clin Pharmacol Ther 2005;78(4):412–21.

53. Blais MC, Bianco D, Goggs R, et al. Consensus on the Rational Use of Antithrombotics in Veterinary Critical Care (CURATIVE): Domain 3-Defining antithrombotic protocols. J Vet Emerg Crit Care 2019;29(1):60–74.

54. Dixon-Jimenez AC, Brainard BM, Brooks MB, et al. Pharmacokinetic and pharmacodynamic evaluation of oral rivaroxaban in healthy adult cats. J Vet Emerg Crit Care 2016;26(5):619–29.

55. Brainard BM, Kleine SA, Papich MG, et al. Pharmacodynamic and pharmacokinetic evaluation of clopidogrel and the carboxylic acid metabolite SR 26334 in healthy dogs. Am J Vet Res 2010;71(7):822–30.

56. Johnson GJ, Leis LA, Dunlop PC. Thromboxane-insensitive dog platelets have impaired activation of phospholipase C due to receptor-linked G protein dysfunction. J Clin Invest 1993;92(5):2469–79.

57. Santilli F, Rocca B, Cristofaro RD, et al. Platelet cyclooxygenase inhibition by low-dose aspirin is not reflected consistently by platelet function assays:implications for aspirin resistance. J Am Coll Cardiol 2009;53(8):667–77.

58. Levy JH, Dutton RP, Hemphill JC, et al. Multidisciplinary approach to the challenge of hemostasis. Anesth Analg 2010;110(2):354–64.

59. Frederick LG, Suleymanov OD, King LW, et al. The protective dose of the potent GPIIb/IIIa antagonist SC-54701A is reduced when used in combination with aspirin and heparin in a canine model of coronary artery thrombosis. Circulation 1996;93(1):129–34.

60. Lunsford KV, Mackin AJ. Thromboembolic therapies in dogs and cats: an evidence-based approach. Vet Clin North Am Small Anim Pract 2007;37(3): 579–609.

61. Mills DC, Puri R, Hu CJ, et al. Clopidogrel inhibits the binding of ADP analogues to the receptor mediating inhibition of platelet adenylate cyclase. Arterioscler Thromb 1992;12(4):430–6.

62. Gurbel PA, Bliden KP, Butler K, et al. Randomized double-blind assessment of the ONSET and OFFSET of the antiplatelet effects of ticagrelor versus clopidogrel in

patients with stable coronary artery disease: the ONSET/OFFSET study. Circulation 2009;120(25):2577–85.

63. Taubert D, Kastrati A, Harlfinger S, et al. Pharmacokinetics of clopidogrel after administration of a high loading dose. Thromb Haemost 2004;92(2):311–6.

64. Hogan DF, Fox PR, Jacob K, et al. Secondary prevention of cardiogenic arterial thromboembolism in the cat: The double-blind, randomized, positive-controlled feline arterial thromboembolism; clopidogrel vs. aspirin trial (FAT CAT). J Vet Cardiol 2015;17(Suppl 1):S306–17.

65. Li RH, Stern JA, Ho V, et al. Platelet activation and clopidogrel effects on ADP-induced platelet activation in cats with or without the A31P mutation in MYBPC3. J Vet Intern Med 2016;30(5):1619–29.

66. Smith RL, Gillespie TA, Rash TJ, et al. Disposition and metabolic fate of prasugrel in mice, rats, and dogs. Xenobiotica 2007;37(8):884–901.

67. Niitsu Y, Sugidachi A, Ogawa T, et al. Repeat oral dosing of prasugrel, a novel P2Y12 receptor inhibitor, results in cumulative and potent antiplatelet and antithrombotic activity in several animal species. Eur J Pharmacol 2008;579(1–3): 276–82.

68. van Giezen JJ, Berntsson P, Zachrisson H, et al. Comparison of ticagrelor and thienopyridine P2Y(12) binding characteristics and antithrombotic and bleeding effects in rat and dog models of thrombosis/hemostasis. Thromb Res 2009; 124(5):565–71.

69. Lev EI, Patel RT, Guthikonda S, et al. Genetic polymorphisms of the platelet receptors P2Y(12), P2Y(1) and GP IIIa and response to aspirin and clopidogrel. Thromb Res 2007;119(3):355–60.

70. Saltzman AJ, Mehran R, Hooper WC, et al. The relative effects of abciximab and tirofiban on platelet inhibition and C-reactive protein during coronary intervention. J Invasive Cardiol 2010;22(1):2–6.

71. Aird WC. Vascular bed-specific thrombosis. J Thromb Haemost 2007;5(Suppl 1): 283–91.

72. Wolberg AS, Rosendaal FR, Weitz JI, et al. Venous thrombosis. Nat Rev Dis Primers 2015;1:15006.

73. Smith JN, Negrelli JM, Manek MB, et al. Diagnosis and management of acute coronary syndrome: an evidence-based update. J Am Board Fam Med 2015;28(2): 283–93.

74. Smith SA. The cell-based model of coagulation. J Vet Emerg Crit Care 2009; 19(1):3–10.

75. Mackman N. New insights into the mechanisms of venous thrombosis. J Clin Invest 2012;122(7):2331–6.

76. Lowe GD. Common risk factors for both arterial and venous thrombosis. Br J Haematol 2008;140(5):488–95.

77. Cooley BC, Herrera AJ. Cross-modulatory effects of clopidogrel and heparin on platelet and fibrin incorporation in thrombosis. Blood Coagul Fibrinolysis 2013; 24(6):593–8.

78. Brighton TA, Eikelboom JW, Mann K, et al. Low-dose aspirin for preventing recurrent venous thromboembolism. N Engl J Med 2012;367(21):1979–87.

79. Castellucci LA, Cameron C, Le Gal G, et al. Efficacy and safety outcomes of oral anticoagulants and antiplatelet drugs in the secondary prevention of venous thromboembolism: systematic review and network meta-analysis. BMJ 2013; 347:f5133.

80. Boothe DM. Therapeutic drug monitoring. In: Boothe DM, editor. Small animal clinical pharmacology and therapeutics. 2nd edition. Philadelphia: WB Saunders; 2012. p. 112–27.

81. Sharp CR, de Laforcade AM, Koenigshof AM, et al. Consensus on the Rational Use of Antithrombotics in Veterinary Critical Care (CURATIVE): Domain 4-Refining and monitoring antithrombotic therapies. J Vet Emerg Crit Care 2019;29(1): 75–87.

82. Mischke R, Jacobs C. The monitoring of heparin administration by screening tests in experimental dogs. Res Vet Sci 2001;70(2):101–8.

83. Allegret V, Dunn M, Bedard C. Monitoring unfractionated heparin therapy in dogs by measuring thrombin generation. Vet Clin Pathol 2011;40(1):24–31.

84. Lynch AM, deLaforcade AM, Sharp CR. Clinical experience of anti-Xa monitoring in critically ill dogs receiving dalteparin. J Vet Emerg Crit Care 2014;24(4):421–8.

85. Wiinberg B, Jensen AL, Rozanski E, et al. Tissue factor activated thromboelastography correlates to clinical signs of bleeding in dogs. Vet J 2009;179(1):121–9.

86. Morassi A, Bianco D, Park E, et al. Evaluation of the safety and tolerability of rivaroxaban in dogs with presumed primary immune-mediated hemolytic anemia. J Vet Emerg Crit Care 2016;26(4):488–94.

87. Brainard BM, Buriko Y, Good J, et al. Consensus on the Rational Use of Antithrombotics in Veterinary Critical Care (CURATIVE): Domain 5-Discontinuation of anticoagulant therapy in small animals. J Vet Emerg Crit Care 2019;29(1):88–97.

88. Hogan DF, Andrews DA, Green HW, et al. Antiplatelet effects and pharmacodynamics of clopidogrel in cats. J Am Vet Med Assoc 2004;225(9):1406–11.

Use of Human Intravenous Immunoglobulin in Veterinary Clinical Practice

Nicole Spurlock, DVM[a],*, Jennifer Prittie, DVM[b]

KEYWORDS

- Human immunoglobulin • Immunosuppression • Veterinary autoimmune disease
- hIVIG • Immune-mediated thrombocytopenia

KEY POINTS

- The immunomodulatory properties of human intravenous immunoglobulin (hIVIG) are not well understood but may involve blockade of the Fc receptors, neutralization of autoantibodies, complement inhibition, and downregulation of cytokine synthesis.
- Veterinary applications for administration of hIVIG include immune-mediated hemolytic anemia and thrombocytopenia, myasthenia gravis, cutaneous autoimmune diseases, and sudden acquired retinal degeneration syndrome.
- Potential complications associated with hIVIG administration to veterinary patients include acute hypersensitivity, including fever, facial edema, urticaria, vomiting, diarrhea, respiratory difficulty, and hypotension.
- Current literature suggests hIVIG may be beneficial as part of multimodal immunosuppression against immune-mediated thrombocytopenia and autoimmune cutaneous disease in veterinary patients.

INTRODUCTION

Immunoglobulin products contain purified, concentrated immunoglobulin collected from human plasma. Products are used in both humans and companion animals to support immune deficiencies and also to temper exuberant immune responses.[1–4]

At least 1000 healthy, screened donors are pooled for extraction of hIVIG.[5] Immunoglobulins are washed with solvents and/or detergents and are then filtered to remove aggregates, plasmin, kinins, and kallikrein activators.[6,7] Formulations contain more than 90% immunoglobulin G (IgG) but also contain trace amounts of immunoglobulin A (IgA), immunoglobulin M, cluster of differentiation (CD) 8, CD4, and

Disclosure: The authors have nothing to disclose.
a Animal Specialty Emergency Center, 1535 South Sepulveda, Los Angeles, CA 90025, USA;
b 510 East 62nd Street, New York, NY 10065, USA
* Corresponding author.
E-mail address: spurlocknicole@gmail.com

Vet Clin Small Anim 50 (2020) 1371–1383
https://doi.org/10.1016/j.cvsm.2020.07.015
0195-5616/20/© 2020 Elsevier Inc. All rights reserved.

leukocyte antigen.[5] Certain manufacturers alter product pH to discourage bacterial contamination and aggregation.[2] Product half-lives are 21 to 33 days and 7 to 9 days in humans and canines, respectively.[4–8]

HUMAN INTRAVENOUS IMMUNOGLOBULIN AND IMMUNOMODULATION

Immunoregulatory properties are poorly understood. Commercial immunoglobulin preparations are heterogeneous, making it difficult to assign function to individual components. hIVIG modulates the immune system via the following mechanisms:[7–18]

- Fc receptor disruption
- Pathologic autoantibody neutralization
- Complement inhibition
- Fas–Fas ligand (FasL) binding interference
- Cytokine synthesis downregulation

FC RECEPTOR BLOCKADE

Fc receptors are membrane proteins located on neutrophils, natural killer cells, macrophages, eosinophils, mast cells, and platelets. Antibody-antigen complexes bind Fc receptors and initiate phagocytosis. hIVIG transiently blocks Fc receptors, interferes with antigen presentation, and downregulates the immune response.[4,9–12,16] In humans, Fc blockade is concentration dependent and immediate.[6] Clinical effects are generally evident within 3 days of initiation of therapy.[6] Rapid therapeutic response has been observed in canines treated with hIVIG as well, with studies reporting immunosuppression within 24 to 48 hours of drug administration.[8,17]

In addition to physically blocking Fc receptors, hIVIG initiates self-inhibition in inflammatory cells.[18] In the presence of hIVIG, macrophages upregulate inhibitory receptors, which block Fc receptors normally activated by immune complexes.[18] As a result, macrophages do not release inflammatory mediators, which may mitigate ensuing tissue damage.[18]

AUTOANTIBODY NEUTRALIZATION

Stimulation of the immune system depends on lock-and-key antibody-antigen interaction. Anti-idiotype antibodies in hIVIG solutions bind to both antigen binding sites and non–binding site idiotopes on B-cell immunoglobulin or circulating autoantibody.[6,18] Via this mechanism, hIVIG can help regulate the immune response, possibly neutralizing pathogenic autoantibodies.[6,18] This mechanism is less effective in companion animals, because interspecies antibody binds poorly and rarely yields anti-idiotypic antibodies.[6,18]

COMPLEMENT INHIBITION

hIVIG also inhibits the complement cascade.[4] Circulating complement initiates apoptosis after binding to IgG-antigen complexes on cell membranes. Transfused immunoglobulin binds C3b and C4b and subsequently inhibits generation of the membrane attack complex, C5b-C9,[18] which prevents complement-IgG interaction and limits tissue damage.[4,18]

FAS–FAS LIGAND MEDIATION

Fas receptors are located on the surface of various cells and are part of the tumor necrosis factor superfamily.[7] Interactions between Fas and FasL trigger proinflammatory cytokines.[7] FasL transmits apoptotic signals and precipitate cellular death in keratinocytes. Infused hIVIG blocks Fas-FasL interaction and prevents epidermal apoptosis.[8,9]

CYTOKINE DOWNREGULATION

Cytokines bind to target cell membrane receptors and stimulate immune activity. In the presence of hIVIG, mononuclear cells and activated T cells produce fewer proinflammatory cytokines (interleukin-1 [IL-1], tumor necrosis factor-β, and INFa-γ) in response to lipopolysaccharide or bacterial superantigens.[4,18] In addition, the same cells are stimulated to produce the antiinflammatory cytokine, IL-1 receptor antagonist.[4,18]

OTHER IMMUNOMODULATORY EFFECTS

Other immunoregulatory properties of hIVIG have been suggested. Studies document immunoglobulin modulation of adhesion molecules as well as B and T cells.[18] Mechanisms are nebulous, and involve modifications of both innate and adaptive immunity.[18] Some actions of immunoglobulin seem dependent on dose and/or the specific inflammatory condition in question.[18] Regardless, is likely that properties of hIVIG are synergistic and not mutually exclusive.[18]

HUMAN INTRAVENOUS IMMUNOGLOBULIN IN HUMAN MEDICINE

The US Food and Drug Administration (FDA) has approved the use of immunoglobulin in humans for the following conditions[9,10]:

- Immune-mediated thrombocytopenia purpura (ITP)
- Chronic lymphocytic leukemia
- Common variable immunodeficiency
- Chronic inflammatory demyelinating polyneuropathy
- Primary humoral immunodeficiency
- Kawasaki disease
- Pediatric human immunodeficiency virus type 1 infection
- Multifocal motor neuropathy

Off-label use of hIVIG is widespread, and reportedly beneficial for more than 30 immunologic conditions, including Guillain-Barré syndrome, necrotizing fasciitis, and toxic epidermal necrolysis (TEN).[11–13]

New immunoglobulin research is focusing on difficult-to-treat conditions, including Alzheimer disease, polyradiculoneuritis, cardiomyopathy, pregnancy loss, transplant rejection, and sepsis. Investigators have also uncovered antiangiogenic properties associated with immunoglobulin, which may aid in treatment of metastatic neoplasia.[14]

In 2000, researchers conducted a multicenter study comparing efficacy and risk between approved and off-label transfusion of hIVIG.[15] Complication rates were comparable between groups, and adverse events were generally mild. However, patients treated for approved conditions had better outcomes. Researchers concluded that hIVIG therapy is effective and safe, but that judicious use is indicated given lack of clinical trials, associated cost, and limited product availability.[15]

VETERINARY APPLICATION

hIVIG has long been touted as an effective immunomodulator for companion animals, but evidence-based data are lacking. hIVIG has so far been evaluated for the following conditions:

- Immune-mediated hemolytic anemia (IMHA)
- ITP
- Evans syndrome (ES)
- Cutaneous autoimmune disease
- Myasthenia gravis (MG)
- Sudden acquired retinal degeneration syndrome (SARDS)

Immune-mediated hemolytic anemia Veterinarians first used hIVIG to augment glucocorticoid therapy in refractory IMHA.[16–19] Multiple medications are available for second-tier immunosuppression, but often take days or weeks to become effective.[17–21]

Circulating hIVIG immediately blocks Fc receptors, transiently blunting immune activity. Investigators postulated that temporary immunosuppression could stabilize critical patients with IMHA, allow time for standard therapies to become effective, and decrease mortality.[21–24]

Early retrospective reviews suggested improved outcome after immunoglobulin administration in canine IMHA. However, retrospective reviews lack power, and few prospective studies are available.

A 1997 prospective study evaluated hIVIG therapy in 10 dogs with IMHA dogs that were unresponsive to traditional immunosuppressive therapy.[24] In all dogs, packed cell volume (PCV) rapidly improved after hIVIG infusion. Two dogs were subsequently removed from the study for blood transfusion after hIVIG. Five of 8 remaining dogs showed clinical improvement after hIVIG treatment; 3 dogs lived more than 12 months after discharge. Although the investigators concluded that hIVIG may be useful for short-term stabilization of dogs with IMHA, results were questionable because the study lacked a control population and involved multiple immunosuppressive drugs administered concurrently.

A 2009 prospective, blinded, randomized clinical trial evaluated efficacy of hIVIG therapy in 28 dogs with IMHA.[21] Canines received multiple doses of hIVIG or placebo over 3 consecutive days. After 72 hours, glucocorticoids were added to the treatment protocol. No other immunosuppressive drugs were administered. Length of hospitalization, number of blood transfusions required, and overall survival time did not differ between groups. The small study size likely affected results, but researchers concluded that the benefits of hIVIG therapy in dogs with IMHA are not great enough to justify the cost of therapy.[20,21]

At this time, the evidence for use of hIVIG in veterinary patients with IMHA is not convincing. Until additional prospective, clinical trials are completed, hIVIG use for canine IMHA cannot be recommended.

PRIMARY IMMUNE-MEDIATED THROMBOCYTOPENIA

Glucocorticoids are considered gold standard for management of veterinary ITP, with therapeutic improvement expected within 1 week of initiation. Patients with refractory ITP often receive vincristine in addition to steroids, and show improvement within 5 days.[25] Although classic immunosuppressive drugs are ultimately successful for most patients with ITP, significant blood loss can occur before medications reach efficacy.[25] Immunoglobulin therapy is used in humans to bolster platelet count during the acute phase of ITP. In humans, immunoglobulin therapy is linked to fewer blood transfusions, shortened hospitalization time, and improved outcome.[3,4,25,26] Conservation of resources and shorter length of hospitalization may offset the cost of hIVIG, making transfusion attainable.[25]

In 2007, Bianco and colleagues[26] investigated hIVIG infusion in 5 dogs with ITP that had uncontrollable hemorrhage. Participants received 1 hIVIG infusion as well as glucocorticoids. Four of 5 dogs improved after hIVIG: mean platelet count increased from 2.5×10^9/L to 62.7×10^9/L within 24 hours. Dogs responding to immunoglobulin therapy did not require packed red blood cell (pRBC) transfusion after hIVIG. Despite promising results, the small study population and retrospective nature make it difficult to draw meaningful conclusions.

The same group later launched a prospective, controlled study evaluating early hIVIG intervention in canine ITP.[27] Researchers compared outcomes between dogs receiving prednisone monotherapy and those given 1 infusion of hIVIG with prednisone. After day 7, additional immunosuppressive drugs were allowed at clinician discretion. Investigators evaluated platelet recovery time, transfusion requirements, length of hospitalization, and cost of therapy. Thrombocytopenia improved in patients receiving hIVIG (platelet count $>40 \times 10^9$/L) 4 days before the placebo group. Further, thrombocytopenia resolved in dogs treated with hIVIG ($>160 \times 10^9$/L) a median of 5 days before the control group. hIVIG-treated animals were discharged an average of 4 days earlier than animals receiving placebo. Importantly, there was no significant difference in overall cost between groups. Investigators concluded that a single hIVIG infusion, administered within 24 hours of glucocorticoid therapy, improves platelet recovery and decreases length of hospitalization in canines with ITP.

Although hIVIG administration seems to improve outcome in canine ITP compared with glucocorticoid monotherapy, an advantage of hIVIG compared with standard secondary immunosuppressive drugs has not been shown. In 2013, a prospective, randomized study evaluated 20 dogs with ITP that received hIVIG or vincristine in addition to corticosteroids.[28] Multimodal immunosuppression yielded faster recovery than steroids alone, but no advantage of hIVIG therapy compared with vincristine was found. Median platelet recovery time and length of hospitalization were identical between groups (2.5 and 4 days, respectively). Mean cost of therapy was significantly higher in the hIVIG group, and immunoglobulin administration did not decease the requirement for pRBC transfusion. Investigators concluded that, because of cost, ease of administration, and availability, vincristine is superior to hIVIG as adjunctive therapy for the acute phase of canine ITP.

Although further research is warranted, existing data suggest that hIVIG is an effective but costly intervention for canine ITP.

EVANS SYNDROME

ES is a condition in which IMHA and ITP occur simultaneously. A 2009 report describes use of hIVIG in a diabetic dog with ES for whom glucocorticoid therapy was considered contraindicated.[29] Before hIVIG, severe anemia (PCV 12%) and thrombocytopenia (platelets$<2.0 \times 10^9$/L) were recorded. Following therapy with leflunomide and a single hIVIG infusion, platelet count was 51×10^9/L. The platelet count was 116×10^9/L at 24 hours and normalized shortly thereafter. In contrast, PCV did not improve after hIVIG, and multiple pRBC transfusions were required. The dog represented 1 week after discharge, with anemia (PCV 19%) but only mild thrombocytopenia (platelets 136×10^9/L). One additional pRBC transfusion was administered.

No further relapses occurred over the next 10 months. These findings further support use of hIVIG for management of ITP but not IMHA.

CUTANEOUS DISEASE

Dermatologic autoimmune diseases, such as erythema multiforme (EM), Stevens-Johnson syndrome (SJS), and TEN can result as a reaction to drug administration. These disorders are typified by full-thickness epidermal detachment and systemic disease, and can be extremely painful with guarded prognoses.[29–35] Pemphigus foliaceus (PF) is an additional autoimmune disorder (the most common in veterinary patients) and is characterized by destruction of desmosomes, blistering, and pustule formation.[29] These conditions are often unresponsive to standard immunosuppressive medications. Immunoglobulin is widely incorporated into treatment protocols in sick people with cutaneous autoimmune disorders.[32–35] Two retrospective studies evaluating hIVIG administration in select patient cohorts showed high remission (>80%) in patients with pemphigus and resolution of epidermal detachment and decreased mortality in patients with TEN, respectively.[29–35]

Veterinary studies suggest hIVIG may also benefit companion animals with cutaneous autoimmune disease. A 2004 case report of a dog that developed SJS after trimethoprim-potentiated sulfadiazine administration documented complete disease resolution after a single infusion of hIVIG.[35] This patient was referred for a 14-day history of mucocutaneous ulceration, nasal planum and footpad sloughing, and diffuse macular eruption after failing therapy with antimicrobials and topical fusidic acid/betamethasone gel. *Pseudomonas aeruginosa* infection precluded methylprednisolone treatment in this dog. hIVIG (0.5 g/kg) was subsequently administered over 7 hours. Lesions improved visibly within 12 hours of infusion, and resolved completely within a week.

A 2006 report describes successful treatment of necrotic dermatitis with hIVIG in 2 critically ill dogs.[8] Both dogs developed clinical signs after multiple-drug exposure, and continued to decline following standard immunosuppressive therapy. hIVIG (1 g/kg) was administered to each patient twice, 24 hours apart, whereas steroids were temporarily discontinued because of concerns for infection. Appreciable improvement in dermal lesions and systemic stability occurred within 72 hours, and both dogs ultimately recovered. No reactions occurred, despite serial hIVIG infusion. Patients were followed for 3 years without evidence of relapse.

Immunoglobulin therapy may also benefit dogs with PF. Pemphigus is generally treated with prednisone, and adjunctive treatments (cyclosporine or azathioprine) are added as needed. PF is notoriously difficult to control, and relapse is common. A 2006 study describes effective management of PF with hIVIG added to standard immunosuppressive protocol.[29] Clinicians elected serial hIVIG infusion rather than steroid therapy because of risk of sepsis. The treatment protocol consisted of daily hIVIG for 4 days (total dose 2 g/kg). Significant improvement occurred after hIVIG infusion, and the dog was deemed stable enough for prednisone and azathioprine therapy on day 5. One additional 0.5-g/kg hIVIG infusion was administered 3 weeks later and 2 additional 0.5-g/kg treatments 24 hours apart 9 weeks after discharge for disease relapse. The patient again improved, and was released with maintenance hIVIG scheduled for weeks 12, 22, 26, and 31. No immediate or delayed infusion reactions were recorded. The dog remained asymptomatic for 4 months after discharge before being lost to follow-up. This report is the first to detail serial hIVIG infusion for sustained remission of canine autoimmune disease. Further, results challenge the longstanding belief that multiple hIVIG infusions are not tolerated in dogs.

Only 1 report exists describing the use of hIVIG in cats. Byrne and Giger[36] describe successful hIVIG therapy in a kitten that developed EM after being vaccinated. Before referral, the kitten developed progressive systemic malaise and skin lesions that progressed despite topical moisturizer, lime sulfur, antibiotics, and prednisone therapy. Clinicians administered 2 1-g/kg hIVIG treatments 24 hours apart. Significant healing occurred within 4 days; lesions were largely resolved by day 8. No signs of relapse were present when rechecked 8 weeks later.[36]

Although encouraging, observational case reports lack statistical power and studies do not provide evidence-based data. Immunoglobulin therapy holds great promise for management of veterinary cutaneous autoimmune disease, but cannot be fully recommended until controlled clinical studies are completed.

MYASTHENIA GRAVIS

Acquired MG is characterized by localized or fulminant weakness secondary to autoimmune destruction of postsynaptic acetylcholine (Ach) receptors.[37] Anticholinesterase inhibition is the cornerstone of therapy and works by increasing Ach available to bind receptors.[37] Therapy has variable efficacy, because salvaged Ach competes with circulating autoantibodies for a dwindling number of receptors.[37] Spontaneous resolution is common in patients with MG, but prognosis remains guarded because many animals succumb to complications before remission.[37] As such, immunosuppressive therapy is often used to hasten recovery and improve outcome.

No consensus exists regarding immunomodulation for MG. Strategies often involve prednisone, azathioprine, cyclosporine, and/or mycophenolate mofetil.[37,38] Although not approved by the FDA, anecdotal reports in human medicine tout hIVIG infusion as effective therapy against MG.[38]

A 2009 report chronicles outcomes after administration of hIVIG in 2 dogs with MG. One dog received a single hIVIG infusion, whereas the other received a series of infusions over several weeks.[39] Anaphylaxis occurred during the final infusion in the series, but resolved after discontinuation of the infusion and administration of corticosteroids and diphenhydramine. Muscle strength increased appreciably in both dogs within 48 hours, but both relapsed within weeks. Researchers surmised that benefits of hIVIG in canines with MG are transient and debatable at best.

SUDDEN ACQUIRED RETINAL DETACHMENT SYNDROME

SARDS is an enigmatic disorder resulting in acute, painless canine blindness. Immunoglobulin-producing plasma cells in retinal tissue may generate autoantibodies that cause irreversible retinopathy in patients with SARDS.[40,41] No viable treatment options for SARDS exist: antiinflammatory, antimicrobial, and immunosuppressive therapies have all proved to be ineffective.[41,42] Human immune-mediated retinopathy is similarly difficult to treat, but partial return of vision is reported after immunoglobulin treatment.[42]

Investigators at Iowa State examined hIVIG therapy for treatment of SARDS in 2007.[43] Eight dogs with SARDS received immunoglobulin infusions (0.5 g/kg) over 6 hours on days 1 and 3. Vision (assessed via photoreceptor-mediated pupil response and visual maze behavior) remained crude to nonexistent. Given the high cost of hIVIG and lack of meaningful return of vision, hIVIG cannot be recommended for treatment of SARDS. A list of studies and potential uses for hIVIG in veterinary patients is provided in **Table 1**.

Table 1
Human intravenous immunoglobulin use in veterinary patients

Condition	Study Design	hIVIG Dose	Adverse Effects
IMHA	Blinded, randomized controlled, prospective trial (28 dogs)[21]	0.5 g/kg over 6 h for 3 consecutive days	Swelling at catheter site (2 of 28) Volume overload (1 of 28)
ITP	Retrospective case series (5 dogs)[26] Prospective, randomized, placebo-controlled trial (18 dogs)[27]	0.28–0.76 g/kg over 6 h, once 0.5 g/kg over 6 h, once	None None (followed for 6 mo)
ES	Case report (1 dog)[44]	1.3 g/kg over 8 h, once	None
Cutaneous drug reactions	Case reports (2 dogs,[8] 1 kitten[36])	1 g/kg over 4 h for 2 consecutive days (all subjects)	None
PF	Case report (1 dog)[29]	0.5 g/kg over 5 h on 4 consecutive days. Protocol repeated 3 wk after discharge 0.5 g/kg again administered over 4 h 9 wk after discharge on 2 consecutive days Maintenance hIVIG infusions administered on weeks 12, 22, 26, and 31	None
SARDS	Case series (8 dogs)[42]	0.5 g/kg over 7 h, once	None
MG	Case series (2 dogs)[37]	Dog 1: 0.5 g/kg over 6 h, once Dog 2: 0.5 g/kg over 6 h for 2 consecutive days. Two additional 0.5-g/kg doses administered 12 and 17 d after discharge	Dog 1: none Dog 2: erythema and anxiety during third transfusion, anaphylaxis during fourth transfusion 0

Data from Refs. [21,26,27,29,36,37,42, 44]

COMPLICATIONS OF HUMAN INTRAVENOUS IMMUNOGLOBULIN ADMINISTRATION

Immunoglobulin transfusion is generally well tolerated in people, with complication rates ranging from 5% to 15%.[43] Hypersensitivity reaction is the most common adverse effect reported.[43,45] Other undesirable potential effects include thromboembolism (TE), renal failure, hypotension, aseptic meningitis, intravascular fluid overload, transient neutropenia, and serum sickness.[43,45–47] The same list of potential complications applies for veterinary patients, but risk of infusion reaction is higher because hIVIG is a xenoprotein. However, few studies report complications after peri-hIVIG transfusion in veterinary patients.[8,16,18–24,29,35–37]

HYPERSENSITIVITY AND ANAPHYLAXIS

Acute hypersensitivity is also the most common complication of hIVIG infusion in companion animals. Clinical signs of hypersensitivity to hIVIG include pyrexia, flushing, facial edema, tachycardia, vomiting, diarrhea, dysrhythmias, dyspnea, hypotension, and seizures.[43,45–47] Most acute hypersensitivity reactions are transient and mild, but anaphylaxis can develop.[43,45] As with most transfusions, rate of hIVIG administration is correlated with complication rate. Slow initiation coupled with gradual increase in the rate of administration decrease the risk of adverse reaction substantially. Further, clinical signs of hypersensitivity often resolve after slowing or temporarily discontinuing the infusion.[48,49]

Type III hypersensitivity reactions are possible following hIVIG transfusion. Delayed hypersensitivity can cause antigen-antibody complex deposition in renal basement membranes and glomerulonephritis. This finding has yet to be documented in veterinary patients.[43,45]

THROMBOEMBOLIC DISEASE

Although considered safe in veterinary patients, research has shown that hIVIG administration stimulates inflammation, promotes hypercoagulability, and leads to increased risk of thromboembolic damage.[50] hIVIG also activates platelets, further stimulating clot formation.[49] This finding is especially pertinent when considering immunoglobulin therapy for patients with prothrombotic conditions such as IMHA. Given the procoagulable properties of hIVIG and lack of evidence supporting its use (for IMHA) in veterinary medicine, the risk/benefit ratio must be considered before hIVIG administration to any prothrombotic critically ill animal. Although TE has not been documented in veterinary patients treated with immunoglobulin, many clinicians advocate prophylactic antithrombotic therapy whenever hIVIG is administered.[48–50] Hyperviscosity also promotes hypercoagulability.[46] Many immunoglobulin preparations are hyperosmolar; rapid administration can disrupt capillary flow and encourage microthrombi formation.[46] Human guidelines advocate infusion rates of less than 400 mg/kg over 8 hours to avoid abrupt increase in viscosity.[50]

RENAL FAILURE

Acute renal failure is a rare complication of immunoglobulin therapy in humans. Renal injury is strongly linked to sucrose used as a stabilizer in some immunoglobulin preparations, which leads to osmotic damage to proximal tubules and subsequent cellular swelling, tubular occlusion, and marked cytoplasmic vacuolization.[13,51] Azotemia occurs within 5 days of therapy but is sometimes transient.[51] Sucrose-free immunoglobulin products (containing agents such as albumin, glucose, maltose, glycine, or D-sorbitol for stabilization) are widely available and exponentially safer[13,51]; however, these formulations still carry a small risk of tubular damage secondary to high solute load.[13,47,52] To avoid glycemic disruption, human patients with diabetes mellitus are often treated with sucrose-containing hIVIG products. In these cases, infusion rates of less than 3 mg/kg/min are recommended.[4,13]

MISCELLANEOUS CONDITIONS

Mild and transient pseudohyponatremia secondary to plasma hyperproteinemia is documented after hIVIG infusion in humans.[47] Intravascular fluid overload commonly occurs in humans after large-volume infusion or in patients with preexisting heart disease.[45–47] Dosing and transfusion rate must be carefully considered in patients with underlying heart disease. Very infrequently, dose-related aseptic meningitis develops 6 to 48 hours after hIVIG infusion in people.[52] Pathophysiology remains unclear. This finding is not reported in veterinary patients.[52]

VETERINARY ADMINISTRATION GUIDELINES

Immunoglobulin products are available in liquid, lyophilized, and freeze-dried forms.[45,48] A variety of diluents are used for reconstitution, which allows flexibility in final concentration and osmolality.[45,48] Liquid immunoglobulin requires refrigeration and has a shorter shelf life than powdered formulations.[47,48] Immunoglobulin should be warmed to room temperature before administration.[48] A dedicated peripheral line is required for administration of hIVIG, and an in-line filter is recommended during transfusion. Filter size requirements vary with manufacturers' recommendations.[48,49]

No dosing guidelines exist for hIVIG in companion animals. Studies report doses from 0.5 to 2.2 g/kg, with 1 g/kg most commonly administered.[8,16–22,24,35–40] Infusions are started at a slow rate (0.01 mL/kg/min) and gradually increased every 30 to 60 minutes to a maximum maintenance fluid rate of 0.08 mL/kg/min.[48,49] Comprehensive monitoring is imperative during administration, and signs of allergic reaction warrant discontinuation of infusion and administration of an antihistamine.[48,49] Many patients tolerate completion of the infusion at a lower rate.[48,49] Infusion time in veterinary studies ranges from 4 to 8 hours.

Multiple transfusions are commonly administered in humans, but the safety of repeat xenotransfusion in companion animals is questionable.[5–9] Several veterinary studies document serial intravenous immunoglobulin infusions without complication, but others report anaphylaxis after repeat administration.[31,34,37]

Current literature suggests hIVIG may be beneficial as part of multimodal immunosuppression against ITP and autoimmune cutaneous disease in veterinary patients. Efficacy against other immune-mediated diseases is debatable and hIVIG cannot be recommended for treatment of IMHA, ES, MG, and SARDS. Adverse effects associated with hIVIG occur infrequently in companion animals, and infusion is considered safe. hIVIG is expensive, but cost may be offset by decreased length of hospitalization. More controlled clinical trials are warranted to fully determine the utility of hIVIG for treatment of veterinary autoimmune disease and to establish standard dosing and transfusion guidelines.

REFERENCES

1. Berger M, Richard E. From subcutaneous to intravenous immunoglobulins and back. In: Etzioni A, Ochs HD, editors. Primary immunodeficiency disorders: a historic and scientific perspective. 1st edition. Oxford (United Kingdom): Elsevier Academic Press; 2014. p. 283–4.

2. Kazatchkine M, Kaveri S. Immunomodulation of autoimmune and inflammatory diseases with intravenous immune globulin. N Engl J Med 2001;345(10):747–55.

3. Lemieux R, Bazin R, Neron S. Therapeutic intravenous immunoglobulins. Mol Immunol 2005;42(7):839–48.

4. Emmi L, Chiarini F. The role of intravenous immunoglobulin therapy in autoimmune and inflammatory disorders. Neurol Sci 2002;23(Suppl 1):S1–8.

5. World Health Organization. Appropriate uses of human immunoglobulin in clinical practice: memorandum from an IUIS/WHO meeting. Bull World Health Organ 1982;60(1):43–7.

6. Bayry J, Misra N, Latry V, et al. Mechanisms of action of intravenous immunoglobulin in autoimmune and inflammatory diseases. Transfus Clin Biol 2003;10(3):165–9.
7. Yanada Y, Arakaki R, Saito M, et al. Dual role of Fas/FasL-mediated signal in peripheral immune tolerance. Front Immunol 2017;8:403.
8. Trotman T, Phillips H, Fordyce H, et al. Treatment of severe adverse cutaneous drug reactions with human intravenous immunoglobulin in two dogs. J Am Anim Hosp Assoc 2006;42(4):312–20.
9. Knezevic-Maramica I, Kruskall M. Intravenous immune globulins: an update for clinicians. Transfusion 2003;43(10):1460–80.
10. Immune Globulin Intravenous (IGIV) indications. FDA Website; 2018. Available at: fda.gov. Accessed October 1, 2020.
11. Katz J. Intravenous Immunoglobulin. Medscape. 2018. Available at: https://emedicine.medscape.com/article/210367-overview#a2. Accessed September 1, 2019.
12. de Albuquerque-Campos R, Sato MN, Da Silva DAG. IgG anti-IgA subclasses in common variable immunodeficiency and association with severe adverse reactions to intravenous immunoglobulin therapy. J Clin Immunol 2000;20(1):77–82.
13. Foster R, Suri A, Filate W, et al. Use of intravenous immune globulin in the ICU: a retrospective review of prescribing practices and patient outcomes. Transfus Med 2010;20(6):403–8.
14. Yasuma R, Cicatiello V, Mizutani T, et al. Intravenous immune globulin suppresses angiogenesis in mice and humans. Signal Transduct Target Ther 2016;1 [pii: 15002].
15. Chen C, Danekas L, Ratko TA, et al. A multicenter drug use surveillance in intravenous immunoglobulin utilization in US Academic Health Centers. Ann Pharmacother 2000;34(3):295–9.
16. Scott-Moncrieff J, Regan W, Glickman L, et al. Treatment of nonregenerative anemia with human gamma-globulin in dogs. J Am Vet Med Assoc 1995;206(12):1895–900.
17. Kellerman D, Bruyette D. Intravenous human immunoglobulin for the treatment of immune-mediated hemolytic anemia in 13 dogs. J Vet Intern Med 1997;11(6):327–32.
18. Ballow M. The IgG molecule as a biological immune response modifier: mechanisms of action of intravenous immune serum globulin in autoimmune and inflammatory disorders. J Allergy Clin Immunol 2011;127(2):315–23.
19. Reagan W, Scott-Moncrieff C, Christian J, et al. Effects of human intravenous immunoglobulin on canine monocytes and lymphocytes. Am J Vet Res 1998;59(12):1568–74.
20. Rozanski E, Callan M, Hughes D, et al. Comparison of platelet count recovery with use of vincristine and prednisone or prednisone alone for treatment of severe immune-mediated thrombocytopenia in dogs. J Am Vet Med Assoc 2002;220(4):447–81.
21. Whelan MF, O'Toole TE, Chan D, et al. Use of human immunoglobulin in addition to glucocorticoids for the initial treatment of dogs with immune-mediated hemolytic anemia. J Vet Emerg Crit Care (San Antonio) 2009;19(2):158–64.
22. Gerber B, Steger A, Hassig M, et al. Use of human intravenous immunoglobulin in dogs with primary immune mediated anemia. Schweiz Arch Tierheilkd 2002;144(4):180–5.
23. Scott-Moncrieff J, Regan W. Human intravenous immunoglobulin therapy. Semin Vet Med Surg (Small Anim) 1997;12(3):178–85.

24. Scott-Moncrieff JC, Reagan WJ, Snyder PW, et al. Intravenous administration of human immune globulin in dogs with immune-mediated hemolytic anemia. J Am Vet Med Assoc 1997;210(11):1623–7.

25. Darabi K, Abdel-Whab O, Dzik W. Current usage of Intravenous immune globulin and the rationale behind it: the Massachusetts General Hospital data and a review of the literature. Transfusion 2006;46(5):741–53.

26. Bianco D, Armstrong P, Washabau R. Treatment of severe immune-mediated thrombocytopenia with human IV immunoglobulin in 5 dogs. J Vet Intern Med 2007;21(4):694–9.

27. Bianco D, Armstrong P, Washabau R. A prospective, randomized, double blinded, placebo-controlled study of human intravenous immunoglobulin for the acute management of presumptive primary immune-mediated thrombocytopenia in dogs. J Vet Intern Med 2009;23(5):1071–8.

28. Balog K, Huang A, Sum S, et al. A prospective randomized clinical trial of vincristine versus human intravenous immunoglobulin for acute adjunctive management of presumptive primary immune-mediated thrombocytopenia in dogs. J Vet Intern Med 2013;27(3):536–41.

29. Rahilly LJ, Keating JH, O'Toole TE. The use of intravenous human immunoglobulin in treatment of severe pemphigus foliaceus in a dog. J Vet Intern Med 2006;20(6):1483–6.

30. Jolles S, Hughes J, Whittaker S. Dermatological uses of high-dose intravenous immunoglobulin. Arch Dermatol 1998;134(1):80–6.

31. Hinn AC, Olivery T, Luther PB, et al. Erythema multiforme, Stevens-Johnson Syndrome, and toxic epidermal necrolysis in the dog: clinical classification, drug exposure, and histopathological correlations. J Vet Allergy Clin Immunol 1998; 6:13–20.

32. Prins C, Kerdel F, Padilla R. Treatment of toxic epidermal necrolysis with high dose intravenous immunoglobulins: multicenter retrospective analysis of 48 consecutive cases. Arch Dermatol 2003;139(1):26–32.

33. Stella M, Cassano P, Bollero D. Toxic epidermal necrolysis treated with intravenous high-dose immunoglobulins: our experience. Dermatology 2001; 203(1):45–9.

34. Ahmed AR, Spigelman Z, Cavacini LA, et al. Treatment of pemphigus vulgaris with rituximab and intravenous immunoglobulin. N Engl J Med 2006;355(17): 177–201.

35. Nuttall T, Malham T. Successful intravenous human immunoglobulin treatment of drug-induced Stevens-Johnson syndrome in a dog. J Small Anim Pract 2004; 45(7):357–61.

36. Byrne KP, Giger U. Use of human immunoglobulin for treatment of severe erythema multiforme in a cat. J Am Vet Med Assoc 2002;220(2):197–210.

37. Abelson A, Shelton G, Whelan M. Use of mycophenolate mofetil as a rescue agent in the treatment of severe generalized myasthenia gravis in three dogs. J Vet Emerg Crit Care (San Antonio) 2009;19(4):369–74.

38. Zinman L, Ng E, Bril V. IV immunoglobulin in patients with myasthenia gravis: a randomized controlled trial. Neurology 2007;68(11):837–41.

39. Bellhorn R, Murphy C, Thirkhill C. Anti-retinal immunoglobulins in canine ocular diseases. Semin Vet Med Surg (Small Anim) 1988;3(1):28–32.

40. Keller R, Kania S, Hendrix D. Evaluation of canine serum for the presence of anti-retinal autoantibodies in sudden acquired retinal degeneration syndrome. Vet Ophthalmol 2006;9(3):195–200.

41. Guy J, Aptsisauri N. Treatment of paraneoplastic visual loss with intravenous immunoglobulin: report of 3 cases. Arch Ophthalmol 1999;117(4):471–7.
42. Grozdanic S, Harper M, Kecova H, et al. Antibody-mediated retinopathies in canine patients: mechanism, diagnosis, and treatment modalities. Vet Clin North Am Small Anim Pract 2008;38(2):361–87.
43. Stiehm ER. Adverse effects of human immunoglobulin therapy. Transfus Med Rev 2013;27:171.
44. Bianco D, Hardy M. Treatment of Evans' syndrome with human intravenous immunoglobulin and lefunomide in a diabetic dog. J Am Anim Hosp Assoc 2009;45(3): 147–50.
45. Dunhem C, Dicato M, Ries F. Side effects of intravenous immune globulins. Clin Exp Immunol 1994;97:79–87.
46. Nydegger U, Sturzenegger M. Adverse effects of intravenous immunoglobulin therapy. Drug Saf 1999;43(10):171–85.
47. Orbach H, Katz U, Sherer Y, et al. Intravenous immunoglobulin: adverse effects and safe administration. Clin Rev Allergy Immunol 2005;29:173–85.
48. Murphy E, Martiin S, Valino-Patterson J. Developing practice guidelines for the administration of intravenous immunoglobulin. J Infus Nurs 2005;28:265–72.
49. Kirmse J. The nurse's role in administration of intravenous immunoglobulin therapy. Home Healthc Nurse 2009;27:104–11.
50. Tsuchiya R, Akutsu Y, Scott MA, et al. Prothrombotic and inflammatory effects of intravenous administration of human immunoglobulin G in dogs. J Vet Intern Med 2009;23(6):1164–9.
51. Cayco A, Perazella M, Hayslett J. Renal insufficiency after intravenous immune globulin therapy: a report of two cases and an analysis of the literature. J Am Soc Nephrol 1997;8(11):1788–94.
52. Sekul EA, Cupler EJ, Dalakas MC. Aseptic meningitis associated with high-dose intravenous immunoglobulin therapy: frequency and risk factors. Ann Intern Med 1994;121(4):259–62.

Resuscitation Strategies for the Small Animal Trauma Patient

Anusha Balakrishnan, BVSc

KEYWORDS

- Trauma • Resuscitation • Transfusion • Crystalloid • Colloid • Coagulopathy

KEY POINTS

- Resuscitation of the trauma patient should focus on the global goals of controlling hemorrhage and improving tissue hypoperfusion and minimize ongoing inflammation by balanced use of blood products, hemorrhage control, and minimizing aggressive crystalloid use.
- Crystalloid fluid resuscitation of the traumatized patient with shock should be titrated in careful bolus infusions of 10 mL/kg to 20 mL/kg, administered over 15 minutes to 30 minutes, while closely monitoring for improvement of perfusion parameters or adverse effects.
- Hypertonic saline (7% or 7.5%; 3–5 mL/kg intravenous, over 20 minutes) is beneficial for rapid, small-volume resuscitation in trauma patients, especially those with traumatic brain injury.
- The use of blood products (whole blood, fresh frozen plasma, or packed red blood cells) should be considered in patients presenting with acute hemorrhagic shock after major trauma.
- Hypotensive or damage control resuscitation is a temporary solution until definitive hemostatic control (usually via surgical intervention) is achieved and is not recommended as a long-term treatment approach given the risk of ongoing impairment of tissue perfusion.

Traumatic injuries in small animals are a relatively common cause for presentation to emergency departments. A recent registry report by the American College of Veterinary Emergency and Critical Care Veterinary Committee on Trauma (VetCOT) revealed that blunt force trauma (primarily vehicular trauma and fall from height) was the most common presenting trauma complaint in cats whereas penetrating trauma (primarily bite wounds and lacerations) was the most common source of injury in dogs (52.3%).[1] Overall, the mortality rate reported for traumatic injuries in dogs and cats is low, with the VetCOT registry reporting that 92% of dogs and 82.5% of cats survived to discharge after presenting for evaluation of traumatic injuries.[1]

Cornell University Veterinary Specialists, 880 Canal Street, Stamford, CT 06902, USA
E-mail address: abalakrishnan@cuvs.org

Vet Clin Small Anim 50 (2020) 1385–1396
https://doi.org/10.1016/j.cvsm.2020.07.012
0195-5616/20/© 2020 Elsevier Inc. All rights reserved.

Severe traumatic injury results in a multitude of systemic responses, which can exacerbate the initial tissue damage. The systemic response to trauma involves interaction between the inflammatory, coagulation, and neuroendocrine systems and also is characterized by a weakened immune response toward infection, increasing the risk of sepsis in the posttraumatic state.[2,3]

The approach to resuscitating human and veterinary patients with trauma has evolved greatly over the past decade. Trauma resuscitation should focus on the global goals of controlling hemorrhage and improving tissue hypoperfusion but also minimizing ongoing inflammation and, therefore, morbidity through the concept of "damage-control resuscitation." This approach focuses heavily on the balanced use of blood products, hemorrhage control, and minimizing aggressive crystalloid use.[4] Although these tenets may not be directly applicable to every veterinary patient with trauma, they provide useful guidance when managing the most severely injured subpopulation of these patients.

EMERGENCY ASSESSMENT AND STABILIZATION

Any small animal patient presenting for traumatic injury should be evaluated rapidly by the emergency nursing team and the veterinarian. Ideally, at the time of presentation, permission should be sought from the owner to institute emergency stabilization measures as needed. Triage assessment should include an initial rapid focused visual and brief physical assessment for life-threatening traumatic injuries, including massive hemorrhage, tension pneumothorax, and traumatic brain injury. Additional evaluation of the extent of injuries should be performed in conjunction with initial stabilization efforts.

Triage evaluation should be focused on evaluation of the cardiovascular, respiratory, neurologic, and urinary systems. When patient stability permits, a more thorough physical examination evaluating the gastrointestinal, musculoskeletal, and integumentary systems can be performed to determine the complete extent of injuries.[5]

Systematic evaluation of the trauma patient should focus on the following:

1. Respiratory system: the patient's breathing should be first assessed visually to detect abnormal breathing patterns (such as a restrictive breathing pattern, which may be seen with pleural space disease, such as a pneumothorax, hemothorax, or paradoxic chest wall movements). Patients exhibiting signs of cyanosis or respiratory distress should be stabilized rapidly. Attention also should be paid to any abnormal upper airway noises, such as stridor or stertor, which may be indicative of trauma to the laryngeal or nasopharyngeal regions, respectively. Thoracic auscultation may reveal pulmonary crackles in patients with lung contusions, muffled lung sounds, or occasionally borborygmi in cases of traumatic diaphragmatic hernia. The presence of penetrating thoracic trauma, if there are palpable rib fractures or a flail chest, also should be assessed. The initial physical examination performed at the time of triage may not reveal overt signs of pulmonary contusions, which rapidly worsen over the first 24 hours to 48 hours after trauma or after resuscitation efforts.

When stable, ideally thoracic imaging via radiographs or a CT scan should be performed to evaluate for the complete extent of trauma. As discussed previously, pulmonary contusions may not be radiographically apparent at the time of initial imaging but may develop over the course of the next 24 hours to 48 hours.[6] In addition to subjectively visually monitoring for increased respiratory effort, pulse oximetry and arterial blood gas monitoring can be used to objectively assess for hypoxemia and the ongoing need for supplemental oxygen.

2. Cardiovascular system: the traumatized patient should be assessed for evidence of shock. Hypovolemic shock, manifested by pale mucous membranes, tachycardia, prolonged capillary refill time, poor peripheral pulse quality, and cool extremities, may be common in patients that have experienced significant hemorrhage (either bleeding from external wounds or intracavitary bleeding, such as with a traumatic hemoperitoneum). Cats with significant trauma may present in decompensatory shock and may appear bradycardic instead of tachycardic. The presence of other dysrhythmias, if any, also should be evaluated. Indirect blood pressure (BP) measurement using Doppler plethysmography or oscillometry can serve as a surrogate means of determining the adequacy of tissue perfusion if the systolic BP is greater than 100 mm Hg and the mean arterial BP (MAP) greater than 65 mm A normal BP, however, does not rule out tissue hypoperfusion. Serum lactate, which can be easily obtained via point-of-care testing, is another useful marker for tissue hypoperfusion in the traumatized patient.[7,8]

3. Neurologic system: when possible, initial neurologic assessment should be performed prior to administering any pain medications, such as opioids or other medications, that may influence the findings on a neurologic examination. Initial evaluation should focus on a patient's level of consciousness, posture, ability to ambulate, pupil size, and responsiveness to light. The presence of voluntary motor function and deep pain sensation in the limbs ideally should be evaluated as well, although stabilization of the respiratory and cardiovascular systems should be prioritized prior to a full neurologic exam being performed. When a thorough neurologic examination is able to be performed, scoring systems, such as the modified Glasgow Coma Scale,[9] which has been validated in dogs, can be used to obtain an initial assessment of injury severity as well as monitor serial progression. The presence of shock can have an impact on a patient's level of consciousness and cranial nerve responses, and this must be taken into consideration when interpreting a triage neurologic examination. In addition to traumatic brain injury, spinal trauma also can be present, including the presence of traumatic intervertebral disk herniation and vertebral fractures or luxations.

4. Urogenital system: urinary bladder or other urogenital trauma (such as ureteral avulsion or rupture) resulting in rupture and uroperitoneum can occur after blunt force trauma in dogs and cats. Although a traumatic uroabdomen is a medical emergency that warrants rapid recognition and medical stabilization, surgical intervention ultimately may be required in some of these patients.[10] Initial bedside ultrasonographic evaluation of the abdomen can reveal evidence of urinary tract rupture through the presence of free abdominal fluid. An intact urinary bladder may or may not be able to be visualized in patients with uroabdomen. Diagnostic abdominocentesis can help distinguish peritoneal effusion in a trauma patient from intra-abdominal hemorrhage. Additionally, blood work may reveal evidence of azotemia and hyperkalemia, although these changes may not be immediately evident in the peracute setting.

5. Musculoskeletal and integumentary systems: once more stable, the patient should be closely evaluated for the presence of orthopedic trauma, such as appendicular fractures or luxations, as well as integumentary trauma, such as puncture wounds or lacerations.

EMERGENT STABILIZATION AND FLUID RESUSCITATION OF THE TRAUMA PATIENT

Stabilization efforts should be initiated simultaneously while a patient initially is being examined. Flow-by oxygen therapy should be instituted for any patient with respiratory compromise. Intravenous (IV) access should be obtained and preferably should be the widest bore and shortest length catheter possible to ensure maximal efficiency when delivering IV fluid boluses.[11]

If rapid, large-volume shock fluid administration is required, such as for a trauma patient with massive hemorrhage, multiple large-bore peripheral IV catheters can be placed. When peripheral venous access is difficult to achieve because of severe intravascular volume depletion, jugular venous access can be attempted with a large-bore, short-IV catheter. Care should be taken, however, when manipulating the jugular vein in patients with suspected traumatic brain injury, because this can impede venous return from the brain and cause exacerbation of intracranial hypertension.[12] Occasionally, extremely unstable trauma patients may be presented in cardiopulmonary arrest and a vascular cutdown procedure may be necessary to achieve vascular access. In these cases, ideally a jugular vein or cephalic vein is preferable to saphenous veins. Intraosseous (IO) access is another option in these patients, especially pediatric patients. The proximolateral humerus and proximomedial tibia are excellent choices for easy establishment of IO access. A 20G to 22G hypodermic needle can be used in pediatric patients, and, in adult animals, an IO access drill may be used to provide rapid access.

TRAUMATIC COAGULOPATHY IN VETERINARY PATIENTS

Acute traumatic coagulopathy (ATC) is a well-established phenomenon in human trauma patients that results from a complex interplay of the coagulation and inflammatory systems and has been shown to increase both early and late posttraumatic death in these patients.[13–15] This phenomenon results in prolongation of bleeding and sustained hypoperfusion in the early stages (<24 hours after trauma) and leads to an injurious cascade of systemic inflammation, acute lung injury, and multiple organ failure in the later stages (>24 hours after trauma).[13] Postulated mechanisms for this syndrome include activation of the protein C cascade after massive trauma, damage to the endothelial glycocalyx, endothelial disruption, and depletion of fibrinogen. The consequence of these changes is decreased clot strength and hyperfibrinolysis and ultimately an increase in hemorrhagic tendencies. This increase in hemorrhagic tendencies can be exacerbated by aggressive crystalloid-based resuscitation strategies.[16] Veterinary literature suggests that the incidence of ATC is rare in minimally injured dogs and cats but may have an increased risk of occurrence in more severely injured animals. Veterinary studies have found an increased risk of ATC in trauma patients that present with a low systolic BP and increased admission lactate levels.[17–19] Documentation of ATC in veterinary patients can be performed using either routine bedside coagulation parameter testing or viscoelastic testing, such as thromboelastography. A prothrombin time or activated partial thromboplastin time greater than 1.5 times the reference interval can be considered consistent with ATC when measured on initial presentation. Alternatively, if using viscoelastic testing, maximal amplitude, or G values, which represents global clot strength, less than the reference interval are considered consistent with ATC.

In severely injured patients, the presence of ATC should be a consideration when factoring in initial fluid resuscitation and, ideally, overzealous crystalloid use should be avoided. Management of ATC, aside from tailored fluid therapy with minimal crystalloid use and balanced blood product usage, also includes the use of antifibrinolytic medications, such as tranexamic acid or ε-aminocaproic acid (EACA), which block the lysine binding sites on plasminogen and subsequently inhibit fibrinolysis. Although tranexamic acid has been studied extensively in human trauma patients, EACA recently has been studied in veterinary patients with ATC; a recent case report found that EACA administered at a dose of 33 mg/kg IV, every 6 hours, inhibited fibrinolysis and resulted in rapid clinical improvement in a dog with suspected ATC.[20]

FLUID RESUSCITATION OPTIONS IN THE VETERINARY PATIENT WITH TRAUMA

1. Isotonic crystalloids: these are fluids that have a composition similar to that of the extracellular fluid and primarily contain the inorganic salt sodium chloride (NaCl), with 0.9% NaCl the prototype isotonic crystalloid. Approximately 75% of the volume of sodium-based IV fluids is redistributed rapidly into the interstitium within approximately 20 minutes of administration.

   When used for shock resuscitation, the classic shock dose is approximately 60 mL/kg to 90 mL/kg in dogs and approximately 45 mL/kg to 60 mL/kg in cats, which reflects the approximate blood volumes in each species. Complete shock doses rarely are necessary, however, and excessive volume administration is associated with increased organ dysfunction and mortality, especially in trauma patients.[21,22] A common recommendation in small animals that have sustained trauma is to begin treatment of shock by infusing a bolus of 10 mL/kg to 20 mL/kg, administered over 15 minutes to 30 minutes. The patient should be monitored closely during delivery of the bolus, and it should be slowed or discontinued if any adverse effects are seen or if perfusion parameters improve before the end of the predetermined amount. Considerations that may have an impact on the volume of crystalloids administered as a bolus include the presence of or suspicion for pulmonary contusions (because pulmonary edema and respiratory distress may be worsened after crystalloid administration). Additionally, when ATC is documented or suspected, caution is advised with crystalloid use to avoid diluting out coagulation factors, decreasing blood viscosity, and exacerbating bleeding tendencies. Comorbidities, such as preexisting cardiac disease, also should be taken into account. Aggressive crystalloid resuscitation has been associated with negative outcomes in human patients with blunt trauma,[21] although this has not been demonstrated in veterinary studies.

2. Synthetic colloids: commercially available synthetic colloids typically contain large colloid molecules suspended in an isotonic crystalloid solution. These include derivatives of hydroxyethyl starches, including hetastarch (available as a 6% solution suspended in an isotonic crystalloid solution, such as 0.9% saline [Hespan, Braun, Irvine, CA] or a lactated electrolyte solution [Hextend], Hospira Inc, Lake Forest, IL), pentastarch (Pentaspan, Braun, Irvine, CA), and tetrastarch ([VetStarch, Zoetis, Kalamazoo, MI) or Hydravol, Vedco, St Joseph, MO)]. When synthetic colloids are used for the treatment of shock in trauma patients, the typical dose is 5 mL/kg to 20 mL/kg in the dog and 2.5 mL/kg to 10 mL/kg in the cat. This commonly is administered to effect in incremental boluses over 10 minutes to 20 minutes. Similar considerations for exacerbation of preexisting cardiac disease and pulmonary contusions exist with colloid use. Additional concerns with colloid use include the potential risk for acute kidney injury (AKI), which has been studied in human septic patients[23-29] and some populations of small animals, including critically ill dogs and cats.[30-36] Although there is no definitive evidence to suggest a risk of AKI in dogs and cats with trauma, caution should be exercised when using these fluids. A greater concern in trauma patients is the effect of synthetic colloids on coagulation.[37-42] All colloidal plasma substitutes can interfere with hemostasis either through hemodilution or decreases in the activity of von Willebrand factor and its associated factor VIII activities as well as some degree of platelet

dysfunction.[38] Thus, in trauma patients with significant hemorrhage or concern for ATC, synthetic colloids should be avoided to the extent possible, if other options, such as blood products, are available for use.

3. Hypertonic saline: hypertonic saline solutions are available commercially in variable concentrations of 3% to 23.4%. Hypertonic saline has several beneficial properties that make it an excellent choice for rapid, small-volume resuscitation in trauma patients, especially those with traumatic brain injury. These include immunomodulatory effects, such as decreased neutrophil activation and adherence, stimulation of lymphocyte proliferation, and inhibition of proinflammatory cytokine production by macrophages. Hypertonic saline also improves the rheologic properties of circulating blood, reduces endothelial cell swelling, and helps reduce intracranial pressure in patients with traumatic brain injury.[43–46]

Hypertonic saline is used most commonly as either a 3% or a 7.0% to 7.5% solution. Typically, a 3-mL/kg to 5-mL/kg dose of 7% to 7.5% solution is used for shock resuscitation during trauma. Because hypertonic saline rapidly redistributes into the interstitium within 30 minutes after administration and also causes an osmotic diuresis, its volume expansion effect is short-lived. For this reason, it can be combined with a synthetic colloid.[47] This combined solution, sometimes referred to as turbostarch, is administered at a dose of 3 mL/kg to 5 mL/kg and is prepared by mixing a stock solution of 23.4% hypertonic saline with 6% hydroxyethyl starch in an approximately 1:2 ratio to arrive at a total volume of 3 mL/kg to 5 mL/kg. For example, a 5-mL/kg dose for a 6-kg dog is 30 mL. Therefore, 1 part 23.4% hypertonic saline (10 mL) with 2 parts (20 mL) 6% hydroxyethyl starch creates an approximately 7.5% hypertonic saline/colloid solution. Hypertonic saline can cause transient hypernatremia and hyperchloremia and should be avoided in patients with interstitial dehydration. It should be used cautiously in animals at risk for volume overload or with pulmonary contusions, especially cats.

The use of hypertonic saline and synthetic colloids in veterinary trauma patients is an especially valuable option to consider in military working dogs, where blood product availability is limited, at best. In this population, a majority of cases managed for shock by military personnel have trauma-induced hemorrhagic shock and rapid, effective volume expansion is necessary.[48]

4. Blood products: the use of blood products (whole blood, fresh frozen plasma [FFP], or packed red blood cells [pRBCs]) forms the cornerstone of trauma resuscitation. Fresh whole-blood transfusions carry the benefit of increased levels of clotting factors, fibrinogen, and platelets compared with component therapy. Current recommendations in human trauma resuscitation advocate minimizing or altogether avoiding crystalloid use in patients, especially with more severe trauma, to avoid exacerbating underlying ATC. Aggressive use of FFP is recommended in situations where whole-blood is not easily available with FFP/pRBCs given in the ratio of 1:1. In human trauma patients with severe hemorrhage, the aggressive use of platelet transfusions also is recommended with a ratio of 1:1:1 for FFP:pRBC:platelets to maximize the ability to control bleeding and manage hemorrhagic shock.[49,50]

Typical management of a patient presenting with acute hemorrhagic shock after major trauma includes pRBCs and FFP at a dose of 10 mL/kg to 20 mL/kg. Although transfusions usually are administered over a period of 2 hours to 4 hours, rapidly decompensating patients may require faster infusion rates (ie, 1.5 mL/kg/min over 15–20 minutes). The term, *massive transfusion*, defined as the replacement of a volume of whole-blood or blood components that is greater than the patient's estimated blood volume, may be an approach needed in patient with massive hemorrhage secondary to trauma.[51] This typically involves significant intracavitary bleeding (such as a traumatic hemoperitoneum), although may be relatively uncommon in veterinary medicine because patients with trauma significant enough to cause massive hemorrhage rarely survive and often succumb to their injuries before they can be evaluated by a veterinarian. Massive transfusions carry a much higher risk of adverse transfusion related effects (eg, electrolyte imbalances, acute lung injury, and immunologic reactions). If a patient has been resuscitated only using crystalloids or synthetic colloid fluids, and ongoing monitoring reveals persistent metabolic acidosis, worsening or persistent elevations in serum lactate and base deficit, and abnormal central venous hemoglobin oxygen saturation variables, ongoing tissue ischemia is a concern. These findings may imply that there is a need for additional resuscitative measures, such as blood product transfusions, especially if there is evidence of a decreasing packed cell volume (PCV) when serially monitored.[52]

HYPOTENSIVE RESUSCITATION IN THE TRAUMA PATIENT

Traditional fluid resuscitation for patients with hemorrhagic shock involves resuscitation until a normal systolic BP is achieved. In recent years, however, literature has pointed toward an improved survival (particularly in trauma patients) when a more conservative resuscitation strategy, known as hypotensive resuscitation, is employed in the acute setting during active hemorrhage.[53–56] Restoration of a lower-than-normal systolic BP (approximately 80–90 mm Hg) by avoiding aggressive fluid boluses minimizes rapid increases in intravascular hydrostatic pressure, facilitates control of hemorrhage, and reduces the risk of rebleeding but at the same time ensures preserved blood flow to vital organs, such as the kidney and gastrointestinal tract. It is important to emphasize, however, that hypotensive or damage control resuscitation is a temporary solution until definitive hemostatic control (usually via surgical intervention) is achieved and is not a long-term treatment approach, given the risk of ongoing impairment of tissue perfusion.[53]

MONITORING THE TRAUMA PATIENT

Fluid therapy for the treatment of traumatic shock should be performed under extremely close monitoring and should continue until various resuscitation endpoints have been reached. In general, these endpoints include physical examination parameters, such as normalization of heart rate (between 80 beats per minute [bpm] and 140 bpm in dogs and 180 bpm and 220 bpm in cats), pulse quality (strong and synchronous pulse quality), capillary refill time (<2 seconds), rectal temperature (99oF–101oF), temperature of extremities, and improvement of mentation. Normalization of arterial BP (ideally systolic BP 90–120 mm Hg and MAP 65–85 mm Hg) is another clinical parameter that often is used to guide shock fluid therapy.[12] In patients with traumatic brain injury, maintenance of MAP is a key determinant of cerebral perfusion pressure (as well as ensuring that intracranial hypertension has been addressed). Blood work parameters, such as serial lactate levels (ideally should be <2 mmol/L) and central venous oxygen saturation (65%–70%), when available, can be monitored to ensure improvement with fluid therapy. When possible, urine output monitoring (ideally between 1 mL/kg/h and 4 mL/kg/h) should be performed as an additional tool to gauge adequacy of fluid resuscitation and renal perfusion. Serial monitoring of PCV (ideally >25%) is a useful point-of-care tool to evaluate for ongoing hemorrhage that may require additional intervention, such as surgical hemostasis or blood product therapy.[52]

Respiratory status should be monitored closely in these patients because pulmonary contusions can develop over time and cause rapid clinical deterioration. Pulse oximetry levels (> 95%) or arterial blood gas analysis (Pao_2 >80 mm Hg on room air) are useful indicators of oxygenation. Supplemental oxygen should be provided to patients with evidence of hypoxemia to maintain adequate oxygen levels. In patients with traumatic brain injury or significant thoracic trauma, monitoring CO_2 levels in the blood (venous Pco_2 40–45 mm Hg or arterial Pco_2 30–40 mm Hg) is important to assess adequacy of ventilation. Brainstem injury, cervical spinal trauma, or significant thoracic wall trauma (rib fractures, including flail chest or penetrating chest wall injuries) as well as pleural space trauma (diaphragmatic hernia and pneumothorax) and severe pulmonary contusions all can have an impact on ventilatory function and cause hypercapnia. When Pco_2 levels exceed 60 mm Hg and respiratory acidosis ensues, additional interventions may be required, depending on the cause. If pneumothorax is suspected, thoracocentesis should be initiated immediately because progressive tension pneumothorax can be rapidly fatal.

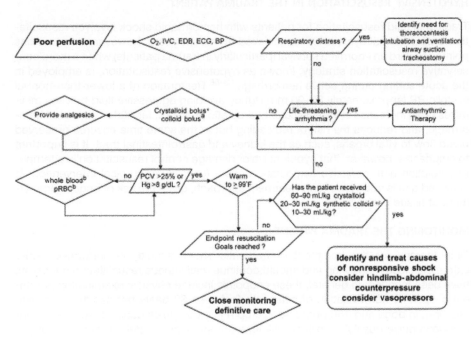

Fig. 1. Resuscitation algorithm for the trauma patient. This resuscitation algorithm is a guide for immediate stabilization and fluid resuscitation of the trauma patient with poor perfusion variables; [a] Buffered isotonic replacement crystalloid (eg, Plasmalyte (Baxter, Deerfield, IL)-7.4 or Normosol-R at a rate of 10–15 mL/kg) and HES (3–5 mL/kg) or Oxyglobin (dog: 3 mL/kg–5-mL/kg boluses up to 30 mL/kg; cat: 1-mL/kg–3-mL/kg boluses up to 10 mL/kg). [b] Calculation of volume of blood transfusion to administer (dog: weight [lb] × 40 × [desired PCV − patient PCV]/donor PCV = milliliters to administer; cat: weight [lb] × 30 × [desired PCV − patient PCV]/donor PCV = milliliters to administer). For the cat, 60 mL/kg, and for the dog, 90 mL/kg; and for the cat, 10 mL/kg, and, for the dog, 30 mL/kg. ECG, electrocardiogram; EDB, emergency database (PCV, total protein, blood glucose, venous blood gas, electrolyte panel, lactate, and blood urea nitrogen); HES, hetastarch; Hg, hemoglobin; IVC, IV catheter; O_2, oxygen. *From* Rudloff E, Kirby R. Fluid resuscitation and the trauma patient. Vet Clin North Am Small Anim Pract. 2008;38(3):645-52; with permission.

If neurologic injury, in particular traumatic brain injury, is suspected, the patient should be monitored for signs of intracranial hypertension, including dull mentation that may not improve with initial fluid therapy, cranial nerve deficits, and Cushing reflex (characterized by a combination of hypertension and reflex bradycardia). If intracranial hypertension is suspected, therapeutic options in veterinary patients include the administration of hyperosmolar fluids, such as mannitol (0.25–1.0 g/kg administered IV over 15–20 minutes) and hypertonic saline (7%–7.5%, administered either in a crystalloid base or combined with a synthetic colloid, as outlined previously).[12] Additionally, other simple interventions that can minimize intracranial hypertension include positioning the head, such that it is elevated at a 15o to 30o angle from the horizontal axis to increase venous drainage from the brain without deleterious changes in cerebral oxygenation, and avoiding the use of constrictive collars or wraps, including jugular catheters, which may obstruct the jugular veins and elevate intracranial pressure (Fig. 1).

SUMMARY

Traumatic injuries are common in dogs and cats. Emergency stabilization and resuscitation of these patients require rapid and thorough evaluation and recognition of potential life-threatening injuries as well as a focus on ameliorating the deleterious systemic responses to trauma. Optimizing tissue perfusion and close ongoing monitoring are crucial to maximizing good outcomes in this patient population.

DISCLOSURE

The author has nothing to disclose.

REFERENCES

1. Hall KE, Boller M, Hoffberg J, et al. ACVECC-Veterinary Committee on Trauma Registry Report 2013-2017. J Vet Emerg Crit Care 2018;28(6):497-502.

2. Lord JM, Midwinter MJ, Chen YF, et al. The systemic immune response to trauma: an overview of pathophysiology and treatment. Lancet 2014;384(9952): 1455-1465.

3. Lenz A, Franklin GA, Cheadle WG. Systemic inflammation after trauma. Injury 2007;38(12):1336-1345.

4. Harris T, Davenport R, Mak M, et al. The evolving science of trauma resuscitation. Emerg Med Clin North Am 2018;36(1):85–106.

5. Reineke E. Triage. In: Silverstein DS, Hopper K, editors. Small animal critical care medicine. 2nd edition. St Louis (MO): W.B. Saunders; 2015. p. 1–5.

6. Oppenheimer LU, Craven KD, Forkert LU, et al. Pathophysiology of pulmonary contusion in dogs. J Appl Physiol Respir Environ Exerc Physiol 1979;47(4): 718–28.

7. deLaforcade A, Silverstein DC. Shock. In: Silverstein DS, Hopper K, editors. Small animal critical care medicine. 2nd edition. St Louis (MO): W.B. Saunders; 2015. p. 26–30.

8. Cooper E. Hypotension. In: Silverstein DS, Hopper K, editors. Small animal critical care medicine. 2nd edition. St Louis (MO): W.B. Saunders; 2015. p. 46–50.

9. Platt SR, Radaelli ST, McDonnell JJ. The prognostic value of the modified Glasgow Coma Scale in head trauma in dogs. J Vet Intern Med 2001;15(6):581–4.

10. Stafford JR, Bartges JW. A clinical review of pathophysiology, diagnosis, and treatment of uroabdomen in the dog and cat. J Vet Emerg Crit Care 2013; 23(2):216–29.

11. Reddick AD, Ronald J, Morrison WG. Intravenous fluid resuscitation: was Poiseuille right? Emerg Med J 2011;28(3):201–2.

12. Sande A, West C. Traumatic brain injury: a review of pathophysiology and management. J Vet Emerg Crit Care 2010;20(2):177–90.

13. Simmons JW, Powell MF. Acute traumatic coagulopathy: pathophysiology and resuscitation. Br J Anaesth 2016;117(suppl 3):iii31–43.

14. Meledeo MA, Herzig MC, Bynum JA, et al. Acute traumatic coagulopathy: The elephant in a room of blind scientists. J Trauma Acute Care Surg 2017; 82(6S-Suppl 1):S33–40.

15. Cohen MJ, Kutcher M, Redick B, et al. Clinical and mechanistic drivers of acute traumatic coagulopathy. J Trauma Acute Care Surg 2013;75(1 Suppl 1):S40–7.

16. Davenport RA, Guerreiro M, Frith D, et al. Activated protein C drives the hyperfibrinolysis of acute traumatic coagulopathy. Anesthesiology 2017;126(1):115–27.

17. Gottlieb DL, Prittie J. Evaluation of acute traumatic coagulopathy in dogs and cats following blunt force trauma. J Vet Emerg Crit Care 2017;27(1):35–43.

18. Holowaychuk MK, Hanel RM, Darren Wood R, et al. Prospective multicenter evaluation of coagulation abnormalities in dogs following severe acute trauma. J Vet Emerg Crit Care 2014;24(1):93-104.

19. Abelson AL, O'Toole TE, Johnston A, et al. Hypoperfusion and acute traumatic coagulopathy in severely traumatized canine patients. J Vet Emerg Crit Care 2013;23(4):395–401.

20. Yoo SH, Venn E, Sullivan L, et al. Thromboelastographic evidence of inhibition of fibrinolysis after ε-aminocaproic acid administration in a dog with suspected acute traumatic coagulopathy. J Vet Emerg Crit Care 2016;26(5):737–42.

21. Kasotakis G, Sideris A, Yang Y, et al. Aggressive early crystalloid resuscitation adversely affects outcomes in adult blunt trauma patients: an analysis of the Glue Grant database. J Trauma Acute Care Surg 2013;74(5):1215–21.

22. Jones DG, Nantais J, Rezende-Neto JB, et al. Crystalloid resuscitation in trauma patients: deleterious effect of 5L or more in the first 24h. BMC Surg 2018;18(1):93.

23. Langeron O, Doelberg M, Ang ET, et al. Voluven®, a lower substituted novel hydroxyethyl starch (HES 130/0.4), causes fewer effects on coagulation in major orthopedic surgery than HES 200/0.5. Anesth Analg 2001;92(4):855–62.

24. Strauss RG, Pennell BJ, Stump DC. A randomized, blinded trial comparing the hemostatic effects of pentastarch versus hetastarch. Transfusion 2002;42(1): 27–36.

25. Bunn F, Trivedi D, Ashraf S. Colloid solutions for fluid resuscitation. Cochrane Database Syst Rev 2011;(3):CD001319.

26. Roberts I, Alderson P, Bunn F, et al. Colloids versus crystalloids for fluid resuscitation in critically ill patients. Cochrane Database Syst Rev 2004;(4):CD000567.

27. Perner A, Haase N, Wetterslev J, et al. Comparing the effect of hydroxyethyl starch 130/0.4 with balanced crystalloid solution on mortality and kidney failure in patients with severe sepsis (6S-Scandinavian Starch for Severe Sepsis/Septic Shock trial): study protocol, design and rationale for a double-blinded, randomized clinical trial. Trials 2011;12:24.

28. Schortgen F, Girou E, Deye N, et al. The risk associated with hyperoncotic colloids in patients with shock. Intensive Care Med 2008;34(12):2157–68.

29. Bayer O, Reinhart K, Sakr Y, et al. Renal effects of synthetic colloids and crystalloids in patients with severe sepsis: a prospective sequential comparison. Crit Care Med 2012;39(6):1335–42.

30. Hayes G, Benedicenti L, Mathews K. Retrospective cohort study on the incidence of acute kidney injury and death following hydroxyethyl starch (HES 10% 250/0.5/5:1) administration in dogs (2007-2010). J Vet Emerg Crit Care 2016;26(1):35–40.

31. Bae J, Soliman M, Kim H, et al. Rapid exacerbation of renal function after administration of hydroxyethyl starch in a dog. J Vet Med Sci 2017;79(9):1591–5.

32. Sigrist NE, Kalin N, Dreyfus A. Changes in serum creatinine concentration and acute kidney injury (AKI) grade in dogs treated with hydroxyethyl starch 130/0.4 from 2013 to 2015. J Vet Intern Med 2017;31:434–41.

33. Zersen KM, Mama K, Mathis JC. Retrospective evaluation of paired plasma creatinine and chloride concentrations following hetastarch administration in anesthetized dogs (2002-2015): 244 cases. J Vet Emerg Crit Care 2019;29(3):309–13.

34. Yozov ID, Howard J, Adamik K. Retrospective evaluation of the effects of administration of tetrastarch (hydroxyethyl starch 130/0.4) on plasma creatinine concentrations in dogs (2010-2013): 201 dogs. J Vet Emerg Crit Care 2016;26(4):568–77.

35. Boyd CJ, Claus MA, Raisis AL, et al. Evaluation of biomarkers of kidney injury following 4% succinylated gelatin and 6% hydroxyethyl starch 130/0.4 administration in a canine hemorrhagic shock model. J Vet Emerg Crit Care 2019;29(2):132–42.

36. Sigrist NE, Kalin N, Dreyfus A. Effects of hydroxyethyl starch 130/0.4 on serum creatinine concentration and development of acute kidney injury in nonazotemic cats. J Vet Intern Med 2017;31(6):1749–56.

37. Ekseth K, Abildgaard L, Vegfors M, et al. The in vitro effects of crystalloids and colloids on coagulation. Anaesthesia 2002;57(11):1102–8.

38. Mortier E, Ongenae M, De Baerdemaeker L, et al. In vitro evaluation of the effect of profound hemodilution with hydroxyethyl starch 6%, modified fluid gelatin 4% and dextran 40 10% on coagulation profile measured by thromboelastography. Anaesthesia 2005;52(11):1061–4.

39. Falco S, Bruno B, Maurella C, et al. In vitro evaluation of canine hemostasis following dilution with hydroxyethyl starch (130/0.4) via thromboelastometry. J Vet Intern Med 2012;22(6):640–5.

40. Fenger-Eriksen C, Tonnesen E, Ingerslev J, et al. Mechanisms of hydroxyethyl starch induced dilutional coagulopathy. J Thromb Haemost 2009;7(7):1099–105.

41. Classen J, Adamik KN, Weber K, et al. In vitro effect of hydroxyethyl starch 130/0.4 on canine platelet function. Am J Vet Res 2012;73(12):1908–12.

42. Gauthier V, Holowaychuk MK, Kerr CL, et al. Effect of synthetic colloid administration on coagulation in healthy dogs and dogs with systemic inflammation. J Vet Intern Med 2015;29(1):276–85.

43. Rizoli SB, Rhind SG, Shek PN, et al. The immunomodulatory effects of hypertonic saline resuscitation in patients sustaining traumatic hemorrhagic shock a randomized controlled double-blinded trial. Ann Surg 2006;243(1):47–57.

44. Bulger EM, Jurkovich GJ, Nathens AB, et al. Hypertonic resuscitation of hypovolemic shock after blunt trauma: a randomized controlled trial. Arch Surg 2008;143(2):139–48.

45. Mortazavi MM, Romeo AK, Deep A, et al. Hypertonic saline for treating raised intracranial pressure: literature review with meta-analysis. J Neurosurg 2012;116(1):210–21.

46. Balbino M, Neto AC, Prist R, et al. Fluid resuscitation with isotonic or hypertonic saline solution avoids intraneural calcium influx after traumatic brain injury associated with hemorrhagic shock. J Trauma Inj 2010;68(4):859–64.

47. Bentsen G, Breivik H, Lundar T, et al. Predictable reduction of intracranial hypertension with hypertonic saline hydroxyethyl starch: a prospective clinical trial in critically ill patients with subarachnoid hemorrhage. Acta Anaesthiol Scand 2004;48(9):1089–95.

48. Lagutchik M, Baker J, Balser J, et al. Trauma management of military working dogs. Mil Med 2018;183(suppl 2):180–9.

49. Como JJ, Dutton RP, Scalea TM, et al. Blood transfusion rates in the care of acute trauma. Transfusion 2004;44(6):809–13.

50. Repine TB, Perkins JG, Kauvar DS, et al. The use of fresh whole blood in massive transfusion. J Trauma 2006;60(6 Suppl):S59–69.

51. Jutkowitz AL, Rozanski EA, Moreau JA, et al. Massive transfusion in dogs: 15 cases (1997-2001). J Am Vet Med Assoc 2002;220(11):1664–9.

52. Rudloff E, Kirby R. Fluid resuscitation and the trauma patient. Vet Clin North Am Small Anim Pract 2008;38(3):645–52.

53. Holcomb JB, Jenkins D, Rhee P, et al. Damage control resuscitation: directly addressing the coagulopathy of trauma. J Trauma 2007;62(2):307–10.

54. Duchesne JC, McSwain NE, Cotton BA, et al. Damage control resuscitation: the new face of damage control. J Trauma 2010;69(4):976–90.

55. Morrison AC, Carrick MM, Norman MA, et al. Hypotensive resuscitation strategy reduces transfusion requirements and severe postoperative coagulopathy in trauma patients with hemorrhagic shock: preliminary results of a randomized controlled trial. J Trauma 2011;70(3):652–63.

56. Balakrishnan A, Silverstein DC. Shock fluids and fluid challenge. In: Silverstein DS, Hopper K, editors. Small animal critical care medicine. 2nd edition. St Louis (MO): W.B. Saunders; 2015. p. 321–7.

Use of Thromboelastography in Clinical Practice

Andrew G. Burton, BVSc[a], Karl E. Jandrey, DVM, MAS[b],*

KEYWORDS

- Coagulation • Hemostasis • Clinical pathology • Blood • Monitoring

KEY POINTS

- Viscoelastic testing with whole blood may provide information on in vivo hemostasis.
- Viscoelastic testing allows the identification of fibrinolysis, unlike many other assessments of hemostasis.
- The data achieved from viscoelastic tests can provide functional assessments of fibrin formation, clot strength, platelet function, as well as fibrinolysis.
- Many diseases are accompanied or identified by altered hemostasis. Viscoelastic tests can be an important adjunct for individualized clinical decision making.
- The use of activators and the introduction of point-of-care viscoelastic instruments is increasing the utility of these tests in clinical practice.

INTRODUCTION

Hemostasis is a complex physiologic process that culminates in the production of a fibrin clot. Classic models of hemostasis suggest that a cascade of coagulation factor interactions drive clot formation. However, the complex interactions between blood cells, platelets, endothelial cells, and soluble plasma factors described in the cell-based model of coagulation[1] highlight the potential limitations of standard plasma-based coagulation tests such as prothrombin time (PT) or activated partial thromboplastin time (aPTT). Viscoelastic testing, such as thromboelastography (TEG) or thromboelastometry, is performed on whole-blood samples, which include both soluble plasma factors as well as tissue factor and phospholipid-bearing blood cells and platelets. Therefore, viscoelastic tests may provide a closer representation of in vivo hemostasis. In addition, this methodology allows identification of fibrinolysis, and can provide analysis of platelet function.

[a] IDEXX Laboratories, Inc., 3 Centennial Drive, North Grafton, MA 01536, USA; [b] Clinical Small Animal Emergency and Critical Care, Department of Surgical and Radiological Sciences, School of Veterinary Medicine, University of California, Davis, One Shields Avenue, 1104C Tupper Hall, Davis, CA 95616, USA
* Corresponding author.
E-mail address: kejandrey@ucdavis.edu

Vet Clin Small Anim 50 (2020) 1397–1409
https://doi.org/10.1016/j.cvsm.2020.08.001
0195-5616/20/© 2020 Elsevier Inc. All rights reserved.

In recent years, viscoelastic testing has become increasingly accessible and popular in emergency and critical care settings and can provide important information for the diagnosis and management of patients with hemostatic disorders. This article discusses the principles and interpretation of viscoelastic testing, its application to small animal emergency and critical care medicine, and potential advantages and disadvantages of these tests.

METHODOLOGY
Samples

Original viscoelastic analyzers were designed as bedside tests, using nonanticoagulated (native) whole blood, and were analyzed within minutes of collection. This approach is impractical in a laboratory or clinical setting, and the use of citrated blood samples has been validated in dogs and cats.[2,3] Importantly, a comparison study reported that results from TEG performed on citrated and native blood are not comparable.[4]

Instrumentation

The most common viscoelastic testing systems used in veterinary medicine include TEG (Haemonetics Corp., Haemoscope division, Niles, IL) and ROTEM (rotation thromboelastometry, Pentapharm GmbH, Munich, Germany). TEG and ROTEM systems use a pin, attached to a torsion wire, suspended in a cylindrical cup. An aliquot of 0.36 mL of blood is added to the cup (prewarmed to 37°C). In TEG systems, movement is initiated by the cup, which rotates around the static pin at an angle of 4.45° every 10 seconds. In contrast, in ROTEM systems, it is the pin that oscillates within a static cup. As a clot forms, the pin and cup are joined by fibrin strands. In the TEG system, this causes the pin and cup to rotate together, and the change in torque is transmitted through the torsion wire and converted to an electrical signal. In ROTEM systems, the formation of fibrin strands between the cup and pin reduce the pin's oscillation, which is measured by the angle of deflection of a light beam.[5] In both systems, these changes are graphed as change in clot strength (measured in millimeters on the Y axis) against time (measured in minutes on the X axis).

Activators

In veterinary medicine, citrated samples are most frequently used for laboratory or clinic-based viscoelastic testing, using a contact activator such as kaolin or Celite. Recently, assays using tissue factor to assess the intrinsic pathway, or tissue factor with kaolin for more rapid analysis, have been used.[6]

Point-of-Care Testing

A novel, point-of-care viscoelastic device, viscoelastic coagulation monitor (VCM;VCM Vet, Entegrion, Inc, Research Triangle Park, NC) uses frosted glass discs held in parallel on flexible plastic arms within a cartridge. The narrow space between these discs holds the blood sample introduced via capillary action from a detachable sample cup. This surface triggers coagulation through contact activation. The plastic arms interact with optical sensors within the analyzer to assess the differences in proportional movement between stationary and oscillatory arms, and difference in these movements over time is calculated via device software and graphically displayed. Similar to the other viscoelastic technologies, the VCM measures fibrinolysis as the percentage decrease in the amplitude of the trace at various time points after the measurement of maximal clot strength (indicated as lysis parameters).

The VCM has the potential to reach broader veterinary audiences because it does not require sample manipulation. As soon as a native whole-blood sample is loaded to the cartridge, the sample is monitored in real time in a self-contained automated system. It uses small amounts of fresh whole blood (0.25–0.5 mL) directly from the patient, and is less expensive and requires less technical skill compared with TEG and ROTEM. VCM reference intervals have been established for both dogs and cats.[a,b]

INTERPRETATION OF VISCOELASTIC TEST RESULTS

Viscoelastic testing results in the formation of a trace of clot strength against time, from which multiple variables can be derived that allow for in-depth interpretation of coagulation status. The graph documents the progression from platelet aggregation, through clot formation, all the way to fibrinolysis and dissolution of the fibrin clot. Similar variables are measured by TEG and ROTEM; however, different terminology is used to describe these points in the tracing. These values are summarized in **Fig. 1** and **Table 1**, and are discussed in detail later.

Reaction Time/Clotting Time

The first stage of clot formation evaluated in viscoelastic testing is initial fibrin formation, reported as the reaction time (R) in TEG or clotting time (CT) in ROTEM systems. These values represent the point where fibrin polymers are first produced after clot initiation. R and CT can be expressed either in time (minutes) or distance (millimeters), and most commonly are reported as the time in minutes from clot initiation, to when the amplitude of the curve is 2 mm above baseline using citrated blood.

R and CT are affected by clotting factors within the intrinsic pathway including factor (F) VIII, FX, FXI, and FXII, as well as inhibitor activity. Prolongation of R or CT is associated with hypocoagulable states (eg, deficiencies in the aforementioned clotting factors), whereas a shortened R or CT is associated with a hypercoagulable state. The time at which R or CT are measured is the point at which standard plasma-based clotting assays such as PT or aPTT would end. Studies have shown variable correlation between results of R and CT from viscoelastic testing and results of standard coagulation assays. In a study that compared a control population with dogs admitted to an intensive care unit (ICU) with diseases known to affect coagulation status, there was a significant correlation between R and PT.[7] In contrast, another study found that dogs with decreased PT and aPTT had significantly more thrombus formation, but there was no correlation with TEG variables, although 19 out of 25 (76%) dogs with shortened PT and aPTT also had a shortened R.[8] In another study, there was also a trend toward shortened R times in patients with evidence of thrombosis on postmortem.[9]

Clot Kinetics/Clot Formation Time

After initial clot formation, the speed and strength of clot development is reported as clot kinetics (K) in TEG or clot formation time (CFT) in ROTEM systems. These values reflect the time taken to reach a predetermined level of clot strength, from initiation of

---

[a] Buriko Y, Silverstein D. Establishment of normal reference intervals in dogs using viscoelastic coagulation monitor (VCM) and validation of the VCM device using thromboelastography (TEG). European Veterinary Emergency and Critical Care Congress, Venice, Italy, June 2018. J Vet Emerg Crit Care 2018; 28: S27.

[b] Rosati T, Jandrey K, Burges J, et al. Establishment of a reference interval for a novel viscoelastic coagulometer and comparison to thromboelastography in healthy cats. European Veterinary Emergency and Critical Care Congress, Venice, Italy, June 2018. J Vet Emerg Crit Care 2018; 28: S34.

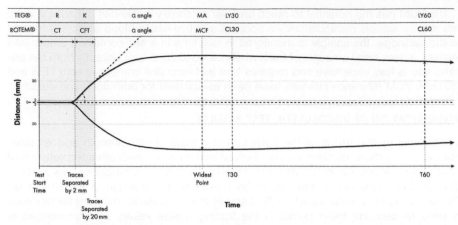

Fig. 1. A representative example of a viscoelastic trace showing the most common parameters and comparison between TEG and thromboelastometry (ROTEM). The X axis (time) shows critical points during the analysis where measurements are benchmarked. The Y axis is distance of the trace from baseline in millimeters (the amplitude). R (reaction time) or CT (clotting time) is reached when the amplitude reaches 2 mm. The K (clot kinetics) or CFT (clot formation time) is measured at 20-mm amplitude, a predetermined clot strength. The α (alpha) angle is formed from the line tangent between these first 2 points. The α angle represents the speed of fibrin formation and cross-linkage. Maximum amplitude (MA) or maximum clot firmness (MCF) is the widest point on the trace. The LY (lysis) or CL (clot lysis) times are measured at 30 minutes (T30) and 60 minutes (T60) after, and are indicated by the percentage of the MA/MCF.

clot formation at 2 mm, to when the curve reaches an amplitude of 20 mm. A shortened K or CFT is associated with hypercoagulability, whereas prolonged K or CFT is associated with hypocoagulability.

The K and CFT values are affected by platelet concentration and function, thrombin, fibrinogen, activity of FII and FVIII, and hematocrit (HCT). One study showed a significant increase in CFT after induction of in vivo reduced red cell mass (via phlebotomy), which was not confirmed by other coagulation variables, suggesting decreased HCT may artifactually result in hypercoagulable tracings using viscoelastic testing.[10] This possibility is further supported by the results of a study whereby in vitro manipulation of blood to create different reductions in HCT (45%, 20%, and 10%) were either corrected for viscosity with alginate or diluted with equal volumes of saline. This method resulted in hypercoagulability (with a shortened K) when using saline to decrease viscosity, but hypocoagulability when using alginate to correct for changes in viscosity associated with reduced HCT.[11] This phenomenon has also been reported in a population of diseased dogs with naturally occurring anemia.[12]

Alpha Angle

The alpha angle (α) is the angle formed between the baseline and a line tangent to the curve at the point of R or CT. Both TEG and ROTEM systems use this terminology and definition. The α is a reflection of the speed of clot formation as well as the kinetics of fibrin formation and cross-linkage. It is therefore closely related to the K or CFT values, and thus is influenced largely by the same factors. An increased α is associated with hypercoagulability, whereas a decreased α is associated with hypocoagulability. In a study of human patients with trauma, the alpha angle from rapid TEG results (tissue

Table 1
Thromboelastography and thromboelastometry (rotational thromboelastometry) system variables and interpretation of results

TEG	ROTEM	Units	Interpretation Hypercoagulable	Interpretation Hypocoagulable	Affected by
Reaction time	Clotting time	Minutes	Shortened	Prolonged	Clotting factors (FVIII, FIX, FXI, FXII)
Clot kinetics	Clot formation time	Minutes	Shortened	Prolonged	Platelet concentration, platelet function, FII, FVIII, fibrinogen concentration, HCT
Alpha angle	Alpha angle	Degrees	Increased	Decreased	Platelet concentration, platelet function, FII, FVIII, fibrinogen concentration, HCT
Maximum amplitude	Maximum clot firmness	Millimeters	Increased	Decreased	Fibrinogen concentration, platelet concentration and function, thrombin concentration FXIII, HCT
G (shear elastic modulus)	G (shear elastic modulus)	Dynes/cm^2	Increased	Decreased	Fibrinogen concentration, platelet concentration and function, thrombin concentration, FXIII, HCT
—			Hyperfibrinolysis	Hypofibrinolysis	—
LY30/60	CL30/60	Percent	Increased	Decreased	Clot inhibitor concentration

Abbreviation: HCT, hematocrit.

factor activated) had the greatest single factor sensitivity (compared with other TEG parameters and conventional clotting tests) in predicting transfusion need in cases of moderate blunt trauma.[13]

Maximum Amplitude/Maximum Clot Firmness

The maximum height of the curve is referred to as the maximum amplitude (MA) in TEG or the maximum clot firmness (MCF) in ROTEM systems. MA depends on platelet concentration and function, as well as fibrinogen concentration and is directly correlated to platelet and fibrin interactions, which determines the ultimate strength of the fibrin clot.

Shear Elastic Modulus

The shear elastic modulus (denoted by G in both TEG and ROTEM systems) measures overall coagulation status as hypocoagulable (decreased G), normocoagulable (normal G), or hypercoagulable (increased G). It is derived by the formula $G = 5000 \times MA/(100 - MA)$, and depends only on MA, but increases exponentially compared with MA, permitting more sensitive resolution at high amplitudes.

Clot Lysis

The final variable of the viscoelastic testing procedure reflects fibrinolytic-induced dissolution of the fibrin-platelet bonds formed between the pin and cup. The percentage return of MA to baseline is an indicator of this process, is evaluated either at 30 or 60 minutes, and is referred to as LY30/LY60 in TEG or CL30/CL60 in ROTEM systems.

Thromboelastography Platelet Mapping

Platelet mapping is available on the TEG platform to assess platelet function and measures percentage inhibition of platelet function compared with maximal uninhibited platelet function. The assay compares tracings obtained by cleaving and cross-linking fibrinogen (with reptilase and FXIIIa) inhibiting thrombin and platelets, with a tracing obtained by the addition of platelet agonists such that only thrombin is inhibited. The resulting MA is a function of platelet activation and offers a specific representation of platelet function.

Tracings

The following list includes tracing interpretations from TEG/ROTEM systems that are commonly encountered in emergency and critical care medicine. These are depicted visually in **Fig. 2**.

- Normal
- Hypercoagulable
- Hypocoagulable
- Thrombocytopenia/thrombocytopathia
- Hyperfibrinolysis
- Disseminated intravascular coagulation (DIC) stage 1

VISCOELASTIC TESTING IN EMERGENCY AND CRITICAL CARE

The role of viscoelastic testing in veterinary emergency and critical care has grown rapidly over the last 20 years. It detects both hypocoagulable and hypercoagulable states, which has driven a large body of publications in the diagnosis and treatment of many disease states in the past decade. It has also been useful in the monitoring of anticoagulant therapy as well as evaluation of platelet function. A recent study used TEG to guide transfusion in dogs with hypocoagulable disorders.[14] The important application of viscoelastic testing to veterinary emergency and critical care may also be emphasized by a study of dogs admitted to an ICU, which found abnormal TEG tracings in 14 of 27 (52%) patients in whom a wide array of disease states contributed to hemostatic dysfunction.[7] A summary is given next of some important disease conditions in veterinary emergency and critical care medicine where viscoelastic testing has been shown to be helpful to evaluate hemostatic function, as well as to enhance diagnosis and treatment.

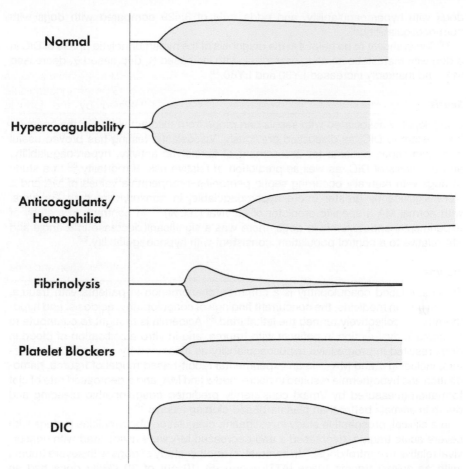

Normal

Hypercoagulability

Anticoagulants/
Hemophilia

Fibrinolysis

Platelet Blockers

DIC

Fig. 2. A series of viscoelastic traces in health and disease shown for comparison and pattern recognition.

Disseminated Intravascular Coagulation

DIC represents a complex and dynamic hemostatic disorder. The classic progression of disease is characterized by early hypercoagulability caused by activation of tissue factor and inhibitor consumption by inflammatory mediators, followed by hypocoagulability caused by consumption of coagulation factors and increased fibrinolysis.[15,16] The ability of TEG to assess global coagulation status, including hypocoagulability, hypercoagulability, and fibrinolysis, makes it a powerful tool for the diagnosis and management of patients with DIC.

Reflecting the pathophysiology outlined earlier, the results of a prospective study of 50 dogs with DIC showed hypercoagulability in 22 of 50 (44%), hypocoagulability in 11 of 50 (22%), and normocoagulability in 17 of 50 (34%) based on G values from recombinant human tissue factor–activated TEG[17]. Dogs with hypocoagulability had 2.38 increase in relative risk of death compared with hypercoagulable dogs. In another study, an increased risk of mortality associated with hypocoagulability based on thromboelastometry (TEM) in dogs with DIC was also found, with an odds ratio of 4.800 compared with dogs with hypercoagulability, and odds ratio of 3.429 compared with dogs with normocoagulability.[18]

TEG was shown to be helpful in the diagnosis of the hyperfibrinolytic phase of DIC in a dog with metastatic hemangiosarcoma, with increased K, decreased α, decreased MA, and markedly increased LY30 and LY60.[19]

Sepsis

Coagulopathy associated with sepsis can range from mild activation of the coagulation system to DIC, as discussed previously. Viscoelastic testing has proved useful in human septic patients for assessment of fibrinolytic activity, hypercoagulability, and diagnosis of DIC, as well as prediction of relative risk of mortality.[20] In a study of dogs with naturally occurring septic peritonitis, preoperative values of MA and α were significantly greater (more hypercoagulable) in nonsurvivors than survivors, with normal MA a specific predictor of survival (100%).[21] In contrast, in a study of experimental endotoxemia in dogs, there was a significant decrease in α angle and MA relative to a control population, consistent with hypocoagulability.[22]

Trauma

Trauma-induced coagulopathy is a common phenomenon in patients with trauma, and, in human medicine, the concurrent findings of coagulopathy, acidosis, and hypothermia are collectively termed the lethal triad.[23] Acidemia is thought to contribute to hemostatic dysfunction in patients with trauma, and in vitro acidification of blood in dogs resulted in progressive hypocoagulability as measured by some TEG parameters, including α and MA.[24] In an experimental rabbit-based model of trauma, hemodilution and hypothermia resulted in decreased α and MA, and a decreased rate of clot formation (measured by Vmax) consistently predicted coagulopathic bleeding and death in animals better than plasma-based clotting assays.[25]

In a clinical, prospective study investigating coagulation abnormalities in dogs with severe acute trauma, decreased α and decreased MA were associated with nonsurvival relative to control dogs.[26] In contrast, in another study of dogs with severe trauma (with an animal trauma triage [ATT] score >5), 10 out of 30 (33%) dogs had an increased G, suggesting hypercoagulability.[27] No dogs in this study were hypocoagulable based on TEG or standard coagulation test results. Hypercoagulability was also found in a population of dogs (4 out of 18 [22%]) and cats (1 out of 19 [5%]) following blunt trauma.[28] This study also documented hypocoagulability, and, in dogs, decreased MA was significantly associated with injury severity based on ATT scores.

Trauma also importantly affects clot degradation. Hyperfibrinolysis is reported commonly in human studies of acute trauma and in animal models of hemorrhagic shock; however, inhibition of fibrinolysis (fibrinolysis shutdown) is also reported and has been documented in animal studies of tissue injury.[29,30]

The complex hemostatic disorders associated with trauma may be influenced by acid-base status, effective circulating volume, inflammatory mediators, body temperature, and therapeutic interventions. Viscoelastic testing may play an increasingly important role in global evaluation of the coagulation status of veterinary patients with trauma.

Immune-Mediated Hemolytic Anemia

Immune-mediated hemolytic anemia (IMHA) has been associated with many hemostatic disorders, including DIC, hypercoagulability, and a predisposition for thromboembolism, including pulmonary thromboembolism (PTE).[31] Viscoelastic testing is therefore a valuable tool in this disease condition for global assessment of coagulation status, and numerous clinical studies have been conducted.

A prospective study of 11 dogs with primary IMHA found a hypercoagulable state relative to a control population, based on lower median K, higher median α, higher median MA, and increased G.[32] A subsequent study with greater numbers of dogs (n = 30) with primary IMHA also reported that dogs were significantly hypercoagulable versus controls, with significantly shorter K, greater α, and greater MA. Interestingly, this study also found that MA was significantly higher at hospital admission in survivors than nonsurvivors, with increased odds of 30-day survival of 1.13 with each unit increase in MA.[33] This counterintuitive finding was also supported by a study whereby no dogs with a normal coagulation index survived, suggesting that dogs that were not hypercoagulable had an increased risk of death.[34]

As noted previously, there is an inverse correlation between HCT and TEG variables K and MA, which may result in artifactual hypercoagulable tracings, possibly hampering interpretation of results in a study of IMHA. As noted in the Goggs and colleagues[33] study, if the MA, for example, were affected solely by the decreased HCT, then it would be expected that the packed cell volume would have been associated with outcome, which was not the case in that study. In addition, IMHA is associated with an inflammatory state, which is a known possible cause of hypercoagulability, and other possible causes may include hyperfibrinogenemia, increased contact pathway activation, platelet hyper-reactivity, or hemolysis. In addition, IMHA can be a secondary disease process to an underlying cause such as neoplasia or infectious disease, which may also affect coagulation.

Neoplasia

Malignant neoplasia has been associated with an increased risk of pulmonary thromboembolism (PTE), although the condition is often diagnosed postmortem.[35] Viscoelastic testing can be helpful to diagnose hypercoagulability, which in turn may predispose to PTE formation; however, this modality has not proved helpful as a stand-alone test in the prediction of PTE formation.[36,37]

One study using tissue factor–activated TEG found hemostatic dysfunction in 28 of 49 dogs (57%) in a cross-section of different neoplasms.[38] Hemostatic dysfunction was significantly more likely in dogs with malignant neoplasia, and most dogs in the study were hypercoagulable (22 out of 49 [45%]). It was interesting to note that all dogs with hypocoagulability (6/ out of 49 [12%]) had malignant neoplasia with evidence of metastatic disease, although patient numbers were small. Another study of 71 dogs with malignant neoplasia also found that hypercoagulability was the most common TEG abnormality, present in 47 out of 71 (66%) patients.[39] In a study of dogs with multicentric lymphoma, 17 out of 27 (63%) were found to be hypercoagulable based on TEG findings of decreased R, shortened K, increased α angle, or increased MA, and these alterations did not resolve in some patients for up to 1 month following clinical remission.[40]

Hemostatic dysfunction is common in veterinary patients with neoplasia, including hypercoagulability, and viscoelastic testing is an important test modality for evaluation of coagulation status in these patients. Further studies may be helpful to investigate any possible prognostic significance to these results.[41]

ADVANTAGES AND DISADVANTAGES OF VISCOELASTIC TESTING

Viscoelastic testing offers numerous advantages for the diagnosis and monitoring of coagulation status in emergency and critical care patients. There are also some

> **Box 1**
> **Advantages and disadvantages of viscoelastic monitoring in small animal critical care**
>
> Advantages
> - More global assessment of hemostasis that better reflects the complex physiology of in vivo coagulation.
> - Rapid turnaround time.
> - Small volume of blood required.
> - Possible to evaluate both hypercoagulability and hypocoagulability.
> - Able to evaluate hypofibrinogenemia and fibrinolysis.
> - TEG system can analyze platelet function.
> - Results reported in both graphical format and numerical measurements, aiding in rapid interpretation of results.
>
> Disadvantages
> - Does not evaluate contribution of endothelium to coagulation.
> - Requirement for close access to machine.
> - Variability in results, especially based on use of different activators.[41]
> - Poor reproducibility, even with the same analyzer subject to standardized testing.[42]
> - Results may be affected by HCT of the patient.
> - May be affected by hypothermia.[43]
> - Low sensitivity to mild coagulation factor deficiencies or mild defects in primary hemostasis.

disadvantages to this test modality that should be considered. These considerations are summarized in **Box 1**.

SUMMARY

Viscoelastic testing offers unique insight into the process of clot initiation, amplification, propagation, and termination through fibrinolysis. The graphical and numeric outputs from these tests are easy and rapid to interpret, and results can be used for both diagnosis and management of disease. However, although viscoelastic testing may provide a more global assessment of coagulation status, it is not intended to replace standard coagulation tests, or be interpreted as a stand-alone test. Viscoelastic testing is most powerful when used in conjunction with other tests of hemostasis. The use of these tests in veterinary emergency and critical care medicine continues to increase and likely will continue to expand with ongoing clinical use and research.

DISCLOSURE

The authors have nothing to disclose.

REFERENCES

1. Hoffman M, Monroe DM 3rd. A cell-based model of hemostasis. Thromb Haemost 2001;85(6):958–65.

2. Bauer N, Eralp O, Moritz A. Establishment of reference intervals for kaolin-activated thromboelastography in dogs including an assessment of the effects of sex and anticoagulant use. J Vet Diagn Invest 2009;21(5):641–8.

3. Marschner CB, Bjørnvad CR, Kristensen AT, et al. Thromboelastography results on citrated whole blood from clinically healthy cats depend on modes of activation. Acta Vet Scand 2010;52:38. Accessed December 14, 2019.

4. Zambruni A, Thalheimer U, Leandro G, et al. Thromboelastography with citrated blood: comparability with native blood, stability of citrate storage and effect of repeated sampling. Blood Coagul Fibrinolysis 2004;15(1):103–7.

5. McMichael MA, Smith SA. Viscoelastic testing: technology, applications, and limitations. Vet Clin Pathol 2011;40(2):140–53.

6. Wang H, Nam A, Song K, et al. Comparison of native and citrated whole blood samples for rapid thromboelastography in Beagles. J Vet Emerg Crit Care 2020;30(1):54–9.

7. Wagg CR, Boysen SR, Bédard C. Thromboelastography in dogs admitted to an intensive care unit. Vet Clin Pathol 2009;38(4):453–61.

8. Song J, Drobatz KJ, Silverstein DC. Retrospective evaluation of shortened prothrombin time or activated partial thromboplastin time for the diagnosis of hypercoagulability in dogs: 25 cases (2006-2011). J Vet Emerg Crit Care (San Antonio) 2016;26(3):398–405.

9. Thawley VJ, Sánchez MD, Drobatz KJ, et al. Retrospective comparison of thromboelastography results to postmortem evidence of thrombosis in critically ill dogs: 39 cases (2005-2010). J Vet Emerg Crit Care 2016;26(3):428–36.

10. McMichael MA, Smith SA, Galligan A, et al. In vitro hypercoagulability on whole blood thromboelastometry associated with in vivo reduction of circulating red cell mass in dogs. Vet Clin Pathol 2014;43(2):154–63.

11. Brooks AC, Guillaumin J, Cooper ES, et al. Effects of hematocrit and red blood cell-independent viscosity on canine thromboelastographic tracings. Transfusion 2014;54(3):727–34.

12. Marschner CB, Wiinberg B, Tarnow I, et al. The influence of inflammation and hematocrit on clot strength in canine thromboelastographic hypercoagulability. J Vet Emerg Crit Care 2018;28(1):20–30.

13. Jeger V, Willi S, Liu T, et al. The Rapid TEG α-Angle may be a sensitive predictor of transfusion in moderately injured blunt trauma patients. ScientificWorldJournal 2012;2012:8217943. Accessed December 14, 2019.

14. Langhorn R, Bochsen L, Willesen JL, et al. Thromboelastography-guided transfusion in dogs with hypocoagulable disorders: a case series. Acta Vet Scand 2019; 61(1):35. Accessed December 17, 2019.

15. Toh CH, Downey C. Back to the future: testing in disseminated intravascular coagulation. Blood Coagul Fibrinolysis 2005;16(8):535–42.

16. Bick RL, Arun B, Frenkel EP. Disseminated intravascular coagulation: clinical and pathophysiological mechanisms and manifestations. Haemostasis 1999;29(2–3): 111–34.

17. Wiinberg B, Jensen AL, Johansson PI, et al. Thromboelastographic evaluation of hemostatic function in dogs with disseminated intravascular coagulation. J Vet Intern Med 2008;22(2):357–65.

18. Barthélemy A, Pouzot-Nevoret C, Rannou B, et al. Prospective assessment of the diagnostic and prognostic utility of rotational thromboelastometry for canine disseminated intravascular coagulation. Vet Rec 2018;183(22):692.

19. Vilar-Saavedra P, Hosoya K. Thromboelastographic profile for a dog with hypocoagulable and hyperfibrinolytic phase of disseminated intravascular coagulopathy. J Small Anim Pract 2011;52(12):656–9.

20. Scarlatescu E, Juffermans NP, Thachil J. The current status of viscoelastic testing in septic coagulopathy. Thromb Res 2019;183:146–52.

21. Bentley AM, Mayhew PD, Culp WT, et al. Alterations in the hemostatic profiles of dogs with naturally occurring septic peritonitis. J Vet Emerg Crit Care 2013;23(1): 14–22.

22. Eralp O, Yilmaz Z, Failing K, et al. Effect of experimental endotoxemia on thromboelastography parameters, secondary and tertiary hemostasis in dogs. J Vet Intern Med 2011;25(3):524–31.

23. Simmons JW, Pittet JF, Pierce B. Trauma-induced coagulopathy. Curr Anesthesiol Rep 2014;4(3):189–99.

24. Burton AG, Burges J, Borchers A, et al. In vitro assessment of the effect of acidemia on coagulation in dogs. J Vet Emerg Crit Care 2018;28(2):168–72.

25. Kheirabadi BS, Crissey JM, Deguzman R, et al. In vivo bleeding time and in vitro thromboelastography measurements are better indicators of dilutional hypothermic coagulopathy than prothrombin time. J Trauma 2007;62(6):1352–9.

26. Holowaychuk MK, Hanel RM, Darren Wood R, et al. Prospective multicenter evaluation of coagulation abnormalities in dogs following severe acute trauma. J Vet Emerg Crit Care 2014;24(1):93–104.

27. Abelson AL, O'Toole TE, Johnston A, et al. Hypoperfusion and acute traumatic coagulopathy in severely traumatized canine patients. J Vet Emerg Crit Care 2013;23(4):395–401.

28. Gottlieb DL, Prittie J, Buriko Y, et al. Evaluation of acute traumatic coagulopathy in dogs and cats following blunt force trauma. J Vet Emerg Crit Care 2017;27(1): 35–43.

29. Brohi K, Cohen MJ, Ganter MT, et al. Acute traumatic coagulopathy: initiated by hypoperfusion: modulated through the protein C pathway? Ann Surg 2007; 245(5):812–8.

30. Moore HB, Moore EE, Lawson PJ, et al. Fibrinolysis shutdown phenotype masks changes in rodent coagulation in tissue injury versus hemorrhagic shock. Surgery 2015;158(2):386–92.

31. Scott-Moncrieff JC, Treadwell NG, McCullough SM, et al. Hemostatic abnormalities in dogs with immune-mediated hemolytic anemia. J Am Anim Hosp Assoc 2001;37(3):220–7.

32. Fenty RK, deLaforcade AM, Shaw SE, et al. Identification of hypercoagulability in dogs with primary immune-mediated hemolytic anemia by means of thromboelastography. J Am Vet Med Assoc 2011;238(4):463–7.

33. Goggs R, Wiinberg B, Kjelgaard-Hansen M, et al. Serial assessment of the coagulation status of dogs with immune-mediated haemolytic anemia using thromboelastography. Vet J 2012;191(3):347–53.

34. Sinnott VB, Otto CM. Use of thromboelastography in dogs with immune-mediated hemolytic anemia: 39 cases (2000-2008). J Vet Emerg Crit Care 2009;19(5): 484–8.

35. LaRue MJ, Murtaugh RJ. Pulmonary thromboembolism in dogs: 47 cases (1986-1987). J Am Vet Med Assoc 1990;187(10):1368–72.

36. Marschner CB, Kristensen AT, Rozanski EA, et al. Diagnosis of canine pulmonary thromboembolism by computed tomography and mathematical modelling using haemostatic and inflammatory variables. Vet J 2017;229:6–12.

37. Goggs R, Chan DL, Benigni L, et al. Comparison of computed tomography pulmonary angiography and point-of-care tests for pulmonary thromboembolism diagnosis in dogs. J Small Anim Pract 2014;55(4):190–7.

38. Kristensen AT, Wiinberg B, Jessen LR, et al. Evaluation of human recombinant tissue factor-activated thromboelastography in 49 dogs with neoplasia. J Vet Intern Med 2008;22(1):140–7.

39. Andreasen EB, Tranholm M, Wiinberg B, et al. Haemostatic alterations in a group of canine cancer patients are associated with cancer type and disease progression. Acta Vet Scand 2012;26:54, 3. Accessed December 17, 2019.

40. Kol A, Marks SL, Skorupski KA, et al. Serial haemostatic monitoring of dogs with multicentric lymphoma. Vet Comp Oncol 2015;13(3):255–66.
41. Smith SA, McMichael M, Galligan A, et al. Clot formation in canine whole blood as measured by rotational thromboelastometry is influenced by sample handling and coagulation activator. Blood Coagul Fibrinolysis 2010;21(7):692–702.
42. Goggs R, Borrelli A, Brainard BM, et al. Multicenter in vitro thromboelastography and thromboelastometry standardization. J Vet Emerg Crit Care 2018;28(3): 201–12.
43. Taggart R, Austin B, Hans E, et al. In vitro evaluation of the effect of hypothermia on coagulation in dogs via thromboelastography. J Vet Emerg Crit Care 2012; 22(2):219–24.

Nutritional Support of the Critically Ill Small Animal Patient

Daniel L. Chan, DVM

KEYWORDS

- Enteral nutrition • Nutritional assessment • Parenteral nutrition

KEY POINTS

- Nutritional support should be fully integrated with the treatment plan of critically ill small animal patients in order to positively affect outcome.
- Nutritional assessment in veterinary patients requires further refinement and with further development and validation, could be better used to predict patient populations most likely to benefit from nutritional support.
- Setting appropriate caloric targets that avoid overfeeding may be vitally important in reducing patient morbidity relating to nutritional interventions and ultimately influence patient outcomes.
- Veterinary studies on critical care nutrition must now move from descriptive studies to prospective controlled trials in order to determine optimal energy and nutrient provision in critically ill patients.

INTRODUCTION

Nutritional support is now considered an essential part of managing critically ill patients, especially if they are malnourished. There are several reasons for critically ill animals to be at high risk for becoming malnourished.[1] Moreover, critically ill animals undergo several metabolic alterations that further increase this risk for malnutrition.[1–5] The risk of malnutrition in this patient population primarily relates to inadequate food intake and catabolic effects of the primary disease. Because malnutrition can occur quickly in these animals, it is vital that we identify animals at risk for malnutrition by carrying out a nutritional assessment and initiating early nutritional support.[6] The goals of nutritional support are to treat malnutrition when present and, just as important, to prevent malnutrition from developing in at-risk patients.

Whenever possible, the enteral route should be used because it is the safest, most convenient, and most physiologically sound method of providing nutritional support. Ensuring the successful nutritional management of critically ill patients involves

Department of Clinical Science and Services, The Royal Veterinary College, University of London, RVC, Hawkshead Lane, North Mymms, Hertfordshire AL97TA, UK
E-mail address: dchan@rvc.ac.uk

Vet Clin Small Anim 50 (2020) 1411–1422
https://doi.org/10.1016/j.cvsm.2020.07.006
0195-5616/20/© 2020 Elsevier Inc. All rights reserved.

identifying those most likely to benefit from nutritional support, making an appropriate nutritional assessment, and implementing a feasible and effective nutritional plan. This review aims to clarify the consequence of inadequate nutritional intake and provide guidance for initiating effective nutritional supportive measures. By improving nutritional management strategies we can ensure critically ill patients have the best chance for recovery.

IMPORTANCE OF NUTRITIONAL SUPPORT

Many of the challenges encountered when managing critically ill patients relate to the presence of organ dysfunction (eg, ileus, diarrhea, azotemia), clinical signs that suggest gastrointestinal intolerance (eg, nausea, regurgitation, vomiting), metabolic complications (eg, acidosis, hyperglycemia, hypokalemia, accelerated lean muscle loss), and the presence of comorbidities (eg, anemia, chronic kidney disease, aspiration pneumonia), all of which can be barriers for effective feeding. Moreover, the lack of proper nutrition will only worsen the nutritional and metabolic state, making it more difficult for these patients to recover.[1] For example, protracted lack of food intake will negatively affect nitrogen balance and accelerate the catabolic state, which is not easily reversed even when feeding is reinstituted.[2] Lack of enteral nutrition will contribute to abnormal gastrointestinal function such as dysmotility and loss of mucosal barrier function.[7,8] Lack of proper nutrition also compromises the body's ability to synthesize important substances such as albumin, which in turn affects drug pharmacokinetics. For these reasons, the importance of proper nutrition cannot be underestimated. There is now growing evidence that with early nutritional support, animals can have improved outcomes.[8-12] Therefore, it is vital that clinicians managing critically ill patients explore ways of initiating early nutritional support whenever possible.

PATHOPHYSIOLOGY OF MALNUTRITION

One of the major metabolic alterations associated with critical illness involves catabolism of body protein in which protein turnover rates may become markedly increased.[1,13] Although healthy animals primarily lose fat when temporarily deprived of sufficient calories (ie, "simple starvation") as may be encountered by fasting animals before surgery, sick or traumatized patients catabolize lean body mass when they are not provided with sufficient calories (ie, "stressed starvation"). During the initial stages of fasting in the healthy state, glycogen stores are used as the primary source of energy. Following depletion of glycogen stores, a metabolic shift occurs toward the preferential use of fat depots, sparing catabolic effects on lean muscle tissue. However, during diseased or stressed states, the inflammatory response triggers alterations in metabolism toward a catabolic state. Glycogen stores are quickly depleted, especially in strict carnivores such as the cat, and this leads to an early mobilization of amino acids from muscle stores. With continued lack of food intake, the predominant energy source is derived from accelerated proteolysis (muscle breakdown), which in itself is an energy-consuming process. Muscle catabolism that occurs during stress provides the liver with gluconeogenic precursors and other amino acids for glucose and acute-phase protein production. The resultant negative nitrogen balance or net protein loss has been documented in critically ill dogs and cats.[2,14] One study estimated that 73% of hospitalized dogs (including postoperative patients) evaluated in 4 different veterinary referral centers were in a negative energy balance.[15] Taken together, these studies highlight the need to ensure critically ill patients receive nutritional support during hospitalization.

The consequences of continued lean body mass losses include negative effects on wound healing, immune function, skeletal and respiratory muscle strength, and ultimately on overall prognosis. In the context of postoperative patients, this could lead to greater risk of surgical wound dehiscence and postoperative infections. Because of the metabolic alterations associated with critical illness, and in part due to an inability or reluctance of many critically ill and postoperative dogs and cats to voluntarily eat sufficient calories, this patient population is at increased risk for developing complications related to their malnourished state. Given the serious sequelae of malnutrition, preservation or reversal of deteriorating nutritional status via nutritional support is paramount. Nutritional support is therefore aimed at minimizing the impact of malnutrition and enhancing rate of recovery.

In dogs, a period as short as 3 days of anorexia has been documented to produce metabolic changes consistent with those seen associated with starvation in people.[16] However, such dogs would not necessarily exhibit any easily detectable abnormalities on clinical assessment that suggest being malnourished. Dogs with overt signs that suggest malnutrition (eg, severe muscle wasting, poor coat quality) usually have a more protracted period of usually weeks to months of disease progression. In healthy cats detectable impairment of immune function can be demonstrated during acute starvation by day 4, and so recommendations to institute some form of nutritional support in any ill cat with inadequate food intake for more than 3 days have been made.[4] Based on growing evidence, we can conclude that there is a need to implement a nutritional intervention (eg, place feeding tube) when a dog or cat has not eaten for more than 5 days.

NUTRITIONAL ASSESSMENT

The successful management of critically ill patients may involve the selection of patients most likely to benefit from nutritional support and the selection of the most appropriate route for providing nutrition. The technique for performing nutritional assessment was designed to use readily available historical and physical parameters to identify malnourished patients who are at increased risk for complications and who will presumably benefit from nutritional intervention.[6] The assessment involves determining whether nutrient assimilation has been restricted because of decreased food intake, maldigestion, or malabsorption, whether any effects of malnutrition on organ function and body composition are evident, and whether the patient's disease process influences its nutrient requirements. The findings of the historical and physical assessment are used to categorize the patient as well nourished, moderately malnourished, or at risk of becoming malnourished or severely malnourished.[6] Checklists have been proposed to allow assessment of a patient's need for instituting nutritional support based on certain risk factors, and a modified checklist is found in **Table 1**. A patient with 2 or more high-risk factors present should receive nutritional support as soon as they are stable. Patients with fewer than 2 high risk factors should be closely monitored and reassessed every few days.

The patient history should be assessed for indications of malnutrition including evidence of weight loss and the time frame in which it has occurred; there should be a determination of the adequacy of dietary intake including the nutritional adequacy of the diet, the presence of persistent gastrointestinal signs, the patient's functional capacity (eg, evidence of weakness, exercise intolerance), and the metabolic demands of the patient's underlying disease state. The physical examination should focus on changes in body composition, presence of edema or ascites, and appearance of the patient's hair coat. With regard to assessing changes in body composition,

Table 1			
Assessment of need for nutritional support			
Parameter	Low Risk	Moderate Risk	High Risk
Food intake <80% RER for <3 d	☑		
Food intake <80% RER for 3–5 d		☑	
Food intake <80% RER for >3 d			☑
Presence of weight loss		☑	
Severe vomiting/diarrhea			☑
Body condition score <4/9			☑
Muscle mass score <2			☑
Hypoalbuminemia		☑	
Expected course of illness <3 d	☑		
Expected course of illness 2–3 d		☑	
Expected course of illness >3 d			☑

A patient with 2 or more high-risk factors present should receive nutritional support as soon as they are stabilized. Patients with fewer than 2 high-risk factors should be closely monitored and reassessed every few days.

Abbreviation: RER, resting energy requirements.

Modified from Perea, SC. Parenteral Nutrition. In: Fascetti AJ, Delaney SJ, eds. Applied Veterinary Clinical Nutrition. Chichester, UK: John Wiley & Sons, Inc., 2012:355; with permission.

it is important to recognize that although metabolically stressed patients experience catabolism of lean tissue, these changes may not be noted using standard body condition scoring systems if the patient has normal or excessive body fat. Because catabolism of lean tissue can have deleterious consequences for outcome, it is important that along with evaluation of body fat, patients undergo evaluation of muscle mass to assess lean tissue status. A muscle mass scoring system that has been used in dogs and cats is outlined in **Table 2**.

The next step of nutritional assessment is to determine whether or not the patient's voluntary food intake is sufficient. To do this one must have a caloric goal in mind, select an appropriate food, and formulate a feeding plan for the patient, which will permit an accurate accounting of how much food is offered to the patient and will allow evaluation of the patient's intake based on how much of the food is consumed.

Providing nutrition via a functional digestive system is the preferred route of feeding, and so particular care should be taken to evaluate whether the patient can tolerate enteral feedings. Even if the patient can tolerate only small amounts of enteral nutrition, this route of feeding should be pursued, as there are benefits even when a portion of energy needs are met.[17] Supplementation with parenteral nutrition should only be

Table 2	
Description of a muscle mass scoring system for dogs and cats	
Score	Muscle Mass
0	On palpation over the spine, muscle mass is severely wasted
1	On palpation over the spine, mass is moderately wasted
2	On palpation over the spine, muscle mass is mildly wasted
3	On palpation over the spine, muscle mass is normal

pursued when the use of enteral nutrition cannot meet at least 50% the patient's nutritional needs (ie, 50% of the patient's resting energy requirement).[18] Based on the nutritional assessment, the anticipated duration of nutritional support, and the appropriate route of delivery (ie, enteral or parenteral), a nutritional plan is formulated to meet the patient's nutritional needs.

It is worth noting that before instituting the nutritional plan, patients should have their hydration status and electrolyte and acid-base disturbances addressed and they should be hemodynamic stable. Commencing nutritional support before these abnormalities are addressed can increase the risk of complications and, in some cases, can further compromise the patient.[19] It should be emphasized that this is *not* counter to the concept of "early nutritional support," which has been documented to result in positive effects in several animal and human studies.[8–11] Early nutritional support advocates feeding as soon as possible after hemodynamic stability is achieved, rather than delaying nutritional intervention by several days.[20,21]

MEETING NUTRITIONAL NEEDS AND SPECIAL CONSIDERATIONS

There is much that remains unclear regarding the nutritional requirements of critically ill animals in general. In certain circumstances assumptions are made that nutritional requirements in animals are similar to that of people afflicted with similar diseases. However, it is important to recognize that there may be significant species and disease differences that make such direct comparisons or extrapolations less applicable. Experimental data suggest that there are dramatic changes in energy requirements in animals with thermal burns[22]; however, this does not seem to apply to clinical cases with critical illnesses. In the absence of definitive data to suggest otherwise, current recommendations are to start nutritional support as soon as it is deemed safe and initially target the resting energy requirements (RER) but to reassess the patient continually, as energy requirements may exceed 2 x RER in some cases. These recommendations align with current recommendations for pediatric critically ill patients.[20,21]

The goal of nutritional support is to optimize protein synthesis and preserve lean body mass. With this in mind, the current recommendation is to feed 5 to 6 g protein per 100 kcal (25%–35% of total energy) in dogs and 6 to 8 g protein per 100 kcal (30%–40% of total energy) in cats.[5] Patients with protein intolerance (eg, hepatic encephalopathy, severe azotemia) should receive reduced amounts of protein (eg, 3–4 g protein per 100 kcal). Similarly, patients with hyperglycemia or hyperlipidemia may also require decreased amounts of simple carbohydrates and fat, respectively. Other nutritional requirements will depend on the patient's underlying disease, clinical signs, and laboratory parameters.

WHEN TO INITIATE FEEDING

As alluded to earlier, for many years conventional therapy actually ignored nutritional needs of critically ill patients. As more and more evidence illustrates the consequences of malnutrition, there has been a gradual change to ensure that all patients received adequate nutrition. Typical delays in starting nutrition decreased from weeks to 10 days, and now the debate has shifted to how many hours from admission should nutrition be delayed. Because more and more research have uncovered the benefits of enteral nutrition and the complications arising from gut atrophy, critical care specialists have begun feeding patients earlier and earlier in the course of hospitalization with good results.

In veterinary medicine a similar transition occurred as well, probably only in the past 20 years. From the ineffective strategies such as force or syringe feeding, warming foods, adding flavor enhancers, to more recent recommendations for early tube feeding in most if not all critically ill patients. Studies in canine patients with parvoviral enteritis, peritonitis, and acute pancreatitis support the premise that early nutritional intervention is at least well tolerated and produces little complications.[8–12] The lack of any serious consequence to initiating feeding early in these patient populations dispels the myth that feeding early is fraught with complications. The overall effect of early nutrition on survival is beyond the limitations of these small trials, unfortunately.

Commencing feeding after tube placement should really be held at least until the animal has recovered from anesthesia. Recumbent animals receiving feedings are at risk of aspiration. Patients with compromised gastrointestinal motility (eg, anesthetized patients, patients on opioids analgesics, patients with ileus) are also at risk for complications and should be monitored closely.

CHOOSING THE MOST APPROPRIATE FEEDING TUBE

Determination of the route of nutritional support is an important step in the nutritional management of critical care patients. Nutritional support is broadly categorized into enteral and parenteral routes. Enteral routes include nasoesophageal, nasogastric esophageal, gastric, and jejunal feeding tubes, whereas parenteral routes include peripheral and central venous catheters. In most veterinary practices, nasoesophageal/nasogastric and esophagostomy feeding tubes are usually the most commonly considered feeding routes. The route selected for each patient will ultimately be influenced by the patient's medical and nutritional status, the anticipated length of time required for nutritional support, and consideration of the advantages and disadvantages presented by each route. **Table 3** summarizes the major advantages and disadvantages associated with each feeding tube.

Nasoesophageal and nasogastric feeding are relatively easy and convenient methods of nutritional delivery for patients who will require short-term nutritional support for fewer than 5 days or for patients who are not candidates for general anesthesia. The distinction between these techniques is whether the tip of the feeding tube remains within the esophagus or whether it is placed in stomach. Concerns regarding possible interference of feeding tubes of the lower esophageal sphincter led to recommendations that feeding tube should terminate into the distal esophagus. However, a recent study found no difference in complication rates between nasoesophageal and nasogastric tube; the importance of where these tubes terminate is unclear.[23] The one advantage afforded by nasogastric tubes is that these provide access for aspirating gastric residual volumes.

In general, nasoesophageal and nasogastric feeding tubes provide the advantages of being relatively easy to place and are inexpensive. However, because of the risk of aspiration, nasoesophageal/nasogastric feeding should not be implemented in patients with protracted vomiting or those that lack a gag reflex. The major disadvantage of nasoesophageal and nasogastric feeding tubes is their smaller diameter (typically 3.5–5 French in cats and 6–8 French in dogs), which limits diet selection to liquid enteral formulas. Liquid formulations may be delivered via continuous or intermittent bolus feedings. Although continuous feeding can be helpful in pets in which high feeding volumes may not be tolerated, a recent study demonstrated that gastric residual volumes and clinical outcome did not differ between the 2 feeding methods.[24]

Placement of an esophagostomy feeding tube requires general anesthesia for placement but is still a relatively quick and simple procedure. Compared with

Table 3
Types of feeding tubes used to provide nutritional support in critically ill patients

Feeding Tube	Typical Duration of Use	Advantages	Disadvantages
Nasoesophageal	Short-term (<5 d)	• Inexpensive • Easy to place • No anesthesia required	• Must use complete liquid diet • Prone to being dislodged or obstructed
Esophagostomy	Extended (wk to mo)	• Inexpensive • Simple to place • Can accommodate high-calorie semi-liquid diets	• Requires brief anesthesia • Prone to becoming obstructed • Incision can become inflamed or infected
Gastrostomy	Extended (wk to mo)	• Can accommodate highcalorie semi-liquid diets	• Requires general anesthesia for placement • Endoscopic placement requires special equipment • Tube displacement may result in peritonitis
Jejunostomy	Long-term (wk)	• Can bypass upper gastrointestinal tract	• Requires general anesthesia • Requires laparotomy and special expertise for placement • Requires complete liquid diet • Tube displacement may result in peritonitis

nasoesophageal/nasogastric feeding tubes, esophagostomy tubes can be used for an extended period of time, with some reported over a year of use. Other advantages include increased comfort for the animal, and an increased tube diameter (12–14 French), allowing for a wider selection of diets that may be fed through the tube.

ESOPHAGOSTOMY TUBES

This modality of nutritional support entails a relatively easy placement technique that is minimally invasive and well tolerated. For guidance in placing esophagostomy tubes the reader is referred elsewhere.[25] Placement of the feeding tube into the midcervical region mitigates complications associated with pharyngostomy tubes including gagging and partial airway obstruction. Esophagostomy tubes can provide at-home nutritional support for weeks to months for patients unable or unwilling to meet nutritional needs orally. The larger diameter of this tube compared with nasoesophageal or jejunostomy tubes allows for a wider selection of diet options including blenderized prescription formulated for specific medical conditions (eg, novel protein diets, fat-restricted diets).

NUTRITIONAL PLAN
Choosing the Most Appropriate Diet

The guiding principle regarding the diet to be used for nutritional support will depend on the individual needs of each patient. The composition of the diet needs to reflect the patient's dietary needs (eg, higher protein requirements in catabolic patients, fat restriction in hyperlipidemic patients). Generally speaking, critically ill patients should be fed a calorically dense diet high in protein and fat. However, patients who have specific contraindications to high protein (eg, chronic kidney failure, hepatic encephalopathy) should be fed a moderately restricted protein diet. In animals with gastrointestinal diseases, there may be a need to restrict the fat content of the diet. The chosen diet must also be able to be fed via feeding tubes. Liquid diets have the advantage that they can be delivered virtually via any feeding tube. However, it is important to consider the caloric density of these liquid diets. Diets that require a large amount of water to be blenderized in order to get through feeding tubes drops the caloric-density of the diet and also means that large volumes of the diet are fed.

Calculating of Energy Requirements

The patient's RER is the number of calories required for maintaining homeostasis while the animal rests quietly. The RER is calculated using the following formula:

$$RER = 70 \times (\text{body weight in kg})^{0.75}$$

For animals weighing between 2 and 30 kg, the following formula gives a good approximation of energy needs:

$$RER = (30 \times \text{body weight in kg}) + 70$$

Traditionally, the RER was then multiplied by an illness factor between 1.0 and 1.5 to account for increases in metabolism associated with different conditions and injuries. Recently, there has been less emphasis on these subjective illness factors and current recommendations are to use more conservative energy estimates to avoid overfeeding; therefore, illness factors are usually not applied when formulating feeding plans of critically ill patients.[26] Overfeeding can result in metabolic and gastrointestinal complications, hepatic dysfunction, increase carbon dioxide production, and weaken respiratory muscles. Of the metabolic complications, the development of hyperglycemia is most common.

Currently, the RER is used as an initial estimate of a critically ill patient's energy requirements. It should be emphasized that these general guidelines should be used as starting points, and animals receiving nutritional support should be closely monitored for tolerance of nutritional interventions. Continual decline in body weight or body condition should prompt the clinician to reassess and perhaps modify the nutritional plan (eg, increasing the number of calories provided by 25%).

IMPLEMENTING NUTRITIONAL PLAN

To implement enteral nutritional support, a feeding tube is typically required. Placement of a feeding tube is recommended whenever voluntary eating by the patient is lacking in sufficient amounts to meet at least 80% RER. Once a feeding tube is in place, a diet preparation that is suitable to meet the nutritional needs of the patient and appropriate for the tube is chosen. Small-bore tubes, such as those typically used for nasoesophageal placement or jejunostomy tubes, require complete liquid diets. Gruel-type diets require larger-bore tubes such as esophagostomy and gastrostomy tubes, and the preparation of these diets may require the use of a kitchen blender. Alternatively, there are veterinary diets that have been especially formulated for use via feeding tubes. Other considerations for choosing a diet include fat and protein contents and caloric density. The next consideration involves the manner in which food is delivered; animals with nasoesophageal, esophagostomy, and gastrostomy tubes tolerate bolus feedings in which the prescribed amount of food is administered over 15 to 20 minutes and fed every 4 to 6 hours. The volumes of food that can be fed per feeding should typically be less than 10 mL/kg; however, some patients will not tolerate being fed no more than 2 mL/kg, whereas some animals can tolerate 30 to 40 mL/kg per feed.

Regardless of the severity of malnutrition, one must remember that the immediate goals of therapy in any critically ill patient should focus on proper cardiovascular resuscitation, stabilization of vital signs, and identification of primary disease process. As steps are taken to address the primary disease, formulation of a nutritional plan should aim to mitigate overt nutritional deficiencies and imbalances. By providing adequate energy substrates, protein, essential fatty acids, and micronutrients, the body can support wound healing, immune function, and tissue repair. A major goal of nutritional support is to minimize metabolic derangements and the catabolism of lean body tissue. During hospitalization, recovery of normal body weight is not the top priority, as this should occur when once the animal is discharged from the hospital and complete their recovery from critical illness at home.

MONITORING AND REASSESSMENT

Body weights should be monitored daily in all patients receiving nutritional support. However, the clinician should take into account fluid shifts when evaluating changes in body weight. For this reason, body condition score assessment is important as well. The use of the RER as the patient's caloric requirement is merely a starting point. The number of calories provided may need to be increased to keep up with the patient's changing needs, typically by 25% if well tolerated. In patients unable to tolerate the prescribed amounts, the clinician should consider reducing amounts of enteral feedings and supplementing the nutritional plan with some form of parenteral nutrition.

With continual reassessment, the clinician can determine when to transition patient from assisted feeding to voluntary consumption of food. The discontinuation of nutritional support should only begin when the patient can consume approximately 75% of its RER without much coaxing.

COMPLICATIONS

Possible complications of enteral nutrition include mechanical complications such as clogging of the tube or early tube removal.[27] Metabolic complications include electrolyte disturbances, hyperglycemia, volume overload, and gastrointestinal signs (eg, vomiting, diarrhea, cramping, bloating).[28–30] In critically ill patients receiving enteral nutritional support, the clinician must also be vigilant for the development of aspiration pneumonia. Monitoring parameters for patients receiving enteral nutrition include body weight, serum electrolytes, tube patency, appearance of tube exit site, gastrointestinal signs (eg, vomiting, regurgitation, diarrhea), and signs of volume overload or pulmonary aspiration.[27]

The complications associated with nasoesophageal feeding tubes are relatively minor and are unlikely to result in significant morbidity. In one study, the most common complications seen with the use of nasogastric feeding tubes were vomiting, diarrhea, and inadvertent tube removal, which occurred in 37% of patients.[31] Other minor complications (eg, irritation of nasal passages, sneezing) can occur during the placement of the tube or as a consequence of the indwelling tube. A recent study comparing complications associated with nasoesophageal versus nasogastric feeding tubes found no difference in complication rates.[23] To prevent inadvertent use of the nasoesophageal tube for anything other than feeding, the feeding tube should be clearly labeled.

Complications associated with esophagostomy feeding tubes are relatively uncommon and typically are minor to moderate. In one retrospective study comparing esophagostomy tubes with percutaneous endoscopic gastrostomy tubes, there was no difference in complication rate or severity.[32] Serious complications such as inadvertent placement in the airway or mediastinum or damage to the major vessels and nerves can be avoided by proper placement technique and by verifying position of the tube radiographically. Midcervical placement minimizes the risk of gagging and partial airway obstruction. Proper tube size and material decrease the risk of esophageal irritation. Proper patient evaluation to ensure the pet can protect his airway in the event of vomiting is critical to lessen the risk of pulmonary aspiration. If the patient vomits, tube placement should be verified to ensure it has not been displaced.

Complications related to the stoma site or mechanical issues with the tube are possible.[25,32] Peristomal cellulitis, infection, or abscess may occur. Peristomal inflammation is a more common complication. It can be managed in mild cases with thorough cleaning and topical antibiotics, whereas more severe cellulitis or abscessation may require systemic antimicrobials and tube removal. These risks can be minimized by ensuring the tube is secured properly and the stoma site is kept clean and protected. Mechanical issues with the tube include premature removal, kinking, or clogging. Risk of premature removal can be minimized by using an appropriately sized tube size for patient comfort. The tube should be securely sutured and wraps should be comfortable. An Elizabethan collar may be needed in some cases. Kinking can occur during tube placement or after vomiting and can be detected radiographically. Completely flushing the tube with water after every use decreases the risk of tube obstruction. The diet used should have the proper consistency to be easily fed through the feeding tube. In addition, the administration of medications through the tube should be avoided or performed with caution, as it could lead to clogging of the tube. Tube obstructions may dislodge with warm water by applying pressure and suction. Other methods include infusing a carbonated beverage or a solution of pancreatic enzyme and sodium bicarbonate.[33]

SUMMARY

Although critically ill patients are often not regarded as in urgent need of nutritional support given their more pressing problems, the severity of their injuries, altered metabolic condition, and necessity of frequent fasting, they are at high risk of becoming malnourished during their hospitalization. Proper identification of these patients and careful planning and execution of a nutrition plan can be key factors in their successful recovery. As our understanding of various disease processes and the interactions with metabolic pathways improve, along with the refinement of nutritional support techniques we can provide, there is indeed great optimism that nutrition can have a significant positive impact on the recovery of critically ill patients.

REFERENCES

1. Gagne JW, Wakshlag JJ. Pathophysiology and clinical approach to malnutrition in dogs and cats. In: Chan DL, editor. Nutritional management of hospitalized small animals. Chichester (West Sussex): John Wiley & Sons, Ltd; 2015. p. 117–27.

2. Mitchel KE. Nitrogen metabolism in critical care patients. Vet Clin Nutr 1998;(Suppl):20–2.

3. Sakurai Y, Zhang X, Wolfe RR. Short-term effects of tumor necrosis factor on energy and substrate metabolism in dogs. J Clin Invest 1993;91(6):2437–45.

4. Freitag KA, Saker KE, Thomas E, et al. Acute starvation and subsequent refeeding affect lymphocyte subsets and proliferation in cats. J Nutr 2000;130(10): 2444–9.

5. Chan DL. Nutritional requirements of the critically ill patient. Clin Tech Small Anim Pract 2004;19(1):1–5.

6. Michel KE. Nutritional assessment in small animals. In: Chan DL, editor. Nutritional management of hospitalized small animals. Chichester (West Sussex): John Wiley & Sons, Ltd; 2015. p. 1–6.

7. Whitehead K, Yonaira Cortes, Eirmann L. Gastrointestinal dysmotility disorders in critically ill dogs and cats. J Vet Emerg Crit Care 2016;26(2):234–53.

8. Mohr AJ, Leisewitz AL, Jacobson LS, et al. Effect of early enteral nutrition on intestinal permeability, intestinal protein loss, and outcome in dogs with severe parvoviral enteritis. J Vet Intern Med 2003;17(6):791–8.

9. Mansfield CS, James FE, Steiner JM, et al. A pilot study to assess tolerability of early enteral nutrition via esophagostomy tube feeding in dogs with severe acute pancreatitis. J Vet Intern Med 2011;25(3):419–25.

10. Hoffberg JE, Koenigshof A. Evaluation of the safety of early compared to late enteral nutrition in canine septic peritonitis. J Am Anim Hosp Assoc 2017; 53(2):90–5.

11. Harris JP, Parnell NK, Griffith EH, et al. Retrospective evaluation of the impact of early enteral nutrition on clinical outcomes in dogs with pancreatitis: 34 cases (2010-13). J Vet Emerg Crit Care 2017;27(4):425–33.

12. Liu DT, Brown DC, Silverstein DC. Early nutritional support is associated with decreased length of hospitalization in dogs with septic peritonitis: A retrospective study of 45 cases (2000-2009). J Vet Emerg Crit Care 2012;22(4):453–9.

13. Biolo G, Toigo G, Ciocchi B, et al. Metabolic response to injury and sepsis: changes in protein metabolism. Nutrition 1997;13(9 Suppl):52S–7S.

14. Michel KE, King LG, Ostro E. Measurement of urinary urea nitrogen content as an estimate of the amount of total urinary nitrogen loss in dogs in intensive care units. J Am Vet Med Assoc 1997;210(3):356–9.

15. Remillard RI, Darden DE, Michel KE, et al. An investigation of the relationship between caloric intake and outcome in hospitalized dogs. Vet Ther 2001;2(4): 301–10.

16. Owen OE, Reichard GA, Patel MS, et al. Energy metabolism in feasting and fasting. Adv Exp Med Biol 1979;111:169–88.

17. Brunetto MA, Gomes MOS, Andre MR, et al. Effects of nutritional support on hospitalized outcomes in dogs and cats. J Vet Emerg Crit Care 2010;20(2):224–31.

18. Chan DL, Freeman LM. Parenteral nutrition in small animals. In: Chan DL, editor. Nutritional management of hospitalized small animals. Chichester (West Sussex): John Wiley & Sons, Ltd; 2015. p. 100–16.

19. Preiser JC, van Zanten AR, Berger MM, et al. Metabolic and nutritional support of critically ill patients: consensus and controversies. Crit Care 2015;19(1):35.

20. Mehta NM, Skillman HE, Irving SY, et al. Guidelines for the provision and assessment of nutritional support therapy in the pediatric critically ill patient: Society of Critical Care Medicine and American Society for parenteral and enteral nutrition. JPEN J Parenter Enteral Nutr 2017;41(5):706–42.

21. Tume LN, Valla FV, Joosten K, et al. Nutritional support for children during critical illness; European Society of Pediatric and Neonatal Intensive Care (ESPNIC) metabolism, endocrine and nutrition section position statement and clinical recommendations. Intensive Care Med 2020;46(3):411–25.

22. Tredget EE, Yu YM. The metabolic effects of thermal injury. World J Surg 1992; 16(1):68–79.
23. Yu MK, Freeman LM, Heinse CR, et al. Comparison of complication rates in dogs with nasoesophageal versus nasogastric feeding tubes. J Vet Emerg Crit Care 2013;23(3):300–4.
24. Holahan M, Abood S, Hauptman J, et al. Intermittent and continuous enteral nutrition in critically ill dogs. A prospective randomized trial. J Vet Intern Med 2010; 24(3):520–6.
25. Eirmann L. Esophagostomy feeding tubes in dogs and cats. In: Chan DL, editor. Nutritional management of hospitalized small animals. Chichester (West Sussex): John Wiley & Sons, Ltd; 2015. p. 29–40.
26. Chan DL. Estimating energy requirements of small animal patients. In: Chan DL, editor. Nutritional management of hospitalized small animals. Chichester (West Sussex): John Wiley & Sons, Ltd; 2015. p. 7–13.
27. Chan DL. Feeding tube complications. In: Drobatz KJ, Hopper K, Rozanski EA, et al, editors. Textbook of small animal emerg medicine. Hoboken (NJ): Wiley Blackwell; 2019. p. 578–81.
28. Justin RB, Hoenhaus AE. Hypophosphatemia associated with enteral alimentation in cats. J Vet Intern Med 1995;9(4):228–33.
29. Pyle SC, Marks SL, Kass PH. Evaluation of complications and prognostic factors associated with administration of total parenteral nutrition in cats:75 cases (1994-2001). J Am Vet Med Assoc 2004;225(2):242–50.
30. Queau Y, Larsen JA, Kass PH, et al. Factors associated with adverse outcomes during parenteral nutrition administration in dogs and cats. J Vet Intern Med 2011;25(3):446–52.
31. Abood SK, Buffington CA. Enteral feeding of dogs and cats:51 cases (1989-91). J Am Vet Med Assoc 1992;201(4):619–22.
32. Ireland LM, Hoenhaus AE, Broussard JD, et al. A comparison of owner management and complications in 67 cats with esophagostomy and percutaneous endoscopically guided feeding tubes. J Am Anim Hosp Assoc 2003;39(3):241–6.
33. Parker VJ, Freeman LM. Comparison of various solutions to dissolve critical care diet clots. J Vet Emerg Crit Care 2013;23(3):344–7.

Update on Anticonvulsant Therapy in the Emergent Small Animal Patient

Heidi L. Barnes Heller, DVM

KEYWORDS

- Anticonvulsant • Benzodiazepine • Diazepam • Seizures • Levetiracetam
- Acute seizure management

KEY POINTS

- Seizures result from an imbalance between excitation and inhibition in the forebrain.
- The goal of acute seizure management is to stop seizures so that neuronal death and systemic complications are limited for the animal.
- The benzodiazepine class of drugs (diazepam, midazolam, and lorazepam) are the most commonly recommended first-line anticonvulsant drugs in veterinary medicine. Benzodiazepine drugs are suspected to control seizures through increased inhibition of the neuronal environment.
- Levetiracetam is a newer anticonvulsant drug that shows promise for acute seizure management, especially when used in combination with diazepam.
- Propofol is a rarely used anesthetic drug, used most commonly to control seizures after surgery for portosystemic shunts.

INTRODUCTION

Seizures have an estimated true prevalence in the general animal population of 0.6% to 0.75%. So, although rare, seizures are one of the most common reasons for presentation to a veterinarian.[1] Regardless of the etiology, seizures can be localized neuroanatomically to the prosencephalon (forebrain). Seizures are caused by hypersynchronous neuronal activity, which results from an imbalance of excitation and inhibition within the neural network.[2] After multiple seizures are confirmed, the disorder may be termed epilepsy if a metabolic or toxic cause is not identified.[3] There are 3 phases to a seizure: (1) preictal phase, (2) ictus, and (3) postictal phase. The preictal phase is the period before the ictus in which animals may display specific behavior or

Disclosure: Parts of this article were previously published in Barnes Heller H. Feline Epilepsy. *Vet Clin North Am - Small Anim Pract.* 2018;48(1):31-43.
Barnes Veterinary Specialty Services, LLC, 1125 Frisch Road, Madison, WI 53711, USA
E-mail address: Barnes@barnesveterinaryservices.com

attitudes that owners can recognize as a preamble to a seizure. These may include hiding or seeking behavior, nausea, vomiting, and aggression. The preictal phase may last for seconds or hours. The ictus, or active seizure, often involves both somatic and autonomic systems. Resolution of the ictus leads to the postictal phase, in which neuronal resetting occurs. Common clinical signs during the postictal phase may include hiding, blindness, and ataxia.

Seizure descriptions are based on the semiology of the clinical signs of the seizure and may be described as focal, complex focal, or generalized. This differs from human epilepsy in which seizures often are categorized based on changes on the electroencephalogram (EEG). In either case, these descriptive terms apply to the ictal phase only. In veterinary medicine, generalized seizures involve bilateral body movements often with impaired consciousness. Agreement about the presence or absence of awareness may be difficult even between veterinarians; therefore, caution should be taken not to over-emphasize the state of awareness when describing a seizure.[4] Focal seizures may manifest as abnormal movement of one part of the body, with or without altered mentation. Complex focal seizures include altered consciousness and often are described as abnormal running behavior or acute changes in mentation with abnormal facial movements and ptyalism.[5,6]

PATHOPHYSIOLOGY OF SEIZURES

The development of a seizure, and the progression after the first seizure, is called epileptogenesis.[7,8] Despite decades of research, understanding and predicting epileptogenesis still is a struggle. Simply stated, seizures occur as a result of an imbalance between excitatory and inhibitory neurotransmitters in the brain.[7] Neurons have a resting membrane potential of -70, which is maintained through a delicate balance of K^+, Na^+, Cl^-, and Ca^{++} ions intracellularly and extracellularly. Excitation, or lessening of the negative intracellular environment of the neuron, occurs via an intracellular shift of positive ions, thus increasing the negative resting membrane potential toward zero. Excitatory neurotransmitters, such as glutamate, are responsible for most excitation in the brain. Inhibition, or dampening down, of neuronal firing occurs with the release of inhibitor neurotransmitters, most commonly γ-aminobutyric acid (GABA), with a resulting increasingly negative intracellular environment. Seizures occur when hypersynchronous firing occurs, possibly from overexcitation, in the prosencephalon. Pharmacologic treatment of seizures targets either modification of ion channels, reducing excitation or decreasing propagation of seizures.

WHY SHOULD SEIZURES BE CONTROLLED?

Prolonged seizures can result in
- Hypertension
- Tachycardia
- Acidosis
- Hyperthermia
- Hypoxia
- Secondary neuronal cell death

These changes adversely affect the brain and also can have systemic effects. The goal of acute seizure management is to stop the seizure as quickly as possible, thereby limiting secondary brain and extracranial organ damage.

ANTICONVULSANT DRUGS
Benzodiazepine

Benzodiazepine drugs (diazepam, midazolam, and lorazepam) were introduced in the 1960s for treatment of status epilepticus in humans. Although the mechanism of action is debated, enhancement of the presynaptic and/or postsynaptic inhibitory neurotransmitter GABA is likely.[9] This suggests the benzodiazepine drugs may not just stop the seizure focus but also disable the spread of seizure activity.[10] Facilitation of GABA at the postsynaptic membrane also may account for the adverse clinical effects of sedation and lethargy observed with this class of drugs.[9]

A 2015 human meta-analysis identified that benzodiazepines are the best first-line intravenous (IV) drugs and identified the therapeutic serum concentration of between 150 µg/mL and 300 µg/mL.[11] A canine or feline therapeutic range has not been established; therefore, the human range often is used. Plasma concentrations as high as 1500 µg/L, however, have been suggested to be therapeutic in animals.[12] A 2018 Cochrane review in children with status epilepticus identified that IV diazepam and lorazepam achieved seizure cessation quickest. Gaining IV access, however, can be time consuming; therefore, alternative routes, including buccal midazolam or rectal diazepam, were considered acceptable first-line choices.[13] To date, there have not been any veterinary studies identifying which drug is best for acute seizure management.

Practitioners also should be aware that chronic administration of phenobarbital, a common long-term anticonvulsant drug, can result in lower the blood concentrations of benzodiazepine drugs. Therefore, these dogs should receive a higher benzodiazepine dosage compared with dogs not previously exposed to chronic phenobarbital administration.[14]

Diazepam

Diazepam has been the main anticonvulsant treatment of veterinary patients.[15–18] It generally is regarded as safe for both dogs and cats and can be administered IV, intranasally, and per rectum. Diazepam is poorly water soluble with high lipid solubility, allowing it to readily cross the blood-brain barrier.[12] Diazepam undergoes marked hepatic metabolism, which produces metabolites nordiazepam, and oxazepam.[19] Both metabolites have reduced anticonvulsant efficacy, compared with the parent compound.[9] Oral administration of diazepam has been linked to acute hepatic necrosis in cats.[20] Oral administration is not recommended for acute seizure management due to the risk of injury to the owner, the long time to peak diazepam concentrations, and diminished anticonvulsant activity.

IV administration of diazepam is the most common route of diazepam administration in emergency seizure treatment.[11,16,17,21] The standard dosage is 0.5 mg/kg IV; however, higher doses may be needed after chronic phenobarbital use.[14] Serum diazepam concentrations have been shown to remain above 300 µg/mL for 30 minutes in dogs, suggesting this may be the period of efficacy.[22] Seizures may reoccur after 30 minutes due to a loss of efficacy, at which time the dosage may be repeated, or administered as a constant rate infusion (CRI), at a dosage of 0.1 mg/kg/h to 0.5 mg/kg/h. Practitioners should note that adverse effects may last longer than the efficacy time. Intramuscular (IM) administration of diazepam has limited clinical usefulness owing to slow systemic absorption as well as frequent pain and necrosis at the injection site.[23,24]

Home care with rectal administration of a commercially available parenteral liquid formulation of diazepam has been recommended for patients at risk for cluster seizures.[25,26] Rectal administration should be placed in the caudal rectum to encourage absorption into the caudal vena cava, thus avoiding hepatic metabolism. The recommended dosage is 1 mg/kg to 2 mg/kg per rectum.[27] Serum benzodiazepine metabolite concentrations have been identified to be greater than 150 μg/mL at a mean of 8 minutes and with a mean time to peak of 14 minutes to 30 minutes utilizing commercially available parenteral liquid formulations.[12,14] These data suggests that rectal administration can result in serum or plasma concentrations sufficient to reach the minimum human therapeutic range within a clinically useful window of time. Compounded suppository formulations of diazepam have not demonstrated reliable serum diazepam concentrations in dogs; therefore, compounded suppositories currently are not recommended.[26] There is a well-accepted rectal diazepam product used in human medicine that has not been evaluated in veterinary patients and is, for now, cost prohibitive for many owners (Diastat AcuDial, Bausch Health, Laval, Quebec, Canada).

In veterinary medicine, intranasal diazepam administration has gained more favor recently due to its relative ease of administration and avoidance of the first-pass effect of hepatic metabolism. Two approaches have been described: (1) nasal drop technique: this requires the administrator to drop a commercially available parenteral solution into the nares over a 30-second period, and (2) a nasal atomizer technique: this utilizes a atomizer specifically designed for attachment to a Luer lock syringe for rapid administration of the same commercially available parenteral solution into the nares.[28] Intranasal diazepam, administered at a dosage of 0.5 mg/kg body weight, resulted in serum diazepam metabolite concentrations greater than 300 μg/mL within 5 minutes with both techniques, making intranasal diazepam administration a practical alternative to IV and rectal administration.[22,28] Care should be exercised when administering intranasal products to avoid inadvertent bite wounds due to the proximity to the mouth.

Midazolam

Midazolam is a water-soluble benzodiazepine drug with a higher binding affinity compared with diazepam; however, bioavailability is between 50% and 70%, depending on the route of administration. Midazolam has a more rapid time to peak concentration and has been found to have superior efficacy in prehospital human studies, when compared with rectal diazepam and IV lorazepam.[19,29] In veterinary medicine, midazolam has been evaluated for IM, IV, rectal, and intranasal administration. Standard doses are 0.2 mg/kg for all administration routes.[15,24,30] Unlike diazepam, IM midazolam does not lead to necrosis at the injection site and has a mean time to maximal concentration of 10 minutes or less.[24] A 2015 Rapid Anticonvulsant Medication Prior to Arrival Trial (RAMPART) clinical trial in humans reported that patients receiving IM midazolam had a shorter time to seizure cessation and less hospitalization compared with patients receiving IV lorazepam.[31] For patients without easy IV access, or at home care, IM midazolam may be a safe alternative.

Recently, attention has been focused on intranasal routes of administration for which midazolam has become especially favored.[15,16,30] Gel formulations increase bioavailability and result in shorter time to maximal concentration (12 minutes vs 18 minutes for the solution) because of increased viscosity. The increased viscosity is proposed to result in slower clearance from the nasal mucosa. Charalambous and colleagues[30] reported intranasal midazolam to be superior to IV midazolam after a multicenter randomized trial in 44 dogs. Intranasal administration was noted to have more rapid seizure cessation rate when accounting for catheter placement for IV administration.[30] Both routes were rapid and effective, however, at controlling seizures in dogs. Intranasal midazolam (with atomizer) showed superior seizure control compared with rectal diazepam in a clinical trial of 38 dogs diagnosed with idiopathic and structural epilepsy.[18] Based on clinical evidence, intranasal midazolam currently is recommended for at-home seizure control.

Rectal midazolam is not recommended due to erratic and unpredictable plasma concentrations at standard dosages.[15,24] Although higher dosages may yield serum concentrations within the human therapeutic range, data to support this suggestion have not been published; therefore, rectal midazolam currently is not recommended.

Lorazepam

Although used less frequently for seizure abatement in veterinary medicine, lorazepam often is used interchangeably with diazepam for management of human status epilepticus.[13,32] Lorazepam is poorly water soluble and less fat soluble and a higher binding affinity than diazepam.[19,33] Administration routes evaluated in animals include IV, IM, intranasal, and rectal. Because lorazepam is metabolized by the liver into an inactive compound, there is a high first-pass effect with rectal administration in dogs; therefore, rectal administration is ineffective for seizure cessation.[33] IM administration results in long peak serum concentrations at 10 minutes, making this route also less desirable for veterinary patients.[6] Intranasal administration, at a dosage of 0.2 mg/kg in 6 dogs, was reported in an abstract. After intranasal administration, therapeutic serum concentrations of lorazepam were obtained in all dogs by 9 minutes, with maintenance of anticonvulsant serum concentrations for 60 minutes.[34] In 1 canine study, IV administration of lorazepam, at a dosage of 0.2 mg/kg, did not result in a significant difference in seizure control or median seizure-free interval compared with IV diazepam, at a dosage 0.5 mg/kg.[35] Although promising as an anticonvulsant, insufficient clinical trials in veterinary medicine have limited the clinical use and understanding of lorazepam.

Levetiracetam

Levetiracetam has received a lot of attention since it was first documented for use in veterinary medicine in 2004.[36] Levetiracetam is suspected of exerting anticonvulsive effects through blockage of presynaptic protein SV2A. It is considered a relatively safe drug, with mild clinical effects that include sedation or gastrointestinal upset.[37] IV levetiracetam, given at dosages of 30 mg/kg to 60 mg/kg and after IV benzodiazepine administration, resulted in cessation of 56% of seizures in a randomized, placebo-controlled, double-masked study of 19 dogs.[38] When levetiracetam is administered with diazepam, seizure control is improved in human epileptic trials compared with either drug alone.[39] This may account for the improved seizure control noted in the canine study rather than a reflection of the efficacy of levetiracetam alone for acute seizure management.

Levetiracetam also has been evaluated for rectal and IM administration. The bioavailability of IM levetiracetam is high; however, the time to maximal concentration is approximately 40 minutes, which limits its clinical usefulness for management of active seizures.[40] Rectal administration of levetiracetam, at dosages of 40 mg/kg, has demonstrated serum concentrations above the minimum human therapeutic range (5 μg/mL) at the first sample times of 10 minutes and 30 minutes.[41,42] Because first sample times were at 10 minutes and 30 minutes, respectively, however, there is a gap of knowledge about when minimal therapeutic serum levetiracetam concentrations are reached.[41,43] A single clinical trial of epileptic dogs was undertaken in which rectal administration of levetiracetam followed administration of diazepam.[42] In this study, significantly more dogs experienced clinical seizure cessation compared with the group receiving benzodiazepine drugs only.[42] It remains unknown in veterinary medicine the efficacy of levetiracetam, without benzodiazepine use; however, the ethical implications of investigating this question may limit investigation.

At home, control of cluster seizures may be improved further through pulse administration of oral levetiracetam.[44] During pulse treatment, patients are administered oral intermediate-release levetiracetam every 8 hours for 1 day to 2 days after seizure abatement. Pulse therapy can be combined with other oral, rectal, or intranasal drug administration protocols at home or with other IV anticonvulsant drug administration in hospital. Pulse therapy is recommended for medium-term seizure control and is not intended for immediate seizure control.

Propofol

Propofol is a common anesthetic drug that has shown to have both proconvulsive and anticonvulsive properties.[45] Propofol's anticonvulsive properties are thought to be secondary to activation of GABA.[45] This drug is recommended for IV use only. Propofol initially was described for seizure control secondary to corrective surgery for portosystemic shunts. Subanesthetic dosages, of 1.0 mg/kg to 3.5 mg/kg for bolus treatment or 0.1 mg/kg/min to 0.25 mg/kg/min for CRI, have been described.[45,46] More recent literature has reported higher initial bolus dosages (2–8 mg/kg IV) for use in dogs and cats with uncontrolled seizures.[44,45] Propofol can cause respiratory suppression. Therefore, bolus dosing should be titrated to the lowest effective dose while attentive respiratory monitoring is performed. Intubation may be required if apnea is encountered during treatment. Propofol withdrawal may result in distal limb twitching, which may be difficult to distinguish from seizure activity. EEG is used in academic practice to differentiate between an ictus and propofol withdrawal; however, other clinical clues, such as mental responsiveness and response to tactile stimuli, may be utilized if EEG is not available. Finally, extended exposure to propofol in cats may result in Heinz body anemia; therefore, a complete blood cell count analysis is recommended every 24 hours during CRI use of propofol.

SUMMARY

Seizures occur from synchronous hyperexcitation in the prosencephalon. The goal with acute seizure management is to stop seizures, thus limiting secondary effects. Prolonged seizures can result in neuronal damage; if adequate ventilation is not maintained, hypoxic damage to the heart may occur; poor perfusion may result in renal failure and hyperthermia may cause rhabdomyolysis, further worsening renal injury. Benzodiazepine drugs currently are the first-line therapy for acute seizure management, with promising research suggesting supplemental levetiracetam may be beneficial as well. After seizures are stopped, clinicians should pursue identification of the underlying cause and initiation of long-term anticonvulsant medication on an individual basis.

REFERENCES

1. Berendt M, Farquhar RG, Mandigers PJJ, et al. International veterinary epilepsy task force consensus report on epilepsy definition, classification and terminology in companion animals. BMC Vet Res 2015;11:182–93.
2. Fisher RS, Van Emde Boas W, Blume W, et al. Epileptic seizures and epilepsy: Definitions proposed by the International League Against Epilepsy (ILAE) and the International Bureau for Epilepsy (IBE). Epilepsia 2005;46(4):470–2.
3. Fisher RS, Acevedo C, Arzimanoglou A, et al. ILAE official report: a practical clinical definition of epilepsy. Epilepsia 2014;55(4):475–82.

4. Packer RMA, Berendt M, Bhatti S, et al. Inter-observer agreement of canine and feline paroxysmal event semiology and classification by veterinary neurology specialists and non-specialists. BMC Vet Res 2015;11(39):1–11.
5. Barnes Heller HL. Feline epilepsy. Vet Clin North Am Small Anim Pract 2018; 48(1):31–43.
6. Pakozdy A, Gruber A, Kneissl S, et al. Complex partial cluster seizures in cats with orofacial involvement. J Feline Med Surg 2011;13(10):687–93.
7. Patterson ENE. Epileptogenesis and companion animals. Top Companion Anim Med 2013;28(2):42–5.
8. Pitkänen A. Therapeutic approaches to epileptogenesis - Hope on the horizon. Epilepsia 2010;51(Suppl. 3):2–17.
9. Brown SA. Anticonvulsant therapy in small animals. Vet Clin North Am Small Anim Pract 1988;18(6):1197–216.
10. Treiman DM. Pharmacokinetics and clinical use of benzodiazepines in the management of status epilepticus. Epilepsia 1989;30:S4–10.
11. Brigo F, Nardone R, Tezzon F, et al. Nonintravenous midazolam versus intravenous or rectal diazepam for the treatment of early status epilepticus : a systematic review with meta-analysis. Epilepsy Behav 2015;49:325–36.
12. Mealey KL, Boothe DM. Bioavailability of benzodiazepines following rectal administration of diazepam in dogs. J Vet Pharmacol Ther 1995;18(1):72–4.
13. McTague A, Martland T, Appleton R. Drug management for acute tonic-clonic convulsions including convulsive status epilepticus in children. Cochrane Database Syst Rev 2018;(1):CD001905.
14. Wagner SO, Sams RA, Podell M. Chronic phenobarbital therapy reduces plasma benzodiazepine concentrations after intravenous and rectal administration of diazepam in the dog. J Vet Pharmacol Ther 1998;21(5):335–41.
15. Eagleson JS, Platt SR, Elder Strong DL, et al. Bioavailability of a novel midazolam gel after intranasal administration in dogs. Am J Vet Res 2012;73(4):539–45.
16. Boothe DM. Anticonvulsant therapy in small animals. Vet Clin North Am Small Anim Pract 1998;28(2):411–48.
17. Patterson ENE. Status epilepticus and cluster seizures. Vet Clin North Am Small Anim Pract 2014;44(6):1103–12.
18. Charalambous M, Bhatti SFM, Van Ham L, et al. Intranasal midazolam versus rectal diazepam for the management of canine status epilepticus: a multicenter randomized parallel-group clinical trial. J Vet Intern Med 2017;31(4):1149–58.
19. Leppik IE, Patel SI. Intramuscular and rectal therapies of acute seizures. Epilepsy Behav 2015;49:307–12.
20. Center SA, Elston TH, Rowland P, et al. Fulminant hepatic failure associated with oral administration of diazepam in 11 cats. J Vet Med Assoc 1996;209(3):618–25.
21. Platt SR. Feline seizure control. J Am Anim Hosp Assoc 2001;37(6):515–7.
22. Platt SR, Randell SC, Scott KC, et al. Comparison of plasma benzodiazepine concentrations following intranasal and intravenous administration of diazepam to dogs. Am J Vet Res 2000;61(6):651–4.
23. Lamson MJ, Sitki-Green D, Wannarka GL, et al. Pharmacokinetics of diazepam administered intramuscularly by autoinjector versus rectal gel in healthy subjects. Clin Drug Investig 2011;51(8):585–97.
24. Schwartz M, Munana K, Nettifee-Osborne J, et al. The pharmacokinetics of midazolam after intravenous , intramuscular , and rectal administration in healthy dogs. J Vet Pharmacol Ther 2012;36(5):471–7.
25. Podell M. The use of diazepam per rectum at home for the acute management of cluster seizures in dogs. J Vet Intern Med 1995;9(2):68–74.

26. Probst CW, Thomas WB, Moyers TD, et al. Evaluation of plasma diazepam and nordiazepam concentrations following administration of diazepam intravenously or via suppository per rectum in dogs. Am J Vet Res 2013; 74(4):611–5.

27. Thomas WB. Idiopathic epilepsy in dogs and cats. Vet Clin North Am Small Anim Pract 2010;40(1):161–79.

28. Musulin SE, Mariani CL, Papich MG. Diazepam pharmacokinetics after nasal drop and atomized nasal administration in dogs. J Vet Pharmacol Ther 2011; 34(1):17–24.

29. Clemency BM, Ott JA, Tanski CT, et al. Parenteral midazolam is superior to diazepam for treatment of prehospital seizures. Prehosp Emerg Care 2015;19(2): 218–23.

30. Charalambous M, Volk HA, Tipold A, et al. Comparison of intranasal versus intravenous midazolam for management of status epilepticus in dogs: A multi-center randomized parallel group clinical study. J Vet Intern Med 2019; 33(6):2707–17.

31. Welch RD, Nicholas K, Durkalski-Mauldin VL, et al. Intramuscular midazolam versus intravenous lorazepam for the prehospital treatment of status epilepticus in the pediatric population. Epilepsia 2015;56(2):254–62.

32. Wu W, Zhang L, Xue R. Lorazepam or diazepam for convulsive status epilepticus: A meta-analysis. J Clin Neurosci 2016;29:133–8.

33. Podell M, Wagner SO, Sams RA. Lorazepam concentrations in plasma following its intravenous and rectal administration in dogs. J Vet Pharmacol Ther 1998; 21(2):158–60.

34. Mariani C, Clemmons R, Lee-Ambrose L, et al. A comparison of intranasal and intravenous lorazepam in normal dogs. J Vet Intern Med 2003;17(3):402.

35. Naeser J, Lichtenberger M, Mariani CL, et al. Clinical comparison of lorazepam vs. diazepam in the control of canine seizures. J Vet Emerg Crit Care (San Antonio) 2004;14(S1):S1–17.

36. Steinberg M, Faissler D. Levetiracetam therapy for long-term idiopathic epileptic dogs. J Vet Intern Med 2004;18(3):410.

37. Charalambous M, Shivapour SK, Brodbelt DC, et al. Antiepileptic drugs' tolerability and safety – a systematic review and meta-analysis of adverse effects in dogs. BMC Vet Res 2016;12(1):79.

38. Hardy BT, Patterson EE, Cloyd JM, et al. Double-masked, placebo-controlled study of intravenous levetiracetam for the treatment of status epilepticus and acute repetitive seizures in dogs. J Vet Intern Med 2012;26(2):334–40.

39. Modur PN, Milteer WE, Zhang S. Sequential intrarectal diazepam and intravenous levetiracetam in treating acute repetitive and prolonged seizures. Epilepsia 2010; 51(6):1078–82.

40. Patterson EE, Goel V, Cloyd JC, et al. Intramuscular, intravenous and oral levetiracetam in dogs: safety and pharmacokinetics. J Vet Pharmacol Ther 2008;31(3): 253–8.

41. Peters RK, Schubert T, Clemmons R, et al. Levetiracetam rectal administration in healthy dogs. J Vet Intern Med 2014;28(2):504–9.

42. Cagnotti G, Odore R, Bertone I, et al. Open-label clinical trial of rectally administered levetiracetam as supplemental treatment in dogs with cluster seizures. J Vet Intern Med 2019;33(4):1714–8.

43. Cagnotti G, Odore R, Gardini G, et al. Pharmacokinetics of rectal levetiracetam as add-on treatment in dogs affected by cluster seizures or status epilepticus. BMC Vet Res 2018;14(1):10–5.

44. De Risio L, Platt SR. Canine and feline epilepsy. Boston: CABI; 2014.
45. Steffen F, Grasmueck S. Propofol for of refractory seizures in dogs and a cat with intracranial disorders. J Small Anim Pract 2000;41(11):496–9.
46. Heldmann E, Holt DE, Brockman DJ, et al. Use of propofol to manage seizure activity after surgical treatment of portosystemic shunts. J Small Anim Pract 1999; 40(12):590–4.

Total Intravenous Anesthesia for the Small Animal Critical Patient

Marc R. Raffe, DVM, MS*

KEYWORDS

- Total intravenous anesthesia • Target controlled infusion • Veterinary medicine
- Emergency and critical care veterinary medicine

KEY POINTS

- Inhalant drugs used for general anesthesia can provide paralysis, a state of unconsciousness, and analgesia, however, also have untoward side effects of decreased cardiac output, vasodilation, and hypotension.
- Total intravenous anesthesia involves use of injectable drugs as intermittent or constant rate infusions to provide balanced analgesia, paralysis and a state of amnesia or unconsciousness, and should be considered for critically ill patients.
- Total intravenous anesthesia can provide rapid induction and recovery from anesthesia as well as decrease postanesthetic nausea and vomiting.
- The combined effects of a sedative–hypnotic drug along with an analgesic drug are synergistic in providing anesthesia.

Anesthesia (from Greek "without sensation") is a state of controlled, temporary loss of sensation or awareness that is induced for medical purposes.[1] It may include analgesia (relief from or prevention of pain), paralysis (muscle relaxation) and amnesia (unconsciousness). A patient under the influence of all these described effects is referred to as being under general anesthesia.[1] The defined criteria may be fulfilled through administration of drugs that produce 1 or more of the listed characteristics. Drug classes used to create anesthesia include inhalation agents, local anesthetics, sedative–hypnotics, tranquilizers, alpha-2 adrenergic drugs, neuromuscular blockers, opioids, and dissociatives.

Anesthesia is unique in that it is not a direct means of treatment; rather, it allows one to perform procedures to treat, diagnose, or cure an ailment that would otherwise be painful or complicated. The best anesthetic, therefore, is the one with the least risk to the patient that still achieves the end points required to complete the proposed

VACCA LLC
* 2770 Hodges Lane, Mounds View, MN 55112-4144.
E-mail address: vaccallc@gmail.com

Vet Clin Small Anim 50 (2020) 1433–1444
https://doi.org/10.1016/j.cvsm.2020.07.007
0195-5616/20/© 2020 Elsevier Inc. All rights reserved.

procedure. Anesthesia drug selection is matched to patient health status to achieve the purpose for anesthesia while maintaining patient safety.[1]

Current anesthesia practice in veterinary medicine includes the use of inhalation anesthesia drugs (isoflurane, sevoflurane, desflurane) to maintain the anesthesia state. These drugs are called "complete anesthetics" in that they provide all the descriptive criteria associated with the general anesthesia. Although inhalant drugs meet all these criteria, it is well-recognized that they do not meet all criteria equally it is well known that sedation and muscle relaxation may be excellent but analgesia is incomplete. Increasing the dose of a single anesthetic drug to meet all criteria may expose the patient to additional risk associated with side effects of that drug. For example, increasing inhalation drug dose results in dose-dependent physiologic destabilization characterized by myocardial depression, vasodilation, hypotension, and depressed control of breathing.

Recognizing that the most challenging anesthesia criterion to achieve is analgesia, recent practice trends have been to reduce inhalation agent level to minimize cardiorespiratory depression by supplementing analgesia with parenterally administered drugs known for their strong analgesic qualities (opioids, ketamine, alpha-2 agonists). Analgesic drugs may be administered as a single dose or intravenously delivered as a constant rate infusion (CRI) after an intravenous loading dose. Use of CRIs have been well-described in the literature and is frequently incorporated into anesthesia protocols. Adding supplemental analgesia to inhalation anesthesia results in better quality of pain control and improves safety by reducing inhalation drug dose. Supplemental drug administration by intravenous route in addition to inhalation anesthesia has several terms including balanced anesthesia and partial intravenous anesthesia.[2]

WHAT IS TOTAL INTRAVENOUS ANESTHESIA?

In human medicine, changes in anesthesia practice to improve quality of anesthesia and patient experience have occurred over the past 2 decades. One goal is to decrease anesthesia recovery time and speed discharge; a second goal is to decrease postanesthesia nausea and vomiting. A third goal is to decrease postoperative opioid use due to addiction concerns. Research, followed by large-scale clinical trials, has shown that anesthesia produced by combination of intravenously administered drugs produces equivalent or better recovery time, postanesthesia analgesia and a reduced incidence of postanesthesia nausea and vomiting.[3,4] The practice of creating and maintaining general anesthesia by administration is described as total intravenous drug. Although TIVA is a recent clinical trend, it is not a new concept. The first documented TIVA report was in the dog in 1656. A combination of opium and spirits was administered to produce anesthesia.[5] Further research languished until the commercial release of propofol, when it was reported that the intravenous combination of propofol and opioid produced general anesthesia. This milestone, coupled with the emerging trend of outpatient anesthesia, fostered investigation into TIVA for providing general anesthesia, residual pain control, decreasing postanesthesia nausea and vomiting, and decreasing recovery time.[3,4]

Conceptually, it is easy to understand TIVA in that anesthesia criteria are fulfilled by parenteral administration of a drug combination instead of administering a single drug (isoflurane, sevoflurane, desflurane) (**Table 1**) By simultaneously delivering several intravenous drugs, each with a specific anesthetic action, the sum of administered drugs, rather than the action of an individual drug, produces general anesthesia. Drug interaction is important in that the aggregate effects of infused drugs need to

Table 1
TIVA drugs: principal characteristics

Drug Class	Name	Analgesia	Unconsciousness	Muscle Relaxation
Opioid	Fentanyl Remifentanil Sufentanil	Yes	No	No
Dissociative	Ketamine	Yes	Yes (dissociation)	No
Sedative–hypnotics	Propofol Alfaxalone Etomidate	No	Yes	Yes
Alpha 2 agonists	Dexmedetomidine	Yes	No (deep sedation)	Yes
Benzodiazepine tranquilizers	Diazepam Midazolam	No	No (sedation)	Yes
Local anesthetics	Lidocaine	Yes	Mild sedation	No
Inhalation Agents	Isoflurane Sevoflurane Desflurane	Yes	Yes	Yes

be complimentary. Synergism, where the combined effect of drugs is greater than expected, is an important strategic goal in formulating TIVA protocols.[4]

TIVA is used in human anesthesia in both inpatient and outpatient settings; its application has been reported in a wide range of patient age and surgical procedures with favorable results.[6–11] TIVA has been refined to better match drug dose with individual patient requirement. Due to biological variation in drug pharmacokinetics, a specific drug dose or infusion rate may not meet individual patient needs. One strategy to address, biological variation is target controlled infusion. By understanding the pharmacokinetic-dynamic (PK-PD) profile of a drug in a large patient population, a statistically appropriate dose can be calculated and delivered across a specified time period. Algorithms have been developed in human medicine and programmed into delivery systems (computers, syringe pumps) to finely control drug delivery and achieve a steady state of drug dose.[12–17] This is beginning to be investigated in veterinary medicine.[13,14]

TIVA is currently not mainstreamed in small animal practice because of perceived complexity and inefficiency in setup time, equipment required, and math skills. With training and experience, these objections can be easily overcome.

TOTAL INTRAVENOUS ANESTHESIA CONCEPTS AND APPLICATION

As noted elsewhere in this article, TIVA is created by administering a combination of parenteral anesthesia drugs which, in sum, produce all criteria described for general anesthesia. To plan a TIVA protocol, one must understand the primary characteristics of selected drugs and ensure that their composite effect fulfills all criteria for general anesthesia. Drugs that work well in TIVA are those that achieve a rapid therapeutic plasma concentration, have a predictable in vivo behavior (PK-PD), and are rapidly metabolized in a consistent fashion so that in vivo accumulation does not occur.[10,14,15,17]

Practical application requires one to understand that, at the beginning of anesthesia, the plasma concentration of the selected drug is zero. To establish a therapeutic drug concentration, a loading or bolus dose of the drug must be intravenously administered. The purpose of loading dose administration is to immediately establish a clinically effective plasma concentration of the drug, which is then sustained by CRI to achieve a drug steady state (**Fig. 1**). Although this seems simple in principle, it can be challenging to achieve because compartmental redistribution, biotransformation, and clearance of a drug begins immediately after administration. The goal is to best match the delivery rate with the drug compartmental redistribution, biotransformation and clearance to achieve a steady-state plasma concentration for the duration of anesthesia.[10,15,17]

In human medicine, common TIVA drug techniques include a sedative-hypnotic drug (usually propofol) in combination with a potent analgesic drug (alfentanil, remifentanil). This combination produces sedation, analgesia and muscle relaxation consistent with general anesthesia. Similar strategies may be adopted in companion animal medicine. Drugs that meet these criteria are described in **Tables 2** and **3**.

Propofol

Propofol is an ideal TIVA drug. Its dosing flexibility produces a spectrum of responses ranging from light to profound sedation and muscle relaxation. It is rapidly, and consistently, metabolized which results in a short in vivo half-life after a single dose or CRI administration. This in vivo behavior translates into a rapid recovery after drug infusion is discontinued. For these reasons, propofol is a foundation drug in both human and veterinary TIVA.[6,15–17]

Alfaxalone

Alfaxalone shows promise for TIVA. It shares many qualities described for propofol and can be useful when used as a CRI. There are outstanding questions regarding PK-PD of CRI infusion; additional studies are underway to better understand its characteristics when CRI administration occurs.

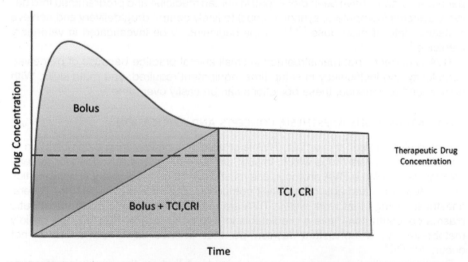

Fig. 1. PK-PD curve for anesthesia drugs. The initial drug concentration is established by a loading or bolus dose given intravenously (*blue area*). A CRI is then started to maintain drug concentration for the duration of anesthesia (*green and yellow areas*). The goal is to maintain drug concentration above therapeutic drug concentration.

Table 2
Examples of TIVA protocols

Drug Protocol	Anesthesia Criteria			Notes
	Sedation	Analgesia	Muscle Relaxation	
Fentanyl + propofol	Y	Y	Y	Limb and jaw muscle tone may be stronger than expected
Remifentanil + propofol	Y	Y	Y	Limb and jaw muscle tone may be stronger than expected
Fentanyl + propofol + dexmedetomidine	Y	Y	Y	Decreased risk of recovery dysphoria
Remifentanil + propofol + dexmedetomidine	Y	Y	Y	Decreased risk of recovery dysphoria
Fentanyl + propofol + lidocaine	Y	Y	Y	Limb and jaw muscle tone may be stronger than expected
Remifentanil + propofol + lidocaine	Y	Y	Y	Limb and jaw muscle tone may be stronger than expected
Fentanyl + alfaxalone	Y	Y	Y	Limb and jaw muscle tone may be present
Remifentanil + alfaxalone	Y	Y	Y	Limb and jaw muscle tone may be present
Fentanyl + alfaxalone + dexmedetomidine	Y	Y	Y	Decreased risk of recovery dysphoria
Remifentanil + alfaxalone + dexmedetomidine	Y	Y	Y	Decreased risk of recovery dysphoria
Fentanyl + dexmedetomidine + ketamine	Y	Y	Y	Decreased risk of recovery dysphoria
Propofol + dexmedetomidine + ketamine	Y	Y	Y	Decreased risk of recovery dysphoria
Propofol + midazolam + ketamine	Y	Y	Y	Mild dysphoria during recovery
Fentanyl + propofol + cis-atracurium	Y	Y	Y	Requires artificial breathing support

Table 3
TIVA drug doses

Drug Class	Drug Name	Initial Loading Dose (Intravenous Administration)	CRI Dose (Intravenous Administration)
Opioid	Fentanyl	5–7 µg/kg	0.02–0.06 µg/kg/min 1–5 µg/kg/h
	Remifentanil	1–3 µg/kg	0.1–0.5 µg/kg/min
Dissociative	Ketamine	0.25–0.50 mg/kg	2–20 µg/kg/min 0.12–1.2 mg/kg/h
Sedative hypnotic	Propofol	2–6 mg/kg	0.1–0.6 mg/kg/min
	Alfaxalone	2–3 mg/kg	0.15 mg/kg/min
Alpha 2 agonist	Dexmedetomidine	0.5–3 µg/kg	0.5–5 µg/kg/h
Benzodiazepine tranquilizer	Diazepam	0.2–0.4 mg/kg	0.2–0.4 mg/kg/h
	Midazolam	0.2–0.4 mg/kg	0.2–0.4 mg/kg/h
Local anesthetic	Lidocaine	1–2 mg/kg	25–50 µg/kg/min
Neuromuscular blocker	Atracurium	0.3–0.5 mg/kg	4–9 µg/kg/min
	Cis-atracurium	0.2 mg/kg	2 µg/kg/min

Opioids

Opioids commonly used in TIVA include fentanyl, alfentanil, sufentanil, and remifentanil. All share the characteristic of producing a rapid effect after an initial loading dose and maintaining steady-state plasma levels during TIVA due to their rapid biotransformation and elimination. In human anesthesia, sufentanil and remifentanil are preferred; unfortunately, they are not commonly used in veterinary TIVA due to cost. The main opioid used in veterinary TIVA is fentanyl. Like remifentanil, it produces a rapid effect after the initial loading dose. Studies evaluating in vivo PK-PD characteristics have found a time delay in developing a steady-state plasma concentration after CRI administration of up to 180 to 240 minutes. This can be noted as change in patient initiating comfort level during the time TIVA is administered if total procedure time is less than 2 hours. If this occurs, the infusion rate is adjusted accordingly to restore patient comfort and physiologic stability.[13]

Ketamine

Ketamine is used in TIVA for its pain control properties. It is used as an adjunct to improve sedation and inhibit pain signal upregulation (wind up) in the central nervous system. At low doses, it produces these effects with minimal psychoactive or physiologic consequences, making it an attractive option. It has a pharmacokinetic long tail, meaning that it can have a recovery time delay when higher doses are administered. This does not seem to be a concern clinically when adjunct doses are administered.[4]

Dexmedetomidine

Dexmedetomidine is used in partial intravenous anesthesia and TIVA protocols owing to its excellent sedation and analgesic qualities. Sedation and moderate analgesia can be achieved at lower doses than those described to produce hemodynamic changes. Dexmedetomidine is an attractive choice because it has residual analgesia and a short recovery after CRI discontinuation. It also has a specific reversal agent if needed.[18,19]

Benzodiazepine Tranquilizers

Diazepam and midazolam are excellent adjunct drugs. Both produce dose-dependent sedation and muscle relaxation. Diazepam and midazolam have complex biotransformation with an extended duration of effect owing to biological activity of first- and second-generation metabolites. This factor makes them less attractive unless a benzodiazepine specific antagonist (flumazenil) is available.[20]

Neuromuscular Blocking Drugs

Neuromuscular blocking drugs can be useful adjuncts if complete skeletal muscle relaxation is required. Newer class members produce excellent neuromuscular relaxation following loading dose and have a predictable, short duration of effect following single dose administration. Cis atracurium is a popular choice owing to its relatively rapid onset (1–2 minutes) and predictable duration (30–35 minutes) of effect.[21]

Lidocaine

Lidocaine is used in TIVA protocols for provision of excellent analgesia at low dose CRI dosing. It has a predictable duration of effect in the dog; in the cat, it may have a longer duration of action owing to interspecies difference in biotransformation and clearance. It is effective in soft tissue procedures including intra-abdominal and intrathoracic techniques, which evokes a high level of visceral pain.

DELIVERY SYSTEMS

To deliver a drug at a constant rate, dedicated delivery devices are required. A dedicated vascular access point for TIVA drug administration must be established. A short tubing length can be interfaced from the vascular access point to a multi-channel infusion manifold or multiple piggy back access points (**Fig. 2**). Individual drug channels are developed by drawing the desired drug quantity into an appropriate size syringe and connecting it via small bore, low-volume, infusion tubing to a manifold connection or piggy back site. The drug syringe is then placed in a motorized syringe pump, which is programmed to deliver the drug at a calculated infusion rate (**Fig. 3**). New-generation syringe pumps are programmed to automate the required calculations by selecting TIVA mode on their control panel. This is convenient, but not required, because manual calculation based on weight and drug infusion rate per time unit is

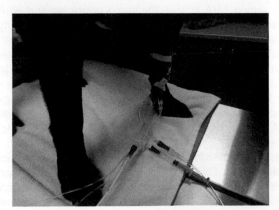

Fig. 2. Example of a multichannel vascular access manifold. Three independent infusions can be administered into a single intravenous catheter.

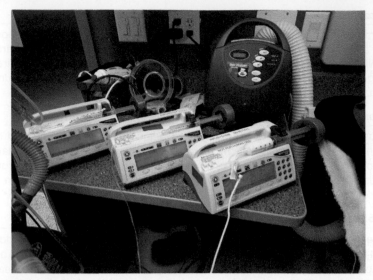

Fig. 3. Example of a TIVA infusion pump set up. Each drug has an individual infusion pump so that drug dose may be independently adjusted as needed.

easily performed. If syringe pumps are not available, the calculated drug dose can be mixed into fluid and infused using a standard intravenous fluid pump or gravity dripped using a drip controller device. These options are not as accurate as syringe pump delivery nor as flexible when dose adjustment is required.

In humans, target controlled infusion is set up using syringe pumps with preprogrammed PK-PD data for individual drugs. This simplifies target controlled infusion because all patient inputs and in vivo responses are known. The operator enters patient information, and the infusion pump automatically calculates and delivers the appropriate TIVA drug dose. There have been several recent articles in veterinary medicine regarding this approach in veterinary anesthesia.[13,14]

MONITORING

Patient monitoring during TIVA applies the same principles and equipment used for inhalation anesthesia. Physical monitoring including reflex integrity, muscle tone, eye position, and absence of pain are identical to other general anesthesia monitoring protocols. Eye position is generally ventromedial in dogs with a prominent third eyelid visible. In cats, eye position may be either ventromedial or central. In either species, ocular reflexes noted by palpebral and eye lash brush reflexes are very sluggish or obtunded. An ear flick reflex may be present in cats. Jaw tone is generally present and is slight or moderate in opening resistance based on the characteristics of the administered TIVA drugs. Skeletal muscle on the front and hind legs should have limited tone and be relaxed.

It is prudent that the anesthetist is knowledgeable about the physiologic characteristics of drugs selected for TIVA use. This point is no different than understanding in vivo characteristics of inhalation anesthesia. Core physiologic values for heart rate, blood pressure, pulse oximetry, and end-tidal carbon dioxide trend similarly to inhalant anesthesia protocols. TIVA drugs do not generally create the degree of vasodilation noted with inhalant anesthetic drugs; thus, blood pressure parameters may be higher compared with isoflurane or sevoflurane. Opioids are hemodynamically neutral, but may cause respiratory depression. A propofol loading dose can cause a transient decrease in blood pressure values and respiratory depression. A slow injection speed for the initial loading dose minimizes this effect. Ketamine may cause an increased heart rate and respiratory depression after administration. Dexmedetomidine may cause slowing of the heart rate.

Central and peripheral nervous systems are monitored by evaluating the level of consciousness coupled with the reflexes as described elsewhere in this article. In addition, a deep pain challenge should be performed to determine if the CRI infusion rate is satisfactory for obtunding somatic and visceral pain. If neuromuscular blocking drugs are used, the level of neuromuscular blockade may be evaluated using commercially available peripheral nerve stimulators.

ADVANTAGES OF TOTAL INTRAVENOUS ANESTHESIA VERSUS INHALATION ANESTHESIA

Several advantages have been reported in human medicine when TIVA is compared with inhalation anesthesia. TIVA is mainstreamed in neuroanesthesia owing to better preservation of neurophysiology and central vascular reflexes compared with inhalation anesthesia.[22] TIVA has demonstrated better recovery quality compared with inhalant anesthesia owing to decreased emergence agitation and dysphoria. Less postoperative nausea and vomiting is noted in patients recovering from TIVA compared with inhalation anesthesia. Multicenter studies have shown a decreased postoperative pain medication requirement in TIVA patients compared with inhalation anesthesia.[23] These observations support the value of TIVA in short duration and/or outpatient anesthesia settings.

Several studies have investigated the potential impact of anesthesia selection on patient survival time. Several reports have compared survival time after TIVA to inhalation anesthesia in cancer surgery. A large, multicenter cohort study demonstrated overall advantage in hazard ratio (survival time) for TIVA compared with inhalation anesthesia. Subgroup analyses of specific cancer types in the same study failed to demonstrate any advantage when TIVA was compared with inhalation anesthesia. Similar results are reported in human patients with breast cancer, where the median survival time for TIVA and inhalation anesthesia patient groups was not statistically different.[24–27] Additional studies are currently underway to determine if outcomes differ between anesthesia techniques for specific medical/surgical conditions.

Environmental pollution and operating room personnel exposure risk from inhalation anesthesia is reduced to zero when TIVA is used. Isoflurane, sevoflurane and desflurane are chemically classified as substituted halogenated hydrocarbons. Chemical analogues include industrial cooling agents (Freon). TIVA decreases exposure to these chemicals, which are environmentally harmful and potentially dangerous to personnel in proximity to their administration. By decreasing patient, veterinary personnel, and environmental exposure, anesthesia is successfully administered with a greener outcome.

DISADVANTAGES OF TOTAL INTRAVENOUS ANESTHESIA VERSUS INHALATION ANESTHESIA

Potential disadvantages of TIVA are personnel training and patient response to parenteral versus inhalation agents. Equipment set up and perceived complexity may be an initial barrier; however, once embraced, set up time is not significantly different from inhalant anesthesia. TIVA does require a comfort level with math calculations that are required for accurate drug delivery. This is slightly more challenging compared with adjusting a vaporizer setting; however, in principle, it is the same concept. Familiarity with delivery devices such as syringe pumps and a comfort level operating these devices is essential. Disposable equipment (intravenous tubing, 3-way valves, vascular manifold) used to deliver TIVA is an additional inventory expense. Additional required supplies, equipment, drugs, and monitors are the same as inhalation anesthesia. The anesthesia machine and breathing circuit is still used for oxygen delivery, carbon dioxide removal, and breathing support during TIVA administration.

TOTAL INTRAVENOUS ANESTHESIA APPLICATION IN EMERGENCY AND CRITICAL CARE MEDICINE

TIVA can be useful in emergency and critical patient care. Diagnostic imaging is a natural fit because the procedures are of a short duration and minimally painful. TIVA is an excellent option for computed tomography scans owing to the procedure's short duration and emphasis on sedation and immobility. Similar goals make TIVA an excellent choice for MRI evaluations. TIVA is especially suited for MRI in that supplies are nonferrous materials and do not pose a hazard under magnetic influence. MRI-compatible infusion pumps are commercially available, making the anesthesia delivery system safe in magnetic fields. TIVA can also be used for ultrasound-guided biopsy of internal organs.

Sedation for emergency procedures is also amenable to TIVA. TIVA is an effective management strategy for patients with severe, refractory status epilepticus, where anesthesia is the best option for seizure control. Rapid induction using propofol followed by a benzodiazepine and propofol TIVA protocol can effectively manage refractory cases. A similar strategy may be elected to control seizures associated with neuroexcitatory toxins during the decontamination period. When TIVA is used for an extended time period, drug tolerance (tachyphylaxis) does occur owing to microsomal enzyme induction associated with constant drug exposure. For this reason, it is important that constant monitoring for drug response and patient stability occur during the TIVA period.

TIVA is an excellent option for short duration anesthesia in emergent patients with incomplete health evaluation. Procedures in which TIVA may be valuable include wound debridement, laceration repair, fracture reduction, splint/bandage application, gastric decompression, and relief of urinary obstruction, because it permits the operator to maintain the patient at a consistent sedation/anesthesia level thereby facilitating time efficiency in task completion. This results in a better quality of sedation/anesthesia with a lower total delivered drug dose compared with intermittent bolus doses. This strategy improves patient safety and decreases recovery time.

TIVA is currently used for ventilator patient management. Sedation protocols for ventilator management use TIVA principles with an emphasis on sedation and analgesia to achieve artificial airway tolerance and prevent ventilator–patient dysynchrony during the support period. Agents and protocols used in ventilator management are identical to other TIVA indications.

SUMMARY

TIVA is an emerging option for creating safe anesthesia and avoiding side effects associated with inhalation class drugs. TIVA use has increased in academic centers to address the need for safe anesthesia in complex cases in which inhalation anesthesia is not indicated. Knowledge regarding TIVA use in companion animal practice is constantly evolving. A greater awareness of TIVA and targeted application has increased use and experience by anesthesia personnel. However, knowledge regarding TIVA in veterinary medicine is in its infancy compared with human medicine, where extensive research on population pharmacokinetics of many injectable anesthetic drugs has been conducted. Future goals include development of pharmacokinetic profiles for parenteral anesthetic drugs in companion animal species and availability of delivery devices that automatically calculate appropriate dose delivery across time for individual patients. Large pool studies for each anesthetic drug will be required to fulfill this vision.[13]

The future is exciting as more information emerges regarding TIVA application in companion animal emergency and critical care practice. The development of TIVA specific delivery equipment, drugs, and patient monitoring techniques will make TIVA and target controlled infusion more attractive options. Development of better ways to determine patient–drug interaction and the ability to monitor TIVA response in real time using closed loop models will decrease the unknowns associated with TIVA and facilitate its wider adoption in veterinary practice.

DISCLOSURE

The author has no commercial or financial conflicts of interest related to the material contained in this article. The author has no research funding which may be a conflict of interest.

REFERENCES

1. Wikipedia: definition of anesthesia. Available at: https://en.wikipedia.org/wiki/Anesthesia.
2. Duke T. Partial intravenous anesthesia in cats and dogs. Can Vet J 2013;54(3):276–82.
3. McIlroy EI, Leslie K. Total intravenous anesthesia in ambulatory care. Anesthesiology 2019;32(6):1–5.
4. Absalom AR, Struys MMRF, editors. An overview of TCI and TIVA. 2nd edition. Ghent (Belgium): Academia Press; 2007.
5. Chong CT. Historical perspectives on total intravenous anaesthesia (TIVA). J Anesth Hist 2018;4:60.
6. Chan V, Skowno J. A practical approach to propofol based total intravenous anaesthesia (TIVA) in children. Paediatric Anaesthesia Tutorial 2018;392:27.
7. Lauder GR. Total intravenous anesthesia will supersede inhalational anesthesia in pediatric anesthetic practice. Paediatr Anaesthes 2015;25(1):52–64.
8. Miller D, Lewis SR, Pritchard MW, et al. Intravenous versus inhalational maintenance of anaesthesia for postoperative cognitive outcomes in elderly people undergoing non-cardiac surgery. Cochrane Database Syst Rev 2018;(8):CD012317.
9. Schraag S, Pradelli L, Alsaleh AJO, et al. Propofol vs. inhalational agents to maintain general anaesthesia in ambulatory and inpatient surgery: a systematic review and meta-analysis. BMC Anesthesiol 2018;18(1):162.
10. Nimmo AF, Absalom AR, Bagshaw O, et al. Guidelines for the safe practice of total intravenous anaesthesia (TIVA): Joint Guidelines from the Association of Anaesthetists and the Society for Intravenous Anaesthesia. Anaesthesia 2019;74(2):211–24.
11. Al-Rifai Z, Mulvey D. Principles of total intravenous anaesthesia: practical aspects of using total intravenous anaesthesia. BJA Educ 2016;16(8):276–80.

12. Struys MR, De Smet T, Glen JB, et al. The history of target-controlled infusion. Anesth Analg 2016;122(1):56–69.
13. Pyendorp BH: Target-controlled infusions in animals- Why aren't we there yet? Proceedings IVECCS 2019, 25-28.
14. Pyendorp BH: Pharmacokinetics in the clinical setting: new insights. Proceedings IVECCS 2019 29-36.
15. Gepts E, Camu F, Cockshott ID, et al. Disposition of propofol administered as constant rate intravenous infusions in humans. Anesth Analg 1987;66(12): 1256–63.
16. Kirkpatrick T, Cockshott ID, Douglas EJ, et al. Pharmacokinetics of propofol (Diprivan) in elderly patients. Br J Anaesth 1988;60(2):146–50.
17. Al-Rifai Z, Mulvey D. Principles of total intravenous anaesthesia: basic pharmacokinetics and model descriptions. BJA Educ 2016;16(3):92–7.
18. Simon BT, Scallan EM, Coursey CD, et al. The clinical effects of a low dose dexmedetomidine constant rate infusion in isoflurane anesthetized cats. Vet J 2018; 234:55–60.
19. Uilenreef JJ, Murrell JC, McKusick BC, et al. Dexmedetomidine continuous rate infusion during isoflurane anaesthesia in canine surgical patients. Vet Anaesth Analg 2008;35(1):1–12.
20. Quandt J. Analgesia, anesthesia, and chemical restraint in the emergent small animal patient. Vet Clin North Am Small Anim Pract 2013;43(4):941–53.
21. Quandt J. Neuromuscular blockers. In: Silverstein D, Hopper K, editors. Small animal critical care medicine. Elsevier; 2009. p. 780–3.
22. Kannabirin N, Bidkar PU. Total intravenous anesthesia in neurosurgery. J Neuroanaesthesiol Crit Care 2018;5:141–9.
23. Stanley SCW, Choi SW, Lee Y, et al. The analgesic effects of intraoperative total intravenous anesthesia (TIVA) with propofol versus sevoflurane after colorectal surgery. Medicine 2018;97(31):116–25.
24. Jin Z, Li R, Lin J, et al. Long-term prognosis after cancer surgery with inhalational anesthesia and total intravenous anesthesia: a systematic review and meta-analysis. Int J Physiol Pathophysiol Pharmacol 2019;11(3):83–94.
25. Yan T, Zhang GH, Wang BN, et al. Effects of propofol/remifentanil-based total intravenous anesthesia versus sevoflurane-based inhalational anesthesia on the release of VEGF-C and TGF-β and prognosis after breast cancer surgery: a prospective, randomized and controlled study. BMC Anesthesiol 2018;18(1):131.
26. Yoo S, Lee HB, Han W, et al. Total intravenous anesthesia versus inhalation anesthesia for breast cancer surgery: a retrospective cohort study. Anesthesiology 2019;130:31–40.
27. Yap A, Lopez-Olivo MA, Dubowitz J, et al. Anesthetic technique and cancer outcomes: a meta-analysis of total intravenous versus volatile anesthesia. Can J Anaesth 2019;66(5):546–61.

Cageside Ultrasonography in the Emergency Room and Intensive Care Unit

Gregory R. Lisciandro, DVM[a,b,*]

KEYWORDS

- AFAST • TFAST • Vet BLUE • Point-of-care ultrasonography

KEY POINTS

- Global Focused Assessment with Sonography for Trauma (FAST) includes the combined use of Abdominal FAST (AFAST), Thoracic FAST (TFAST), and Veterinary Brief Lung Ultrasonography Examination (Vet BLUE) as an unbiased set of data imaging points and should be considered as an extension of the physical examination.
- AFAST and its applied abdominal fluid scoring system and its target-organ approach exceeds a simple binary question of fluid positive or fluid negative.
- TFAST echo views along with the integration of Vet BLUE findings helps formulate a more accurate assessment for cardiac and noncardiac problems.
- TFAST has a set of tenets to ensure an accurate diagnosis of pleural and pericardial effusion and cardiac tamponade.
- Vet BLUE is a proactive, regional, pattern-based approach for pulmonary evaluation and includes its B-line scoring system and its visual lung language for lung assessment.

INTRODUCTION

Veterinary point-of-care ultrasonography (POCUS), which includes Focused Assessment with Sonography for Trauma (FAST) ultrasonography examinations, is defined as a goal-directed ultrasonography examination performed by a veterinary health care provider cageside to answer specific diagnostic questions or guide performance of invasive procedures. Global FAST, a term coined in 2010, is the combination of AFAST (Abdominal FAST), TFAST (Thoracic FAST), and Veterinary Brief Lung Ultrasonography Examination (Vet BLUE [VB]).[1–3] Focused or POCUS examinations are terms used interchangeably, and they target imaging of specific organs or systems.[4]

This article covers how Global FAST and focused ultrasonography examinations (POCUS) may be used advantageously in the emergency room (ER) and intensive care unit (ICU) with the potential to improve small animal patient care.

[a] Emergency and Critical Care, Hill Country Veterinary Specialists, Spicewood, TX, USA;
[b] FASTVet.com, Spicewood, TX, USA
* 1049 Lakeshore Drive, Spicewood, TX 78669.
E-mail address: FastSavesLives@gmail.com

Vet Clin Small Anim 50 (2020) 1445–1467
https://doi.org/10.1016/j.cvsm.2020.07.013
0195-5616/20/© 2020 Elsevier Inc. All rights reserved.

ABDOMINAL FOCUSED ASSESSMENT WITH SONOGRAPHY FOR TRAUMA AND ITS TARGET-ORGAN APPROACH

AFAST uses a standardized approach for abdominal evaluation as a screening test for free fluid/ascites and retroperitoneal fluid, and obvious soft tissue abnormalities of its target organs. Initial AFAST provides a baseline set of data imaging points from which focused ultrasonography organ examinations may be used for more detailed evaluation.[2,5,6] Ultrasonography can identify free fluid and many soft tissue abnormalities and may be advantageous compared with traditional first-line screening based on physical examination, blood and urine testing, and radiography.

AFAST, a modification from the original FAST study, has 5 views: the diaphragmaticohepatic (DH), splenorenal (SR), cystocolic (CC), hepatorenal umbilical (HRU), and hepatorenal fifth (HR5th) bonus view (**Fig. 1**).[1,2,5-9] The HRU remains a misnomer; neither the right kidney nor the liver is imaged, and the probe is not run under the patient but directed into the most gravity-dependent region at the level of the umbilicus, the umbilical pouch. The HRU view is more accurately described as the splenointestinoumbilical view because its target organs are the spleen and small intestine. The liver and right kidney are imaged at the HR5th bonus view, not part of the abdominal fluid scoring system, but this is important for imaging the right kidney, its retroperitoneal space, and adjacent liver. When the patient is in left lateral recumbency, the nomenclature changes, but views are analogous.

AFAST is performed with the patient in standing or sternal position. If AFAST is negative for free fluid, then abdominal fluid scoring in lateral recumbency is unnecessary. When free fluid is detected, the patient is placed in lateral recumbency when safe, followed by waiting 3-minutes to allow ascites to redistribute into gravity-dependent regions before scoring. Standing (or sternal) position is preferable for TFAST and VB, requires less restraint, is lower risk, and is more comfortable for the

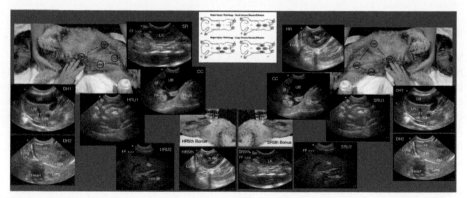

Fig. 1. AFAST and its fluid scoring system in right and left lateral recumbency. The views in right lateral recumbency are performed in this standardized order: DH view, splenorenal (SR) view, cystocolic (CC) view, hepatorenal umbilical (HRU) view, followed by a focused spleen and hepatorenal fifth (HR5th) bonus view. The views in left lateral recumbency are performed in this standardized order: DH view, hepatorenal (HR) view, CC view, SR umbilical (SRU) view, followed by a focused spleen and SR fifth (SR5th) bonus view. The line drawings show the abdominal fluid scoring system and its use for categorizing small-volume versus large-volume bleeder/effusion. CVC, caudal vena cava; DIA, diaphragm; FF, free fluid; GB, gallbladder; LIV, liver; LK, left kidney; RK, right kidney; SI, small intestine; Sp, spleen; UB, urinary bladder. (Courtesy and with permission from Dr. Gregory Lisciandro, Hill Country Veterinary Specialists and FASTVet.com, Spicewood, Texas.)

patient. Dorsal recumbency is not used for any part of Global FAST because of risk of decompensation in a hemodynamically fragile/unstable patient.[1,2,5–11]

ABDOMINAL FOCUSED ASSESSMENT WITH SONOGRAPHY FOR TRAUMA AND ITS MODIFIED ABDOMINAL FLUID SCORING SYSTEM

The AFAST applied abdominal fluid scoring system includes its first 4 views. Originally, each respective view was scored as 0 (negative all 4 views) to 4 (positive all 4 views).[5] However, more recent research has shown that the abdominal fluid scoring system better semiquantitates ascites by scoring smaller positives as 1/2 either by measurement or a visual approach. This change better categorizes dogs and cats with smaller pockets of fluid.[12–14] The gestalt visual approach works well because most pockets of fluid are not borderline between an abdominal fluid score (AFS) of 1/2 and 1 (**Fig. 2**).

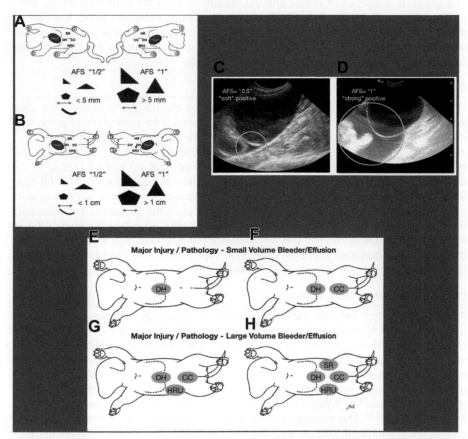

Fig. 2. The AFAST fluid scoring system. (*A* and *B*) Changes in the abdominal fluid scoring system by assigning AFS of 1/2 and 1 depending on the maximum dimension of the free fluid at each respective AFAST view. (*C* and *D*) A visual means to assess scores of 1/2 and 1 at each respective view at the CC view. (*E* and *F*) AFS can categorize patients with AFS less than 3 as small-volume bleeder/effusion versus (*G* and *H*) those with AFS greater than or equal to 3 as large-volume bleeder/effusion. The fifth bonus views, not shown, are scored but not part of the abdominal fluid scoring system. (Courtesy and with permission from Dr. Gregory Lisciandro, Hill Country Veterinary Specialists and FASTVet.com, Spicewood, Texas.)

The measurement approach, based on scoring juvenile and adult dogs and cats, assesses an AFS of 1/2 or 1 by maximum dimensions of less than or equal to 5 mm or greater than 5 mm in cats, and less than or equal to 1 cm or greater than 1 cm in dogs, respectively (see **Fig. 2**).[12–14] Based on total AFS, patients are categorized as small-volume bleeder/effusion (AFS<3) and large-volume/bleeder effusion (AFS ≥ 3).[1,2,5,12–14] Small-volume bleeders are not expected to become anemic directly from their intra-abdominal hemorrhage. Thus, if a patient has an AFS less than 3 and is anemic, then major rule-outs in the acute setting include (1) bleeding elsewhere, thus perform a good physical examination and Global FAST; (2) preexisting anemia, so consider initial packed cell volume; (3) hemodilution; or (4) laboratory error.

ABDOMINAL FOCUSED ASSESSMENT WITH SONOGRAPHY FOR TRAUMA DIAPHRAGMATICOHEPATIC VIEW

The DH view, also part of TFAST and VB, rapidly images the peritoneal cavity, liver, gallbladder, caudal vena cava (CVC) and its associated hepatic veins, the thorax, pleural space, heart, and lung along its pulmonary-diaphragmatic interface.[1,2,7,8,15–17] Enough depth should be used to recognize the triad of gallbladder, CVC, and heart plus the diaphragm (**Fig. 3**).

Gallbladder Wall Edema

Gallbladder wall edema (GBWE), referred to as the double rim sign and halo sign, recognized as sonographic striation, serves as a marker for canine anaphylaxis (AX) and right-sided congestive heart failure, most commonly pericardial effusion.[16,18,19] Integrating Global FAST findings is key for differentiating AX from cardiac disease. When GBWE is recognized, screen for pericardial effusion by looking cranial to the diaphragm (racetrack sign), and, if not present, then evaluate the CVC. A fat (distended) CVC, especially with hepatic venous distension (tree trunk sign), supports other right-sided cardiac problems (dilated cardiomyopathy, pulmonary hypertension, necessitating TFAST echo views), whereas a flat (small) CVC supports canine AX (see **Fig. 3**; **Fig. 4**, **Table 1**).[19,20] The clinician should acknowledge that AX is a life-threatening hypovolemic/distributive shock to best place GBWE in its clinical context because there are many other non-AX causes.[21]

Canine Anaphylactic Hemoabdomen

AX in dogs often induces varying degrees of medically managed hemoabdomen.[19,20,22–26] A typical AX clinical profile includes a healthy dog with acute collapse often accompanied by gastrointestinal signs, with or without witnessed Hymenoptera envenomation, and variable to no cutaneous signs.[18,22,23] Laboratory findings include hemoconcentration, increased liver enzyme levels (alanine transaminase and aspartate transaminase), along with sonographically detected GBWE and hypovolemic/distributive shock.[18,22,23] Warm days and cool nights in spring and fall are also predisposing factors.[19,22] The acquired coagulopathy is caused by the second episode of anaphylaxis, mitigated through the use of glucocorticoids, initially and as a short-tapering protocol over the next 2 to 7 days.[22,23] Hemoabdomen may be tracked by AFAST and AFS; however, Global FAST should be used to integrate information in the thorax as well. Dogs reportedly have no other sites of bleeding, including absent B lines during VB.[19,22,23] When bleeding stops and the coagulopathy, when present, is corrected, expect the AFS to resolve quickly within 24 to 48 hours.[19] Histamine receptor-2 antagonists are continued with glucocorticoids because they also mitigate intra-abdominal bleeding. If a dog with AX inadvertently has exploratory surgery,

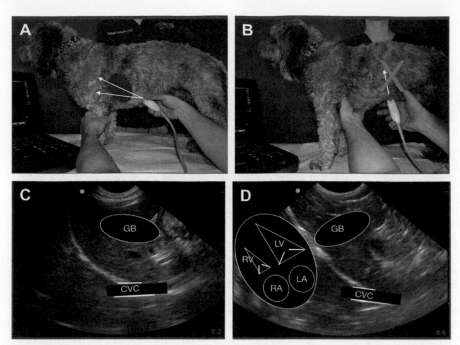

Fig. 3. The DH view and its triad. (*A*) The proper scanning plane to image the triad of landmark structures at the DH view, which includes the gallbladder, heart, and CVC. The white line that represents the diaphragm should come close to the probe head in the near field by rocking the probe close to parallel to the sternum. Contrast with (*B*), where the scanning plane is directed toward the spine, which generally brings too much stomach and gastrointestinal tract into the field of view, each of which is often air filled, obscuring the imaging. (*C* and *D*) The landmark structures shown in the regions they are expected regarding the near and far field. Understanding that the left heart is nearest the diaphragm is helpful in more thoroughly evaluating the heart through the DH view. LA, left atrium; LV, left ventricle; RA, right atrium; RV, right ventricle. (Courtesy and with permission from Dr. Gregory Lisciandro, Hill Country Veterinary Specialists and FASTVet.com, Spicewood, Texas.)

hepatic swelling with no discreet bleeding other than generalized oozing will be observed.[22] Histopathologic results will be nonspecific and, anecdotally, a guarded chance of survival exists perioperatively.[19,22] The acquired coagulopathy is complex and unpredictably variable with traditional coagulation testing of prothrombin time (PT) and activated partial thrombin time (aPTT); however, heparin, a component of mast cells, likely plays a leading role.[22–24] In some patients, a discordance of PT and aPTT exists, where the aPTT is much higher, supporting heparin's role in AX.[22]

Characterization of the Caudal Vena Cava and Its Associated Hepatic Veins

The CVC and its associated hepatic veins are characterized as a noninvasive marker for assessing intravascular volume status.[17,27,28] There are 2 approaches: the eyeball method and actual measurements.[20,27–29] The eyeball method assesses the respirophasic dynamic size changes of the CVC. In normalcy, CVC size changes approximately 35% to 50%. With an increased central venous pressure, the CVC and its associated hepatic veins become distended or fat (tree trunk sign) and size lacks respirophasic change (<10%).[8,17,20,27,30] In contrast, when hypovolemia exists, CVC size becomes small or flat, with size also lacking respirophasic change (<10%) along

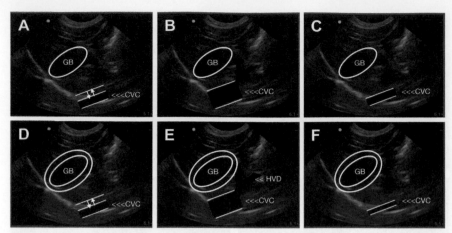

Fig. 4. Characterizing the CVC. (*A–C*) Characterization of the CVC in the presence of a normal gallbladder wall as (*A*) fluid responsive, bounce, with arrows representing change in height, and (*B*) fluid intolerant, fat, along with hepatic venous distension, and (*C*) hypovolemic, flat. (*D–F*) Characterization of the CVC in the presence of a thickened sonographically striated (hyperechoic-anechoic-hyperechoic) gallbladder wall as (*A*) fluid responsive, bounce, with arrows representing change in height; (*B*) fluid intolerant, fat, along with hepatic venous distension, referred to as a cardiac gallbladder, when pericardial effusion and right-sided congestive heart failure are detected; and (*C*) hypovolemic, flat, referred to as an AX gallbladder in the acute setting when the patient profile fits canine AX. There are other causes for gallbladder wall edema that are possible besides right-sided congestive heart failure and canine AX. (*Courtesy and with permission from Dr. Gregory Lisciandro, Hill Country Veterinary Specialists and FASTVet.com, Spicewood, Texas.*)

with inapparent hepatic veins (see **Figs. 4** and **6**).[20,27,30] Absolute measurements for maximum CVC heights for fat and flat at the DH view are easy to remember without requiring calculations (see **Table 1**).[28]

Pleural and Pericardial Effusions

The liver and gallbladder at the DH view advantageously provide an acoustic window into the thorax for detecting pleural effusion (PE) and pericardial effusion (PCE) by avoiding air interference via transthoracic views.[1,2,6–9,16,19,20] The TFAST tenets for accurately diagnosing PE and PCE are described later (**Table 2**).[2,8,19,20]

ABDOMINAL FOCUSED ASSESSMENT WITH SONOGRAPHY FOR TRAUMA SPLENORENAL VIEW

The SR view images both the retroperitoneal space and the peritoneal cavity by imaging the left kidney (and right kidney in cats and some dogs) and the spleen, respectively.[1,2,5–7,15] In right lateral recumbency, this region can be used for the detection of pneumoperitoneum (enhanced peritoneal stripe sign) (see **Fig. 13**).[29,31]

ABDOMINAL FOCUSED ASSESSMENT WITH SONOGRAPHY FOR TRAUMA CYSTOCOLIC VIEW
Urinary Bladder Volume Estimation Formula

Urinary bladder measurements at the AFAST CC view in both dogs and cats are used to estimate urinary bladder volume. Measurements in centimeters using the formula

Table 1
Maximum height at the diaphragmaticohepatic view for characterizing the caudal vena cava

Proposed Reference Values for the CVC Maximum Height Measurements[a] in the Longitudinal Plane at the FAST Subxiphoid View[b] for Dogs and Cats

Size	Body Weight (kg)	Expected CVC Height Measurement (cm) for a Bounce or Fluid-Responsive CVC[d]	Suggested CVC Maximum Height (cm) for a Flat or Hypovolemic, Fluid-Starved CVC[d] (Low Central Venous Pressure)	Suggested CVC Maximum Height (cm) for a Fat or Fluid-Intolerant CVC[d] (High Central Venous Pressure)
Small/toy[c]	<9	0.55 (0.40–0.70)	<0.25	>1.0
Medium	>9<15	0.85 (0.50–1.10)	<0.35	>1.5
Large/giant	>15	0.95 (0.80–1.20)	<0.50	>1.5

[a] Data from the study by Darnis and colleagues[28] and measurements created with permission by Lisciandro G.R. and Vientós -Plotts A.I. These values are unproved but give some guidelines for veterinary clinicians to combine with the eyeball method: bounce (fluid-responsive), fat (fluid-intolerant), and flat (fluid-starved or hypovolemic) CVC.
[b] The subxiphoid view is analogous to the FAST DH view in the longitudinal plane.
[c] Suggested starting point for felines while awaiting current research findings.
[d] Combine absolute height measurements with the eyeball method (bounce, fat, and flat).
Adapted from Lisciandro GR. POCUS: Global FAST for Rapidly Detecting Treatable Forms of Shock, ALS and CPR. In: Lisciandro GR, ed. Point-of-care Ultrasound for the Small Animal Practitioner. 2nd ed. Ames, IA: Wiley-Blackwell;2020:700; with permission.

length (L) times height (H) times width (W) times 0.625 provides a volume estimation in milliliters, and thus, over time, a noninvasive option for estimating urine output.[32]

ABDOMINAL FOCUSED ASSESSMENT WITH SONOGRAPHY FOR TRAUMA HEPATORENAL UMBILICAL VIEW

AFAST fluid scoring is designed to end at the HRU view, being most gravity dependent where fluid would accumulate, and a common site for abdominocentesis (see **Fig. 1**).[1,2,5,19,21] A focused spleen should follow the HRU view, especially in hemoabdomen because of the recently described medically treated canine AX hemoabdomen, first described by the author.[22] The presence of a cavitated mass supports a bleeding splenic mass rather than an AX hemoabdomen, where a cavitated mass would be unexpected.[33] The focused spleen should be considered a rule-in test, being operator dependent.

ABDOMINAL FOCUSED ASSESSMENT WITH SONOGRAPHY FOR TRAUMA FIFTH BONUS VIEW

The AFAST fifth bonus view is not part of the AFS but is important for screening the retroperitoneal space for free fluid and soft tissue abnormalities of the right kidney and adjacent right liver (see **Fig. 1**).[1,2,20,21]

Table 2
Thoracic Focused Assessment with Sonography for Trauma tenets for accurately detecting pleural and pericardial effusion and cardiac tamponade

	Pericardial Effusion			
Imaging Strategies	FAST DH View	TFAST Right PCS View	Thoracic Radiography	Gold Standard
1. Image toward the muscular apex of the heart where no heart chambers that can be mistaken for free fluid	• Racetrack sign	• Bull's eye sign on short axis	• Unreliable test for PCE and for cardiac tamponade	• Ultrasonography and computed tomography
2. Identify all 4 cardiac chambers	—	• TFAST right PCS view: long-axis 4-chamber view	—	—
3. Image the heart in its entirety using the hyperechoic pericardium in the far field as a landmark	—	—	—	—

	Pleural Effusion			
Imaging Strategies	FAST DH View	TFAST Right and Left PCS Views	Thoracic Radiography	Gold Standard
1. Image the heart in its entirety using the hyperechoic pericardium in the far field as a landmark	• Anechoic triangulations: no racetrack sign	• TFAST right and left PCS: anechoic triangulations	Good test	Debatable between ultrasonography, computed tomography, and thoracoscopy
2. TFAST slide moving caudal and cranial to the heart avoiding confounding heart chambers	—	• Curtain sign of pleural effusion	—	—

Courtesy and with permission from Dr. Gregory Lisciandro, Hill Country Veterinary Specialists and FASTVet.com, Spicewood, Texas.

THORACIC FOCUSED ASSESSMENT WITH SONOGRAPHY FOR TRAUMA AND ITS TARGET-ORGAN APPROACH

TFAST, a 5-view examination, screens for PE and PCE, pneumothorax (PTX), and cardiac abnormalities (**Fig. 5**).[1,2,7–9,34] Ideally, TFAST is best performed in a standing (or sternal) position to allow fluid to fall into gravity-dependent pouches and air to rise to non–gravity-dependent regions.[1,2,7–9,35] TFAST echo views screen for volume, contractility, and left-sided and right-sided cardiac problems plus PCE and cardiac

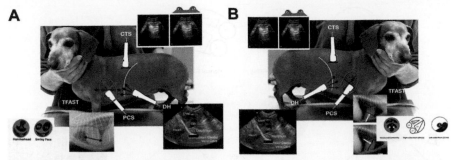

Fig. 5. TFAST protocol. TFAST has 5 acoustic windows performed in a standardized manner. The chest tube site (CTS) is the highest point on the thoracic wall over lung used for PTX. The bilaterally applied pericardial site (PCS) views are used differently from the left (*A*), sliding into the caudal cardiac-diaphragmatic pouch and cranially into the cardiac-cervical pouch for pleural effusion and recognizing the appearance of the heart being much different than the right PCS view (*B*). These views may be used for assessing heart with more advanced skills. From the right PCS view, the TFAST echo views are obtained. The (DH view is used for CVC assessment, pleural and pericardial effusion, lung along the diaphragmatic surface, ascites, and soft tissue changes of the gallbladder and liver. Standing (and sternal) position is advantageous in being generally safer for the patient and creates a gravity-dependent model in which fluid falls into the gravity-dependent PCS and DH views, and air rises to the CTS view. The gator (alligator) sign is used for orientation of all lung ultrasonography to ensure that the intercostal space and lung line, pulmonary-pleural interface, is accurately identified. (Courtesy and with permission from Dr. Gregory Lisciandro, Hill Country Veterinary Specialists and FASTVet.com, Spicewood, Texas.)

soft tissue abnormalities (masses, thrombi, *Dirofilaria*, dilated cardiomyopathy, pulmonary hypertension, and chamber enlargements).[1,2,34–37]

THORACIC FOCUSED ASSESSMENT WITH SONOGRAPHY FOR TRAUMA AND ITS ECHO VIEWS

TFAST echo views are performed with the same orientation every time, so expectations of relevant anatomy are consistent. Proficiency in acquiring short-axis (SAX) and long-axis (LAX) views of the heart from the right pericardial site can be obtained with minimal training (**Fig. 6**).[1,2,8,34,35] The SAX views include the mushroom view for volume and contractility, the left atrial to aortic (LA/Ao) ratio for increased left atrial dilatation or increased filling pressures, and the pulmonary artery to aortic ratio (PA/Ao) for pulmonary hypertension (**Fig. 7**).[34–37] LAX views include the 4-chamber and left ventricular outflow tract views. The different SAX levels of the heart are named for teaching and communication what level is being imaged (see **Fig. 7**).[34,35]

THORACIC FOCUSED ASSESSMENT WITH SONOGRAPHY FOR TRAUMA AND ITS USE FOR PLEURAL AND PERICARDIAL EFFUSION
Pleural Effusion and Pericardial Effusion

The use of the DH view is advantageous because of the acoustic window provided by the liver and gallbladder into the thorax, which avoids the air interference (lung) and confusing heart chambers through transthoracic views. TFAST tenets should be followed to accurately detect PE and PCE and not mistake a heart chamber for either (see **Table 2**).[8,34,35] Cardiac tamponade may be ruled in and ruled out by nonecho views through the characterization of the inferior vena cava in people, and likely the same holds true in small animals.[38–40]

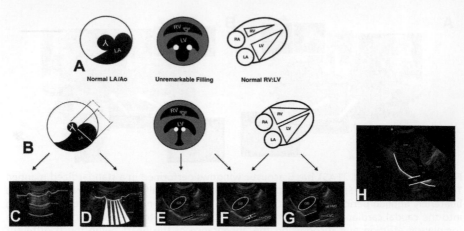

Fig. 6. The TFAST echo views and integrating findings of the lung and CVC. The TFAST echo views are used for volume status and contractility, mushroom view, left-sided cardiac abnormalities, the left atrial to aortic ratio (LA/Ao), and right-sided cardiac problems, and RV/LV ratio. Unremarkable image is shown in (A) in the upper row contrasted to abnormal in (B) in the middle row, which are then correlated to the Global FAST nonecho fallback views of VB and a regional, pattern-based approach for wet versus dry lung in (C) and (D), and the CVC characterization in (E–G) and hepatic venous distension in (H). For example, when left-sided and right-sided enlargement are suspected, the use of the fallback views helps support or refute the presence of left-sided and right-sided congestive heart failure (CHF) and, conversely, when TFAST echo views are too risky, help rule in or rule out CHF, dictating therapy while waiting until the patient is more stable. HV, hepatic veins. (Courtesy and with permission from Dr. Gregory Lisciandro, Hill Country Veterinary Specialists and FASTVet.com, Spicewood, Texas.)

Thoracic Focused Assessment with Sonography for Trauma for Pneumothorax

The transition zone between where lung comes in contact with the thoracic wall and PTX is called the lung point (LP). The LP increases the diagnostic sensitivity of PTX and is used for monitoring and categorizing PTX as trivial, moderate, or severe.[1,9,34,35,41] When PTX is suspected at the chest tube site, the patient is moved to dorsal or sternal recumbency (rather than lateral) to better find the LP. VB is then performed with its caudodorsal lung region considered the upper third, its perihilar lung region the middle third, and its middle lung region the lower third of the thorax (**Fig. 8**).[35] Once lung is observed along the thoracic wall during VB, the probe is moved in smaller increments dorsally to more exactly locate the LP. The LP is most commonly located by the finding of lung sliding or B lines ventral to PTX. However, any VB sign (ie, shred and tissue sign) also provide evidence for the LP when ventral to the PTX. PTX is semiquantitated using the TFAST PTX thirds rule of upper third, trivial; middle third, moderate; and lower third, severe, with the middle and lower thirds warranting treatment (ie, thoracocentesis) (see **Fig. 8**).[1,9,35] Decision-making algorithms have been published.[2,9,35]

New Thoughts: Double Curtain Sign and Reverse Curtain Sign

The imaging of the transition zone of the pleural and peritoneal cavities by the curtain sign is generally avoided because of mistaking abdominal structures for lung disease. However, dynamics of this curtain sign may detect PTX by observing the pleural and peritoneal structures moving toward each other (respiratory asynchrony) rather than

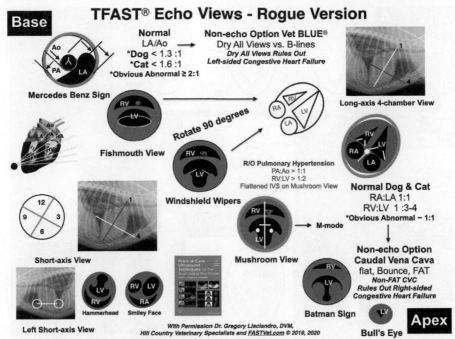

Fig. 7. The TFAST echo chart. The TFAST echo chart contains a lot of clinically relevant information. For learning SAX views, the levels are named from the apex to the heart base as follows: bull's eye, batman, mushroom, windshield wipers, fishmouth, and Mercedes Benz sign (circle in the middle). This system helps distinguish these SAX levels. On mitral valves, the probe is rotated to 90° to the LAX. Shown is the LAX 4-chamber view (LA4CV); however, the left ventricular outflow tract may be easily added being a small movement from the LA4CV. Expected normal values are listed as well as the Global FAST nonecho fallback views. The face of a clock works well for checking probe placement for appropriate scanning planes. On standing or sternal patients, the SAX line is 4 o'clock and the LAX line 1 o'clock from the right TFAST pericardial site view. Note that, from the left side, the heart looks much different from the hammerhead and smiley face views. The probe is also positioned horizontally and slid into the caudal and cranial cardiac pouches, as shown with circle overlays on the radiograph. IVS, interventricular septum; PA, pulmonary artery. (Courtesy and with permission from Dr. Gregory Lisciandro, Hill Country Veterinary Specialists and FASTVet.com, Spicewood, Texas.)

away (respiratory synchrony) during phases of respiration.[42,43] Curtain sign asynchrony has been termed the reverse curtain sign or reverse sliding sign, or a double curtain sign when PTX is located in between lung.[42,43] However, the author has found the dynamic of the reverse curtain sign occurring in paradoxic abdominal breathing in the absence of PTX. Thus, when PTX is suspected, a VB should be performed in standing or sternal position, the LP determined, and semiquantification assessed using the TFAST PTX thirds rule.

VETERINARY BRIEF LUNG ULTRASONOGRAPHY EXAMINATION AND ITS VISUAL LUNG LANGUAGE

The 6 VB signs are (1) dry lung, A lines with lung sliding; (2) wet lung, B lines; and forms of consolidation including (3) shred sign (air bronchogram), (4) tissue sign, (5) nodule sign, and (6) and wedge sign (**Fig. 9**).[10,11,44–48] The use of these signs placed into a

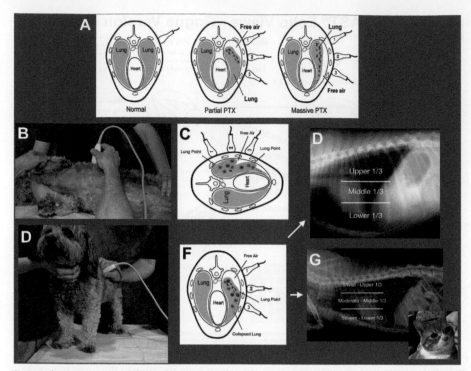

Fig. 8. The LP and the effect of positioning on pneumothorax. (*A*) The normal partial PTX, where the LP is probe 2, and massive PTX where no LP is found. The LP is the transition zone of PTX dorsally and lung recontacting the thoracic wall ventrally as shown in standing or sternal views. (*B* and *C*) PTX may be detected but because probes 1 and 3 are gravity equal, a double LP may be found. (*E* and *F*) Sternal or standing has a clear advantage by making the collapsed lung fall into gravity-dependent regions and the PTX more true for the LP with free air rising into the least gravity-dependent regions of the pleural cavity. PTX may be categorized and tracked using the TFAST thirds rule of upper one-third, trivial-mild; middle one-third, moderate; and lower one-third, massive for dogs (*D*) and cats (*G*). By using this system for recording, clinicians now can assess static, worsening, and resolving PTX. Moreover, the location can help dictate the indication for thoracocentesis with middle and lower thirds as indications for PTX treatment. (Courtesy and with permission from Dr. Gregory Lisciandro, Hill Country Veterinary Specialists and FASTVet.com, Spicewood, Texas.)

pattern-based approach helps screen for common respiratory conditions (**Figs. 10** and **11**).[44–48]

VETERINARY BRIEF LUNG ULTRASONOGRAPHY EXAMINATION AND ITS B-LINE SCORING SYSTEM

The degree of alveolar-interstitial fluid/edema is semiquantitated by counting maximum B lines at each regional VB view (see **Fig. 9**).[10,11,44,46,49] The VB B-line scoring system assesses degree of alveolar-interstitial syndrome by combining B lines per view with total numbers of positive VB views (see **Fig. 9**).[44,48–50] Expect rare to no B lines during VB.[10,11,46] By recording the B-line score at each regional view as well as other findings (ie, shred sign, tissue sign, nodule sign, and wedge sign), VB serves as a monitoring tool for static, resolving, and worsening respiratory conditions. Moreover,

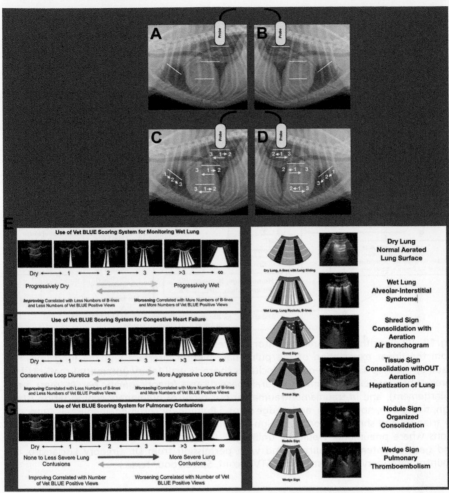

Fig. 9. The VB protocol, its B-line scoring system, and visual lung language. (*A–D*) VB is a regional pattern-based approach in which 3 intercostal spaces are surveyed at each respective regional view of caudodorsal, perihilar, middle, and cranial lung regions bilaterally plus the DH view. The probe is always slid caudally (labeled 2) from the primary intercostal space (ICS) (labeled 1), and then back to the primary and cranially for the final ICS (labeled 3). (*E–G*) Clinically relevant means in using the B-line scoring system in which the maximum score over a single ICS at each of the regional VB views is recorded. The B-line scoring system coupled with numbers of positive regional views helps assess degree of alveolar-interstitial edema and thus guides loop diuretic usage while also assessing severity. The same system may be used for lung contusions and lung hemorrhage. At the bottom right is an echelon of the 6 VB lung language signs from normal aerated lung, dry lung, to wet lung, B lines most commonly representing forms of alveolar-interstitial edema, followed by degrees of consolidation from shred sign, air bronchograms, tissue sign, hepatization of lung, nodule sign, and wedge sign, suggestive of pulmonary thromboembolism when in caudodorsal and perihilar regions. (Courtesy and with permission from Dr. Gregory Lisciandro, Hill Country Veterinary Specialists and FASTVet.com, Spicewood, Texas.)

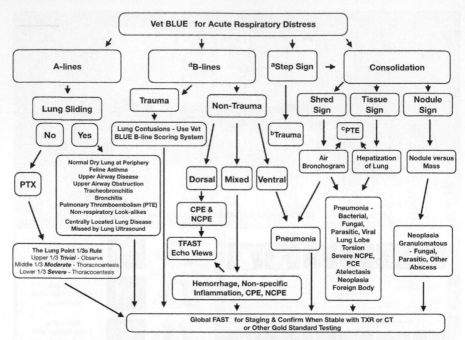

Fig. 10. VB algorithm for acute respiratory distress in dogs and cats. [a] Step sign is a deviation from the linear expectation of the pulmonary-pleural interface and the lung line. [b] In trauma, the step sign's rule-out list includes thoracic wall injury (intercostal tear, rib fractures, subcostal hematoma/mass), pleural space disease (diaphragmatic hernia, mass, heart enlargement), and in trauma/nontrauma various types of pulmonary consolidation (shred sign, tissue sign, nodule sign, and wedge sign). [c] Pulmonary Thromboembolism is supported by triangulated shred sign or tissue sign–like findings at the perihilar and dorsal lung regions where pneumonia would be unlikely. [d] Pseudo–B lines are possible from nodules and gastric contents.[48] (Courtesy and with permission from Dr. Gregory Lisciandro, Hill Country Veterinary Specialists and FASTVet.com, Spicewood, Texas.)

VB is rapid, low impact, and likely a more sensitive imaging modality than lung radiography for many pulmonary conditions.[10,11,50–53] In an imaging study evaluating pulmonary contusions, compared with computed tomography as the gold standard, VB exceeded the sensitivity of thoracic radiography.[54] Absent B lines with dry lung, all VB views rule out left-sided congestive heart failure as well as other lung ultrasonography formats.[10,11,47,49,51,52,54]

VETERINARY BRIEF LUNG ULTRASONOGRAPHY EXAMINATION AND ITS REGIONAL PATTERN-BASED APPROACH

The combined use of VB's B-line scoring system, the visual lung language (VB signs), and their regional distribution in a pattern-based approach help categorize respiratory disease in small animals (see **Figs. 10** and **11**).[44,47–49] In contrast, the absence of B lines during VB in dogs and cats effectively rules out clinically relevant left-sided congestive heart failure and argues against the empiric use of loop diuretics.[10,11,47,49,51,52,54] In cats with respiratory distress, dry lung (A lines with lung sliding) supports feline asthma. For coughing dogs, dry lung commonly supports upper airway disease, heart disease without left-sided congestion, and nonrespiratory

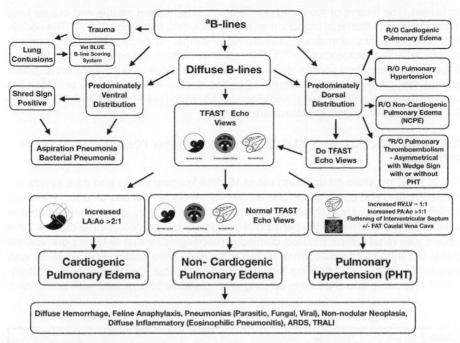

Fig. 11. Algorithm for B lines during VB. [a] Pseudo–B lines are possible from nodules and gastric contents.[48] (Courtesy and with permission from Dr. Gregory Lisciandro, Hill Country Veterinary Specialists and FASTVet.com, Spicewood, Texas.)

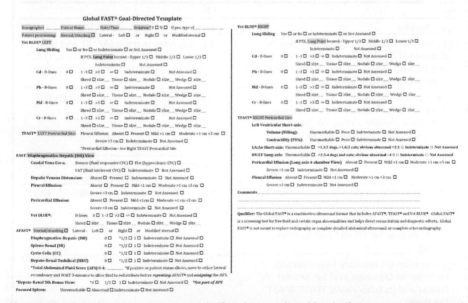

Fig. 12. Goal-directed template example for the standing blend of Vet BLUE, TFAST, and AFAST with focused spleen. Note: if the patient is positive for free fluid during AFAST, then move to lateral recumbency, wait 3 minutes for fluid to redistribute, and then assign an AFAST AFS. (Courtesy and with permission from Dr. Gregory Lisciandro, Hill Country Veterinary Specialists and FASTVet.com, Spicewood, Texas.)

lookalikes. The finding of the shred sign in gravity-dependent middle and cranial lung regions supports bacterial bronchopneumonia including aspiration.[44,47–49] The nodule sign supports granulomatous disease (eg, fungal and parasitic pneumonias), neoplasia, and abscessation.[44,45,47] The regional, pattern-based approach of VB, its B-line scoring system, and its visual lung language serve as a proven, rapid point-of-care respiratory imaging modality to better decide on clinical course, including treatment, subsequent imaging, and diagnostic testing (see **Figs. 10** and **11**). Pseudo B lines have been described elsewhere.[48]

THE GLOBAL FOCUSED ASSESSMENT WITH SONOGRAPHY FOR TRAUMA APPROACH

Global FAST provides an unbiased set of 15 data imaging points and thus avoids selective imaging and confirmation bias as well as satisfaction of search error. There are endless examples of how this occurs, including focused gallbladder examination that detects GBWE but misses the pericardial effusion or right-sided volume overload in a patient with renal failure; focused cardiac ultrasonography that detects poor volume status but misses its cause, intra-abdominal bleed, while challenging a patient with intravenous fluids; and flashing lung for B lines without the VB regional, pattern-based approach, and thus administering loop diuretics to a patient with pneumonia

Table 3
The use of Global Focused Assessment with Sonography for Trauma for the Hs and Ts of treatable forms of shock and advanced life support

Knowing Your Hs and Ts During Cardiopulmonary Resuscitation and Advanced Life Support	
[a]Hs	[a]Ts
Hypothermia	Tension pneumothorax (TFAST and its LP)
Hypotension/hypovolemia (AFAST and its abdominal fluid scoring system; TFAST and its echo views, VB, for Intrathoracic hemorrhage and volume status)	Trauma, hemorrhage (AFAST and its abdominal fluid scoring system; TFAST and VB, for intrathoracic hemorrhage)
Hyperkalemia/hypokalemia (AFAST and its target-organ approach for obvious soft tissue abnormalities, eg, large urinary bladder, and renal pelvic, ureteral, and urethral dilatation)	Thromboembolism, pulmonary (TFAST and VB, wedge sign)
Hypoglycemia	Tamponade, pericardial effusion (TFAST and AFAST-TFAST DH view)
Hydrogen ion (acidosis)	Toxin, canine anaphylaxis (AFAST-TFAST DH view)
Hypocontractility (dilated cardiomyopathy) (TFAST and its echo views)	—
Hypertension (Pulmonary Hypertension, Heartworm Disease/Caval Syndrome) (TFAST and its Echo Views; TFAST-AFAST DH View)	—

[a] The Hs and Ts are rapidly screened for by the physical examination, venous blood gas, and Global FAST approach.

Courtesy and with permission from Dr. Gregory Lisciandro, Hill Country Veterinary Specialists and FASTVet.com, Spicewood, Texas.

or pseudo B lines from nodular disease.[3,54,55] A final example is the canine splenic mass with and without hemoabdomen. The Global FAST approach stages the patient for obvious liver, cardiac, and lung metastases that may or may not be evident radiographically. In dogs that stage negative, the patient becomes more confidently a surgical candidate.[33,56,57]

GOAL-DIRECTED TEMPLATES

Findings must be recorded for multiple reasons, including having patient data for medical records to show what was performed, for future comparison serving as a monitoring tool, and for determining strengths and weaknesses within an institution's Global FAST and POCUS program (**Fig. 12**). Additional examples have been published.[1,2,19–21,35,48,55]

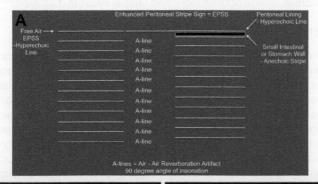

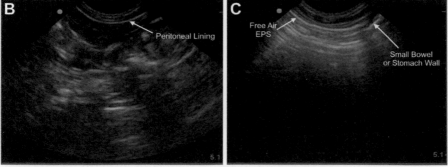

Fig. 13. The enhanced peritoneal stripe sign for detecting pneumoperitoneum. The use of ultrasonography in the least gravity-dependent regions where air would rise may also be applied in the peritoneal cavity. Ultrasonography is very sensitive for detecting free intraperitoneal air. The principle involves identifying the peritoneal lining (*hyperechoic line*). When pneumoperitoneum is suspected, its hyperechoic line is traced to see whether it matches the peritoneal lining. If there is an anechoic step or gap, gastrointestinal (GI) step sign, then the detected air is within the GI tract (*A*). (*B*) The splenorenal view of a patient in right lateral recumbency, in which position air rises (least gravity deponent). In fanning through this region, the enhanced peritoneal stripe sign (EPSS) and the GI step sign are next to one another (*C*). An angle of insonation of 90° to the aerated surface brings out A lines (air reverberation artifacts). A radiograph confirms the pneumoperitoneum. This principle is likewise important when doing VB because air-filled stomach may be easily mistaken for lung disorder. This pitfall is recognized by the anechoic GI step sign. (*Courtesy and with permission from Dr. Gregory Lisciandro, Hill Country Veterinary Specialists and FASTVet.com, Spicewood, Texas.*)

THE USE OF GLOBAL FOCUSED ASSESSMENT WITH SONOGRAPHY FOR TRAUMA FOR THE HS AND TS OF TREATABLE FORMS OF SHOCK AND ADVANCED LIFE SUPPORT

Global FAST screens for treatable forms of shock and is used for basic and advanced life support in questionable or unstable patients (**Table 3**).[3,56–59] Moreover, the Global FAST approach may be used for monitoring anesthetic events and mechanical ventilation.[60,61]

OTHER POINT-OF-CARE ULTRASONOGRAPHY EXAMINATIONS

Focused eye, cardiac, vascular, gastrointestinal, musculoskeletal, nervous system, and so forth as well as detecting pneumoperitoneum (**Fig. 13**) are add-ons that can provide additional important patient information and are easily learned once knowledge of the machine, image optimization, and Global FAST is mastered.[28,29,31,37,62–77]

FINAL COMMENTS

The use of Global FAST and POCUS has the potential to screen for conditions and serve as a monitoring tool rather than traditional means without ultrasonography. Advantages include being point of care, cageside, low impact, rapid, safe, and radiation sparing, and requiring no shaving and/or minimal patient restraint. Moreover, information is real time for detecting free fluid and soft tissue abnormalities of the abdominal, heart, and lung, missed or only suspected by physical examination, basic blood and urine testing, and radiography. A standardized approach along with recording patient data is integral to a successful Global FAST program. Other POCUS should be considered add-on imaging to prevent selective imaging and confirmation bias error, and satisfaction of search error.

DISCLOSURE

The author has nothing to disclose.

REFERENCES

1. Lisciandro GR. Abdominal and thoracic focused assessment with sonography for trauma, triage and monitoring in small animals. J Vet Emerg Crit Care 2011;21(2): 104–22.
2. Boysen SR, Lisciandro GR. The use of ultrasound in the emergency room (AFAST and TFAST). Vet Clin North Am Small Anim Pract 2013;43(4):773–97.
3. Lisciandro GR, Armenise AA. Focused or COAST³ - Cardiopulmonary Resuscitation (CPR), Global FAST (GFAST³), and the FAST-ABCDE Exam. In: Lisciandro GR, editor. Focused ultrasound techniques for the small animal practitioner. Ames (IA): Wiley Blackwell; 2014. p. 269–85.
4. Lisciandro GR, editor. Focused ultrasound for the small animal practitioner. Ames (IA): Wiley Blackwell; 2014.
5. Lisciandro GR, Lagutchik MS, Mann KA, et al. Evaluation of an abdominal fluid scoring system determined using abdominal focused assessment with sonography for trauma in 101 dogs with motor vehicle trauma. J Vet Emerg Crit Care 2009;19(5):426–37.
6. Boysen SR, Rozanski EA, Tidwell AS, et al. Evaluation of a focused assessment with sonography for trauma protocol to detect free abdominal fluid in dogs involved in motor vehicle accidents. J Am Vet Med Assoc 2004;225(8):1198–204.

7. McMurray J, Boysen S, Chalhoub S. Focused assessment with sonography in nontraumatized dogs and cats in the emergency and critical care setting. J Vet Emerg Crit Care 2016;26(1):64–73.

8. Lisciandro GR. The use of the diaphragmatico-hepatic (DH) views of the abdominal and thoracic focused assessment with sonography for triage (AFAST/TFAST) examinations for the detection of pericardial effusion in 24 dogs (2011–2012). J Vet Emerg Crit Care 2016;26(1):125–31.

9. Lisciandro GR, Lagutchik MS, Mann KA, et al. Evaluation of a thoracic focused assessment with sonography for trauma (TFAST) protocol to detect pneumothorax and concurrent thoracic injury in 145 traumatized dogs. J Vet Emerg Crit Care 2008;18(3):258–69.

10. Lisciandro GR, Fosgate GT, Fulton RM. Frequency and number of ultrasound lung rockets (B-lines) using a regionally-based lung ultrasound examination named Vet BLUE (Veterinary Bedside Lung Ultrasound Exam) in dogs with radiographically normal lung findings. Vet Radiol Ultrasound 2014;55(3):315–22.

11. Lisciandro GR, Fulton RM, Fosgate GT, et al. Frequency of B-lines using a regionally-based lung ultrasound examination (the Vet BLUE protocol) in 49 cats with normal thoracic radiographical lung findings. J Vet Emerg Crit Care 2017;27(3):267–77.

12. Romero LA, Lisciandro GR, Fosgate GT, et al. Abdominal FAST (AFAST) and abdominal fluid scores in adult and juvenile dogs. J Vet Emerg Crit Care 2015; 25(S1):S7–8.

13. Lisciandro GR, Fosgate GT, Romero LA, et al. Abdominal FAST (AFAST) and abdominal fluid scores in adult and juvenile cats. J Vet Emerg Crit Care 2015; 25(S1):S8.

14. Lisciandro GR, Fosgate GT, Romero LA, et al. The expected frequency and amount of free peritoneal fluid estimated using the abdominal FAST-applied abdominal fluid scores in clinically normal adult and juvenile dogs. J Vet Emerg Crit Care, in press.

15. Lisciandro GR. Evaluation of initial and serial combination focused assessment with sonography for trauma (CFAST) examinations of the thorax (TFAST) and abdominal (AFAST) with the application of an abdominal fluid scoring system in 49 traumatized cats. Abstract. J Vet Emerg Crit Care 2012;22(S2):S11.

16. Lisciandro GR. The cardiac gallbladder: case series of 13 dogs and 1 cat with sonographically detected gallbladder wall edema. J Vet Emerg Crit Care 2019; 29(S1):S24.

17. Nelson NC, Drost WT, Lerche P, et al. Noninvasive estimation of central venous pressure in anesthetized dogs by measurement of hepatic venous blood flow velocity and abdominal venous diameter. Vet Radiol Ultrasound 2010;51(3):313–23.

18. Quantz JE, Miles MS, Reed AL, et al. Elevation of alanine transaminase and gallbladder wall abnormalities as biomarkers of anaphylaxis in canine hypersensitivity patients. J Vet Emerg Crit Care 2009;19(6):536–44.

19. Lisciandro GR. The Abdominal FAST[3] (AFAST[3]) Exam. In: Lisciandro GR, editor. Focused ultrasound techniques for the small animal practitioner. Ames (IA): Wiley Blackwell; 2014. p. 17–43.

20. Lisciandro GR. POCUS: AFAST-Introduction and Image Acquisition. In: Lisciandro GR, editor. Point-of-Care ultrasound techniques for the small animal practitioner. 2nd edition. Ames (IA): Wiley Blackwell; 2020. p. 57–110.

21. Lisciandro GR. POCUS: AFAST-Clinical Integration. In: Lisciandro GR, editor. Point-of-care ultrasound techniques for the small animal practitioner. 2nd edition. Ames (IA): Wiley Blackwell; 2020. p. 111–48.

22. Lisciandro GR. Abdominal FAST (AFAST)-detected Hemorrhagic Abdominal Effusion in 11 Dogs with Acute Collapse and Gallbladder Wall Edema (Halo Sign) with Presumed Anaphylaxis. J Vet Emerg Crit Care 2016;26(S1):S8–9.

23. Hnatusko AI, Gicking JC, Lisciandro GR. Anaphylaxis-related hemoperitoneum in 11 dogs. J Vet Emerg Crit Care, in press.

24. Caldwell DJ, Petras KE, Mattison BL, et al. Spontaneous hemoperitoneum and anaphylactic shock associated with Hymenoptera envenomation in a dog. J Vet Emerg Crit Care 2018;28(5):476–82.

25. Birkbeck R, Greensmith T, Humm K, et al. Haemoabdomen due to suspect anaphylaxis in four dogs. Vet Rec Case Rep 2019. https://doi.org/10.1136/vetreccr-2018-000734.

26. Lisciandro GR, Lisciandro SC. Sonographic changes of the gallbladder associated with anaphylaxis in dogs (Letter to the Editor). J Vet Emerg Crit Care 2019;29(2):214–5.

27. Ferrada P, Attand RJ, Whelan J, et al. Qualitative assessment of the inferior vena cava: useful tool for the evaluation of volume status in critically ill patients. Am Surg 2012;78(4):468–70.

28. Darnis E, Boysen S, Merveille AC, et al. Establishment of references values of the caudal vena cava by fast-ultrasonography through different views in healthy dogs. J Vet Intern Med 2018;32(4):1308–18.

29. Kim SY, Park KT, Yeon SC, et al. Accuracy of sonographic diagnosis of pneumoperitoneum using the enhanced peritoneal stripe sign in Beagle dogs. J Vet Sci 2014;15(2):195–8.

30. Ferrada P, Vanguri P, Anand RJ, et al. Flat inferior vena cava: indicator of poor prognosis in trauma and acute care surgery patients. Am Surg 2012;78(12):1396–8.

31. Boysen SR, Gambino J. Gastrointestinal tract and pancreas. In: Lisciandro GR, editor. Point-of-care ultrasound for the small animal practitioner. Ames (IA): Wiley Blackwell; 2020.

32. Lisciandro GR, Fosgate GT. Use of urinary bladder measurements from a point-of-care cysto-colic ultrasonographic view to estimate urinary bladder volume in dogs and cats. J Vet Emerg Crit Care 2017;27(6):713–7.

33. Lux CN, Culp WT, Mayhew RD, et al. Perioperative outcome in dogs with hemoperitoneum: 83 cases (2005-2010). J Am Vet Med Assoc 2013;242(10):1385–91.

34. Lisciandro GR. POCUS: TFAST-introduction and image acquisition. In: Lisciandro GR, editor. Point-of-care ultrasound techniques for the small animal practitioner. 2nd edition. Ames (IA): Wiley Blackwell; 2020. p. 297–336.

35. Lisciandro GR. POCUS: TFAST-Clinical Integration. In: Lisciandro GR, editor. Point-of-care ultrasound techniques for the small animal practitioner. 2nd edition. Ames (IA): Wiley Blackwell; 2020. p. 337–88.

36. DeFrancesco TC. Focused or COAST[3]-Echo (Heart). In: Lisciandro GR, editor. Focused ultrasound techniques for the small animal practitioner. Ames (IA): Wiley Blackwell; 2014. p. 189–205.

37. DeFrancesco TC. POCUS: Heart-Abnormalities of Valves, Myocardium, and Great Vessels. In: Lisciandro GR, editor. Point-of-care ultrasound techniques for the small animal practitioner. 2nd edition. Ames (IA): Wiley Blackwell; 2020. p. 403–16.

38. Himelman RB, Kircher B, Rockey DC, et al. Inferior vena cava plethora with blunted respiratory response: a sensitive echocardiographic sign of cardiac tamponade. J Am Coll Cardiol 1988;12(6):1470–7.

39. Candotti C, Arntfield R. Pericardial effusion. In: Soni NJ, Arntfield R, Kory P, editors. Point-of-Care ultrasound. Philadelphia: Elsevier; 2015. p. 130–4.
40. Tchernodrinski S, Arntfield R. Inferior vena cava. In: Soni NJ, Arntfield R, Kory P, editors. Point-of-Care ultrasound. Philadelphia: Elsevier; 2015. p. 135–41.
41. Lichtenstein D, Meziere G, Biderman P, et al. The "lung point": an ultrasound sign specific to pneumothorax. Intensive Care Med 2000;26:1434–40.
42. Hwang TS, Yoon YM, Jung DI, et al. Usefulness of transthoracic lung ultrasound for the diagnosis of mild pneumothorax. J Vet Sci 2018;19(5):660–6.
43. Boysen S, McMurray J, Gommeren K. Abnormal curtain signs identified with a novel lung ultrasound protocol in six dogs with pneumothorax. Front Vet Sci 2019;28:6, 291.
44. Lisciandro GR. The Vet BLUE Lung Scan. In: Lisciandro GR, editor. Focused ultrasound techniques for the small animal practitioner. Ames (IA): Wiley Blackwell; 2014. p. 166–88.
45. Kulhavy DA, Lisciandro GR. Use of a lung ultrasound examination called vet BLUE to screen for metastatic lung nodules in the emergency room. J Vet Emerg Crit Care 2015;25(S1):S14.
46. Lisciandro GR, Romero L, Fosgate GT. The frequency of B-Lines and other lung ultrasound artifacts during Vet BLUE in 91 healthy puppies and kittens. J Vet Emerg Crit Care 2018;28(S1):S16.
47. Ward JL, Lisciandro GR, Ware WA, et al. Lung ultrasound findings in 100 dogs with various underlying causes of cough. J Am Vet Med Assoc 2019;255(5): 574–83.
48. Lisciandro GR. POCUS: Vet BLUE-clinical integration. In: Lisciandro GR, editor. Point-of-care ultrasound techniques for the small animal practitioner. 2nd edition. Ames (IA): Wiley Blackwell; 2020. p. 459–510.
49. Ward JL, Lisciandro GR, Keene BW, et al. Accuracy of point-of-care lung ultrasonography for the diagnosis of cardiogenic pulmonary edema in dogs and cats with acute dyspnea. J Am Vet Med Assoc 2017;250(6):666–75.
50. Ward JL, Lisciandro GR, DeFrancesco TC. Distribution of alveolar-interstitial syndrome in dyspneic veterinary patients assessed by lung ultrasound versus thoracic radiograph. J Vet Emerg Crit Care 2018;28(5):415–28.
51. Rademacher N, Pariaut R, Pate J, et al. Transthoracic lung ultrasound in normal dogs and dogs with cardiogenic pulmonary edema: a pilot study. Vet Radiol Ultrasound 2014;55(4):447–52.
52. Vezzosi T, Mannucci A, Pistoresi F, et al. Assessment of lung ultrasound B-lines in dogs with different stages of chronic valvular heart disease. J Vet Intern Med 2017;31(3):700–4.
53. Dicker SA, Lisciandro GR, Newell SM, et al. Diagnosis of pulmonary contusions with point-of-care lung ultrasonography and thoracic radiography compared to thoracic computed tomography in dogs with motor vehicle trauma: 29 cases (2017–2018). J Vet Emerg Crit Care, in press.
54. Lisciandro GR, Ward JL, DeFrancesco TC, et al. Absence of B-lines on Lung Ultrasound (Vet BLUE protocol) to Rule Out Left-sided Congestive Heart Failure in 368 Cats and Dogs. J Vet Emerg Crit Care 2016;26(S1):S8.
55. Lisciandro GR. POCUS: Global FAST for Patient Monitoring and Staging. In: Lisciandro GR, editor. Point-of-care ultrasound techniques for the small animal practitioner. 2nd edition. Ames (IA): Wiley Blackwell; 2020. p. 685–728.
56. Boston SE, Higginson G, Monteith G. Concurrent splenic and right atrial mass at presentation in dogs with HSA: a retrospective study. J Am Anim Hosp Assoc 2011;47(5):336–41.

57. Lisciandro GR. POCUS: Global FAST for Rapidly Detecting Treatable Forms of Shock and Advanced Life Support. In: Lisciandro GR, editor. Point-of-care ultrasound for the small animal practitioner. 2nd edition. Ames (IA): Wiley Blackwell; 2020. p. 729–56.

58. Andrus P. Cardiac Arrest. In: Soni NJ, Arntfield R, Kory P, editors. Point-of-care ultrasound. Philadelphia: Elsevier; 2014. p. 359–68.

59. Neumar RW, Otto CW, Link MS, et al. Part 8: Adult advanced cardiovascular life support: 2010 American Heart Association guidelines for cardiopulmonary resuscitation and emergency cardiovascular care. Circulation 2010;122(18 Suppl 3): S729–67.

60. Lisciandro GR, Romero LA, Bridgeman CH. Pilot Study: Vet BLUE Profiles Pre- and Post-anesthesia in 31 dogs Undergoing Surgical Sterilization. J Vet Emerg Crit Care 2015;25(S1):S8–9.

61. Lisciandro GR, Fosgate GT. Use of Vet BLUE Protocol for the detection of lung atelectasis and sonographic gallbladder wall evaluation for anaphylaxis and volume overload in 63 dogs undergoing general anesthesia. J Vet Emerg Crit Care 2018;28(S1):S15–6.

62. Cho J. POCUS: Eye. In: Lisciandro GR, editor. Point-of-care ultrasound techniques for the small animal practitioner. 2nd edition. Ames (IA): Wiley Blackwell; 2020. p. 553–78.

63. Rong AJ, Fan KC, Golshani B, et al. Multimodal imaging features of intraocular foreign bodies. Semin Ophthalmol 2019;34(7–8):518–32.

64. Smith JJ, Fletcher DJ, Cooley SD, et al. Transpalpebral ultrasonographic measurement of the optic nerve sheath diameter in healthy dogs. J Vet Emerg Crit Care 2018;28(1):31–8.

65. Loughran KA, Rush JE, Rozanski EA, et al. The use of focused cardiac ultrasound to screen for occult heart disease in asymptomatic cats. J Vet Intern Med 2019; 33(5):1892–901.

66. Gommeren K, Darnis E, Mereveille AC. POCUS: Caudal Vena Cava. In: Lisciandro GR, editor. Point-of-care ultrasound techniques for the small animal practitioner. 2nd edition. Ames (IA): Wiley Blackwell; 2020. p. 541–50.

67. Lisciandro GR. POCUS: vascular-veins and arteries. In: Lisciandro GR, editor. Point-of-care ultrasound techniques for the small animal practitioner. 2nd edition. Ames (IA): Wiley Blackwell; 2020. p. 529–40.

68. Chamberlin S, Sullivan L, Morley PS, et al. Evaluation of ultrasound-guided vascular access in dogs. J Vet Emerg Crit Care 2013;23(5):498–503.

69. Ringold SA, Kelmer E. Freehand ultrasound-guided femoral arterial catheterization in dogs. J Vet Emerg Crit Care 2008;18(3):306–11.

70. Chamberlin S. POCUS: central venous and arterial catheterization. In: Lisciandro GR, editor. Point-of-care ultrasound techniques for the small animal practitioner. 2nd edition. Ames (IA): Wiley Blackwell; 2020. p. 511–28.

71. Boysen SR, Gambino J. POCUS: Gastrointestinal Tract & Pancreas. In: Lisciandro GR, editor. Point-of-care ultrasound techniques for the small animal practitioner. 2nd edition. Ames (IA): Wiley Blackwell; 2020. p. 225–44.

72. Stieger-Varnegas SM. Musculoskeletal - Soft Tissue. In: Lisciandro GR, editor. Point-of-Care ultrasound techniques for the small animal practitioner. 2nd edition. Ames (IA): Wiley Blackwell; 2020. p. 647–62.

73. Stieger-Varnegas SM. Musculoskeletal – Bones and Joints. In: Lisciandro GR, editor. Point-of-Care ultrasound techniques for the small animal practitioner. 2nd edition. Ames (IA): Wiley Blackwell; 2020. p. 663–81.

74. Campoy L, Bezuidenhout AJ, Gleed RD, et al. Ultrasound-guided approach for axillary brachial plexus, femoral nerve, and sciatic nerve blocks in dogs. Vet Anaesth Analg 2010;37(2):144–53.
75. Haro P, Laredo F, Gil F, et al. Ultrasound-guided dorsal approach for femoral nerve blockade in cats: an imaging study. J Feline Med Surg 2013;15(2):91–8.
76. Otero PE, Portela DA, editors. Manual of small animal regional anesthesia: illustrated anatomy for nerve stimulation and ultrasound-guided nerve blocks. 2nd edition. Buenos Aires (Argentina): Inter-Médica S.A.I.C.I; 2019.
77. Carvalho CF. POCUS: Brain-Clinical Integration. In: Lisciandro GR, editor. Point-of-care ultrasound techniques for the small animal practitioner. 2nd edition. Ames (IA): Wiley Blackwell; 2020. p. 595–608.

UNITED STATES POSTAL SERVICE®

Statement of Ownership, Management, and Circulation
(All Periodicals Publications Except Requester Publications)

1. Publication Title	2. Publication Number	3. Filing Date
VETERINARY CLINICS OF NORTH AMERICA: SMALL ANIMAL PRACTICE	003 – 150	9/18/2020

4. Issue Frequency	5. Number of Issues Published Annually	6. Annual Subscription Price
JAN, MAR, MAY, JUL, SEP, NOV	6	$348.00

7. Complete Mailing Address of Known Office of Publication (Not printer) (Street, city, county, state, and ZIP+4®)

ELSEVIER INC.
230 Park Avenue, Suite 800
New York, NY 10169

Contact Person
Malathi Samayan

Telephone (Include area code)
91-44-4299-4507

8. Complete Mailing Address of Headquarters or General Business Office of Publisher (Not printer)

ELSEVIER INC.
230 Park Avenue, Suite 800
New York, NY 10169

9. Full Names and Complete Mailing Addresses of Publisher, Editor, and Managing Editor (Do not leave blank)

Publisher (Name and complete mailing address)

DOLORES MELONI, ELSEVIER INC.
1600 JOHN F KENNEDY BLVD. SUITE 1800
PHILADELPHIA, PA 19103-2899

Editor (Name and complete mailing address)

STACY EASTMAN, ELSEVIER INC.
1600 JOHN F KENNEDY BLVD. SUITE 1800
PHILADELPHIA, PA 19103-2899

Managing Editor (Name and complete mailing address)

PATRICK MANLEY, ELSEVIER INC.
1600 JOHN F KENNEDY BLVD. SUITE 1800
PHILADELPHIA, PA 19103-2899

10. Owner (Do not leave blank. If the publication is owned by a corporation, give the name and address of the corporation immediately followed by the names and addresses of all stockholders owning or holding 1 percent or more of the total amount of stock. If not owned by a corporation, give the names and addresses of the individual owners. If owned by a partnership or other unincorporated firm, give its name and address as well as those of each individual owner. If the publication is published by a nonprofit organization, give its name and address.)

Full Name	Complete Mailing Address
WHOLLY OWNED SUBSIDIARY OF REED/ELSEVIER, US HOLDINGS	1600 JOHN F KENNEDY BLVD. SUITE 1800 PHILADELPHIA, PA 19103-2899

11. Known Bondholders, Mortgagees, and Other Security Holders Owning or Holding 1 Percent or More of Total Amount of Bonds, Mortgages, or Other Securities. If none, check box ► ☐ None

Full Name	Complete Mailing Address
N/A	

12. Tax Status (For completion by nonprofit organizations authorized to mail at nonprofit rates) (Check one)
The purpose, function, and nonprofit status of this organization and the exempt status for federal income tax purposes:
☒ Has Not Changed During Preceding 12 Months
☐ Has Changed During Preceding 12 Months (Publisher must submit explanation of change with this statement)

PS Form **3526**, July 2014 (Page 1 of 4 (see instructions page 4)) PSN: 7530-01-000-9931 PRIVACY NOTICE: See our privacy policy on www.usps.com.

13. Publication Title	14. Issue Date for Circulation Data Below
VETERINARY CLINICS OF NORTH AMERICA: SMALL ANIMAL PRACTICE	JULY 2020

15. Extent and Nature of Circulation		Average No. Copies Each Issue During Preceding 12 Months	No. Copies of Single Issue Published Nearest to Filing Date
a. Total Number of Copies (Net press run)		544	511
b. Paid Circulation (By Mail and Outside the Mail)	(1) Mailed Outside-County Paid Subscriptions Stated on PS Form 3541 (Include paid distribution above nominal rate, advertiser's proof copies, and exchange copies)	345	329
	(2) Mailed In-County Paid Subscriptions Stated on PS Form 3541 (Include paid distribution above nominal rate, advertiser's proof copies, and exchange copies)	0	0
	(3) Paid Distribution Outside the Mails Including Sales Through Dealers and Carriers, Street Vendors, Counter Sales, and Other Paid Distribution Outside USPS®	135	135
	(4) Paid Distribution by Other Classes of Mail Through the USPS (e.g., First-Class Mail®)	0	0
c. Total Paid Distribution (Sum of 15b (1), (2), (3), and (4))		480	464
d. Free or Nominal Rate Distribution (By Mail and Outside the Mail)	(1) Free or Nominal Rate Outside-County Copies included on PS Form 3541	48	31
	(2) Free or Nominal Rate In-County Copies Included on PS Form 3541	0	0
	(3) Free or Nominal Rate Copies Mailed at Other Classes Through the USPS (e.g., First-Class Mail)	0	0
	(4) Free or Nominal Rate Distribution Outside the Mail (Carriers or other means)	0	0
e. Total Free or Nominal Rate Distribution (Sum of 15d (1), (2), (3) and (4))		48	31
f. Total Distribution (Sum of 15c and 15e)		528	495
g. Copies not Distributed (See Instructions to Publishers #4 (page 43))		16	16
h. Total (Sum of 15f and g)		544	511
i. Percent Paid (15c divided by 15f times 100)		90.9%	93.73%

* If you are claiming electronic copies, go to line 16 on page 3. If you are not claiming electronic copies, skip to line 17 on page 3.

16. Electronic Copy Circulation	Average No. Copies Each Issue During Preceding 12 Months	No. Copies of Single Issue Published Nearest to Filing Date
a. Paid Electronic Copies ►		
b. Total Paid Print Copies (Line 15c) + Paid Electronic Copies (Line 16a) ►		
c. Total Print Distribution (Line 15f) + Paid Electronic Copies (Line 16a) ►		
d. Percent Paid (Both Print & Electronic Copies) (16b divided by 16c × 100) ►		

☒ I certify that 50% of all my distributed copies (electronic and print) are paid above a nominal price.

17. Publication of Statement of Ownership
☒ If the publication is a general publication, publication of this statement is required. Will be printed ☐ Publication not required.
in the NOVEMBER 2020 issue of this publication.

18. Signature and Title of Editor, Publisher, Business Manager, or Owner	Date
Malathi Samayan	9/18/2020

Malathi Samayan - Distribution Controller

I certify that all information furnished on this form is true and complete. I understand that anyone who furnishes false or misleading information on this form or who omits material or information requested on the form may be subject to criminal sanctions (including fines and imprisonment) and/or civil sanctions (including civil penalties).

PS Form **3526**, July 2014 (Page 3 of 4) PRIVACY NOTICE: See our privacy policy on www.usps.com

Moving?

Make sure your subscription moves with you!

To notify us of your new address, find your **Clinics Account Number** (located on your mailing label above your name), and contact customer service at:

Email: journalscustomerservice-usa@elsevier.com

800-654-2452 (subscribers in the U.S. & Canada)
314-447-8871 (subscribers outside of the U.S. & Canada)

Fax number: 314-447-8029

Elsevier Health Sciences Division
Subscription Customer Service
3251 Riverport Lane
Maryland Heights, MO 63043

*To ensure uninterrupted delivery of your subscription, please notify us at least 4 weeks in advance of move.

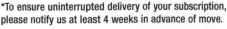

Moving?

Make sure your subscription moves with you!

To notify us of your new address, find your Clinics Account Number located on your mailing label above your name, and contact customer service at:

Email: journalscustomerservice-usa@elsevier.com

800-654-2452 (subscribers in the U.S. & Canada)
314-447-8871 (subscribers outside of the U.S. & Canada)

Fax number: 314-447-8029

Elsevier Health Sciences Division
Subscription Customer Service
3251 Riverport Lane
Maryland Heights, MO 63043